CLINICS IN SURGICAL GASTROENTEROLOGY

Concise Clinical GI Surgery Manual
for Practical Examinations:
DNB/MCh Surgical Gastroenterology,
DNB/DM Medical Gastroenterology,
DNB/ MS General Surgery,
DNB/ MCh Surgical Oncology

Second Edition

CLINICS IN SURGICAL GASTROENTEROLOGY

A Concise Clinical GI Surgery Manual

Second Edition

Dr Prashant R Rao

M.B.B.S, MS, DNB (General Surgery), MNAMS, FMAS, FIAGES
DrNB-SS (Surgical Gastroenterology)

Senior Consultant GI-HPB Cancer & Laparoscopic Surgeon

Founding Member & AP
Department of Surgical Gastroenterology (NBEMS Accredited)
LTMMC & GH, Sion, Mumbai

Author of: "#1 Best-Seller Clinics in Surgical Gastroenterology"
"Concise Cancer Manual" & "Concise Biostatistics Manual"

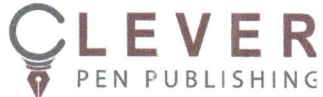

CLEVER
PEN PUBLISHING

Second Edition: 2024

First Edition: 2021

© **Clever Pen Publishing**

All rights reserved. No part of this publication may be reproduced, stored in a retrieval system, or transmitted in any form or by any means, electronic, mechanical, photocopying, recording or otherwise, without the prior written permission of the publisher.

This book has been published in good faith that the material provided by the author is a compilation of the original works done by great people. Every effort is made to ensure accuracy of the material, but the publisher, printer and author will not be held responsible for any inadvertent error(s). In case of any dispute, all legal matters will be settled under Mumbai jurisdiction only.

Published by:

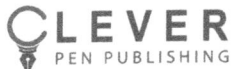

Clever Pen Publishing
D-2 Neelkanth Business Park Co-op. Premises Society Ltd.
Nathani Road
Vidyavihar (West)
Mumbai 400086
Mob.: 09867214519

Email: cleverpen9@gmail.com
Website: www.cleverpen.in

ISBN 978-93-92215-98-8

Printed & Bound in India

Dedicated

to

My Dear Parents

My lovely and ever supportive wife Sarika

&

My dearest son

Preface to the Second Edition

Thank you for making 'Clinics in Surgical Gastroenterology' the #1 Best-Seller. This has inspired the entire team to work harder to make the book even better.

This book has been prepared keeping in mind the format of MBBS, DNB/ MS (general surgery), DNB/MCh (surgical gastroenterology and surgical oncology) and DNB/ DM (Medical Gastroenterology) exams. We have tried to cover all the important GI surgical cases which would be kept as long or short cases in surgery practical examinations.

Format for history taking, justification for each component in history and format for examination for each disease has been provided. The highlight of the book is that an example case has also provided for each disease. This will give the reader an idea of how to present the case of a particular disease in the exams. Format for presenting the summary and diagnosis has also been provided. In cases where a single diagnosis is not possible, a schema has been provided which will help the candidate reach a specific diagnosis or present a sequence of differential diagnosis.

This is followed by section on 'How to Proceed', where we have described how to investigate a specific patient for his/ her disease and the sequence in which the investigations need to be performed, what is to be looked for in each investigation and how to stage or grade the disease. Finally, appropriate management options and strategies are discussed in detail.

This book is completely illustrated and, in this edition, we have added many more concept building diagrams and clinical images to improve understanding in the subject.

Another important highlight of this book is chapter on Trials and literature in GI Surgery where we have done our best to compile all the important and pertinent literature, landmark trials and studies in GI surgery in one place. The general consensus for controversies in GI surgery has also been discussed. This will help our reader with Evidence based decision making. This chapter has been thoroughly updated in this edition.

We surely believe that this is a one of its kind book in the field of GI surgery which has helped multiple students pass their examinations and later in their clinical practice.

With this new edition we hope it continues to do so.

I apologize in advance in case the reader comes across a mistake or shortcoming. I shall be more than happy to receive comments, criticism and feedback via email which shall help in improving the book.

Happy reading & All the Best!!

Dr Prashant R. Rao

gisurgeon.prashantrao@gmail.com

Preface to the First Edition

After more than a year of hard work it gives me immense pleasure to introduce 'Clinics in Surgical Gastroenterology'.

After having given numerous exams at various levels (graduate, post graduate [both MS and DNB] and then super-speciality), going through multitude of books, having had extensive discussions with my teachers, students, senior and junior colleagues and after conducting a few exams myself, I have come to understand what an exam going student needs from a book to help him/ her pass the practical exams. Clinical Surgical gastroenterology (a.k.a GI surgery) is an important part of the curriculum for students preparing for General surgery, Surgical gastroenterology, Medical gastroenterology and Surgical oncology exams. There are some wonderful books on clinical surgery by eminent authors, however few or none exclusively focusses on clinical GI surgery. With this in mind I set out to author this book with the aim to fill up the lacunae and to help the students in their exam preparation.

University practical examinations generally consists of presenting long cases, short cases followed by ward rounds and table vivas (instruments, operative techniques etc.), with majority of the marks being reserved for long cases. Hence one must perform his or her best during this session. While acquiring history from a patient, the candidate must understand that each disease has its own specific set of presenting symptoms, the elaboration of which is important to reach to a specific clinical diagnosis. Similarly, there are specific signs which the candidate must look for and mention during clinical examination. Also, he/ she must be prepared to justify each point mentioned in the presentation when asked for by the examiner. This book has been accordingly prepared with the intention to help our colleagues acquire a thorough history and perform an optimum examination to reach to a specific diagnosis. It has been prepared keeping in mind the format of MBBS, DNB/ MS (general surgery), DNB/MCh (surgical gastroenterology and surgical oncology) and DNB/ DM (Medical Gastroenterology) exams. We have tried to cover all the important GI surgical cases which would be kept as long or short cases in surgery practical examinations. Format for history taking, justification for each component in history and format for examination for each disease has been provided. The highlight of the book is that an example case has also provided for each disease. This will give the reader an idea of how a case of a particular disease may be presented in the exams. This may be used as a template by the reader to modify it as needed to match the history given by his/ her patient and their examination finding. Format for presenting the summary and diagnosis has also been provided. In cases where a single diagnosis is not possible, a schema has been provided with which the candidate may reach a specific diagnosis or present a sequence of differential diagnosis. Additionally, a general schema of history taking, examination and work-up in a GI case has been described in chapter 2.

Once the candidate has crossed the hurdle of presenting appropriate history, examination, summary and diagnosis, the next question that the examiner tends to ask is 'how will you proceed?'. To cover this we have described how to investigate a specific patient for his/ her disease and the sequence in which the investigations need to be performed, including what is to be looked for in each investigation and how to stage or grade the disease. Finally, appropriate management options and strategies are discussed in detail.

In super-speciality exams the candidates are also expected to know pertinent literature including landmark trials which is required for Evidence based decision making. Additionally, for diseases like Carcinoma Gall bladder, Corrosive esophageal injury, Bile duct injury-the Indian contribution to the available literature is immense. For this reason, I have tried my best to compile all the important and pertinent literature, landmark trials and studies in GI surgery in one place. The general consensus for controversies in GI surgery has also been discussed. I am sure that this will help the exam going students immensely. Finally tips for exam going candidates have been provided to help them boost their confidence while appearing for the exams.

The idea behind preparing this book was to provide the exam going students a comprehensive but concise and simple but complete textbook on clinical GI surgery and I hope it gets fulfilled. Apart from exams I'm sure it will also help surgeons in their day to day clinical practice. I apologize in advance in case the reader comes across a mistake or shortcoming. I shall be more than happy to receive comments, criticism and feedback via email which shall help in improving the book.

Thank you all & Happy reading!!

Dr Prashant R. Rao

gisurgeon.prashantrao@gmail.com

Foreword

It gives me immense pleasure to write the foreword for the Second edition of the #1 Best Selling Book **'Clinics in Surgical Gastroenterology'**. This is the third book authored by Dr Prashant R Rao who I have known now for more than a decade now. He is a Skilled Gastro-Surgeon, Acclaimed Author and Excellent Academician.

This is a completely illustrated book describing all cases in GI Surgery in detail, in a point wise lucid manner covering, history taking, justification of each component in history, detailed examination format, sample-case format, summary, diagnosis and how to proceed in each of these case scenarios. I am sure that the exhaustive coverage in these varied sections of GI cases in a single book will be of great convenience and assistance to readers. It is a complete package!

In addition, to cover the ever growing and rapidly increasing research related information, there is a unique chapter on trials in GI surgery. The author has also shared valuable tips for students in form of a very relevant chapter based on his experience and that of his students.

I am sure this book will be an asset and a ready reckoner to final year MBBS, MS/DNB General Surgery, MCh/DNB GI Surgery, Onco Surgery, DM/DNB Gastroenterology and readers of surgery at large. Manual like the current one makes you understand finer nuances, remember it and reproduce as and when required. I wholeheartedly applaud Dr. Prashant's efforts and earnestly hope that the readers are benefited. My best wishes to you Prashant.

Dr. Mohan A. Joshi
Dean
Lokmanya Tilak Municipal Medical College and Hospital
Sion
Mumbai.

Foreword

It's my absolute pleasure to introduce this book that developed from a concept we discussed over a cup of coffee! In the first iteration, Dr Prashant successfully produced a niche surgical bestseller by filling a void that exists between a handbook of clinical methods alone (which we have examples by Das, Bailey and Browse) and a detailed reference textbook. Here is a handy volume primarily aimed at the exam going superspecialty postgraduate but lucid enough to be well understood by a general surgery postgraduate and can spoonfeed even the advanced undergraduate. It is a ready reckoner to explain why each clinical symptom or sign is sought. It even gives a model example of a case taking including how to document the elements of a succinct summary.

The chapters are problem based but offers solutions too on how to proceed logically through the order of investigations (and what to look for) rather than a bland battery of tests. The application of each investigation is deftly woven into the treatment options and ancillary approaches like sequencing of (Neo) adjuvant therapy, when to stent, details of pivotal trials, surgical techniques and follow up.

It can be a quick one stop shop for surgical peers with limited time on their hands and pique their interest enough to read the originals for details if required. It plugssome of the lacunae found in heavy multi author books and bridges the correlation of practical clinical methods with fundamental basis of management.

He has successfully condensed important moments of bedside clinics and discussions scattered throughout literature, and painstakingly compiled them in a brief but precise manner. There were moments of personal involvement to see fragments of knowledge that I've shared with him also feature here!

The current edition has been updated and profusely illustrated and improved based on feedback from peers! I think it would be a handy and quick reference for the advanced surgical learner of gastroenterology.

Dr Puneet Dhar
Professor & Head
Department of Surgical Gastroenterology
Amrita Hospital
Faridabad

Acknowledgement

My sincere thanks and gratitude to:

- My Guide Dr Mohan A Joshi, Dean, Lokmanya Tilak Municipal Medical College and General Hospital, Sion, Mumbai, for his teachings, guidance in preparing the book and for agreeing to write the Foreword for the book.
- Dr Puneet Dhar, Professor and Head, Department of Surgical Gastroenterology, Amrita Hospital, Faridabad, for his teachings, giving me the impetus to write this book, providing constant guidance throughout the process till its completion and for agreeing to write the Foreword for the book.
- Dr Vinay K Kapoor, Professor, Department of Surgical Gastroenterology, MGMCH, Jaipur for providing inputs and feedback in improving the book.
- Dr S Sudhindran, Professor and Head, Department of Surgical Gastroenterology, Amrita Institute of Medical Sciences, Kochi, Kerala for his teachings and providing inputs and feedback in improving thebook.
- Dr Chetan Kantharia, Professor and Head, Department of Surgical Gastroenterology, Seth GS Medical College and KEM Hospital, Mumbai for his teachings and providing inputs and feedback in improving the book.
- Dr Avinash Supe, Professor and Ex-Dean Seth GS Medical college and KEM Hospital, Mumbai, for his teachings and providing inputs and feedback in improving the book.
- Dr Sarika Mayekar Rao, Assistant Professor, Department of Plastic surgery, Lokmanya Tilak Municipal Medical College and General Hospital, Sion, Mumbai for helping with the diagrams and proofreading of the book.
- Dr Prakash Kurumboor, Dr Satheesh Iype, Dr Shaji Ponnambathayil, Dr NP Kamalesh, Dr Pramil Kaniyarakkal, Dr Deepak George, Dr Rohan Shetty, Dr Kartik Kulshrestha and Dr Prasanna BK from PVS Memorial Hospital, Kochi, Kerala for their teachings, constant support and guidance.
- Dr S Prabhakar (Professor and Head), Dr KS Sethna (Professor) and all my seniors, colleagues and friends from the Department of Surgery, Lokmanya Tilak Municipal Medical College and General Hospital, Sion, Mumbai, for all their teachings, support and guidance. Special thanks to my resident surgeons for their feedback which has helped improve the book.
- Dr Sachin Bhojankar, Dr Sampat Kumar from the Department of Surgical Gastroenterology, Lokmanya Tilak Municipal Medical College and General Hospital, Sion, Mumbai for their help & support.
- Dr RY Prabhu and the remaining colleagues from Department of Surgical Gastroenterology, Seth GS Medical College and KEM Hospital, Mumbai for their teachings, constant support and guidance.
- Dr Meghraj Ingle (Professor and Head), Dr Kailash Kolhe (Assistant Professor), Department of Medical Gastroenterology, Lokmanya Tilak Municipal Medical College and General Hospital, Sion, Mumbai, for providing clinical images.

- Dr Anagha Joshi (Professor and Head), Dr Vikrant Firke (Assistant Professor), Department of Radiology, Lokmanya Tilak Municipal Medical College and General Hospital, Sion, Mumbai, for providing radiological images.

- Dr Aditya Kulkarni, Consultant GI Surgeon, Pune, for his contribution in chapter on trials in GI surgery and providing clinical images

- Dr Amit Chopde, Consultant GI Surgeon, Mumbai for his contribution in chapter on trials in GI surgery.

- My colleagues from Department of Anaesthesia, Medical Gastroenterology, Radiology and Interventional Radiology at Lokmanya Tilak Municipal Medical College and General Hospital, Sion, Mumbai.

- Dr Paresh Vohra, Assistant Professor, Department of Surgery, B J Government Medical College, Pune, for his help with proof reading.

- Surgical Gastroenterology Residents from all over India who have given their valuable feedback and helped improve the book.

- I would also like to thank Mr. Rajesh Bhalani and Mrs. Harsha Shah from, Clever Pen Publishing, Mumbai for their constant support, encouragement and their sincere efforts in speedily publishing an excellent quality book.

- DTP operator for his sincere efforts in preparing the book and fulfilling my expectations with regards to the diagrams.

- My teachers throughout my medical education. My students from whom I daily learn something new.

- My parents, in-laws, family and friends for their constant support and guidance.

- And lastly, my patients.

Contents

1. How to use this Book 1
2. General format for History Taking, Examination and Work-Up in a GI Case 3
3. Case of Dysphagia due to Carcinoma Esophagus, Achalasia Cardia 31
4. Case of Dysphagia due to Corrosive Esophageal Injury 56
5. Case of Gastric Outlet Obstruction due to Carcinoma Stomach 76
6. Case of Surgical Obstructive Jaundice 101
7. Case of Chronic Pancreatitis 144
8. Case of Non-Cirrhotic Portal Hypertension 163
9. Case of Bile Duct Injury 191
10. Case of Inflammatory Bowel Disease 214
11. Case of Rectal & Left Colonic Carcinoma 239
12. Case of Lump in Abdomen & How to Proceed in a Case of HCC, Ileo-Cecal TB and Right Colonic Malignancy 262
    - Lump in Right Upper Quadrant of Abdomen 265
    - How to Proceed in a Case of Hepatocellular Carcinoma 271
    - Lump in Epigastrium 284
    - Lump in Left Upper Quadrant of Abdomen 287
    - Lump in Right Lower Quadrant of the Abdomen 290
    - How to proceed in a Case of Ileo-Cecal Tuberculosis 293
    - How to proceed in a Case of Right Colonic Malignancy 300
    - Lump in Left Lower Quadrant of Abdomen 306
13. Literature/Trials in GI Surgery which an Exam-Going Resident Must Know 307
    - Introduction 307
    - Esophageal & GEJ Cancer 308
    - Gastric Cancer 312
    - Colo-rectal Cancer 316
    - Pancreatic Cancer 321
    - Biliary Cancer 330
    - Hepato-cellular Cancer & Liver Resection 334
    - Corrosive Injury 337
    - Non Cirrhotic Portal Hypertension 339
    - Bile Duct Injury 340
    - Pancreatitis 344
    - Inflammatory Bowel Disease 346
    - Miscellaneous 347
14. Tips for Exam Going Candidates 350
15. Compilation of Important Tables 354

Feedback

Help Us Improve

Scan the QR code
and give your feedback
Or
You can email us your feedback on
- ☞ bhalanipublishers@gmail.com
- ☞ cleverpen9@gmail.com
- ☞ gisurgeon.prashantrao@gmail.com

1 How to Use this Book

Introduction

- This book has been prepared with the intention to help our surgical colleagues to acquire a thorough history and perform an optimum examination to reach to a specific diagnosis. This shall not only help you in your day to day practice but will also help you with case presentation in surgery practical examinations.
- This has been prepared keeping in mind the format of MBBS, DNB/MS (General Surgery), DNB/MCh (Surgical Gastroenterology and Surgical Oncology) and DM/DNB (Medical Gastroenterology) exams.
- We have tried to cover all the important GI surgical cases which would be kept as long or short cases in Surgery Practical Examinations.
- Each chapter (except chapters 2, 12, 13 and 14) in this book will have the following sections:
  - General Format for History Taking
  - Justification for Each Component in History
  - Format for Examination
  - Example Case
  - Summary
  - Diagnosis
  - How to Proceed

General Format for History Taking

- In this section we have tried to cover the general format of acquiring and presenting history for a specific case in a point wise manner.
- Each point in history has a specific significance, which will be described in the next section.

Justification of Each Component in History

- In this section we have provided the justification or reason behind asking each component in the history.
- While you narrate history in the exam, the examiner will tend to ask "why did you mention this". He/she may do this for a few specific points in history; alternatively a notorious examiner may ask this question for each and every point. This section will help you answer that.

Format for Examination

- In this section we have covered the pertinent findings to look for while examining a specific case.

Example Case, Summary, Presentation of Diagnosis

- In this section we have provided the reader a way in which the history and examination can be presented for a particular case.
- This may be used as a template by the reader to modify it as needed to match the history given by his/her patient and their examination finding.
- This is followed by section on how to summarize the case and present the diagnosis.

How to Proceed

- Here we have in a comprehensive manner tried to describe the way in which patient needs to be further investigated and subsequently managed for his/her specific disease.

Additionally, all the important trials, literature, controversies and general consensus on each subject has been dealt with in chapter 13

2 General format for History Taking, Examination and Work-Up in a GI Case

General Format for History Taking

- Particulars of the patient: Name, Age, Sex, Address, Occupation
- Chief Complaints in brief
- HOPI: History of presenting illness in detail
- History of pain:
  - Site
  - Onset: Insidious or sudden
  - Duration
  - Nature: Intermittent/continuous
  - Character of pain: Dull aching or colicky
  - Intensity: Mild/moderate/severe
  - Radiation of pain
  - Precipitated by meals or not
  - Precipitated by fasting or not
  - Relation with posture
  - Enquire whether there is any recent change in character of pain.
  - Relieving factor: Spontaneous/oral analgesic/intra venous analgesic
- History of nausea and vomiting:
  - Onset
  - Duration
  - Frequency
  - Quantity: Small or large volume, alternatively one could describe quantity in form of cup
  - Contents:
    - Bilious or not
    - Contains food particles or not: If yes then describe if it is undigested/partially digested/completely digested (Chyme)
  - Projectile or not
  - Related to meals or not i.e. post prandial or not
  - Is there a sense of relief after vomiting or not

- History of fever:
    - Duration
    - Onset: Insidious or sudden
    - Grade: Low or high
    - Nature: Intermittent/fluctuating/continuous
    - Associated chills or not.
- History of dyspepsia: Epigastric pain, burning, fullness, bloating
- History of yellowish discoloration of sclera and high colored urine:
    - Duration
    - Onset: Insidious or sudden
    - Nature: Intermittent or persistent or progressive or waxing and waning
    - Painless or painful: Associated with abdominal pain or not
    - Preceded by prodromal symptoms or not.
    - Identified by self or relative
- History of pruritus (itching):
    - Generalized to whole body or localized to a certain body part
    - Present throughout the day or at certain point of the day (as in, more towards the night)
    - Disturbing lifestyle or not; disturbing sleep or not
- History of alteration in bowel habits:
    - Constipation/obstipation or diarrhea
    - Onset: Insidious or sudden
    - Duration
    - Progression
    - History of laxative use.
    - What does he pass:
        - Stool quantity
        - Stool frequency
        - Stool consistency: Loose/soft/semisolid/hard
        - Color
        - Odor
        - Mucus is present or not.

- History of hematemesis:
  - Spontaneous or not
  - Number of episodes
  - Amount of bleed
  - Whether fresh blood or coffee ground
  - Blood clot present or absent
  - Whether there is history of associated melena, hematochezia
- History of bleeding per rectum (PR):
  - Painful or painless
  - Passage of Fresh bright red blood or altered blood
  - With or without blood clots
  - Quantity
  - Separate from stools or mixed with it
- History to suggest anemia due to GI bleed: Fatigue, shortness of breath, postural dizziness or syncope, need for blood transfusion
- History of dysphagia/difficulty in swallowing: Describe the dysphagia in detail,
  - Onset: Insidious or sudden,
  - Nature: Whether it is intermittent, stable or progressive,
  - The grade of dysphagia,
  - If progressive describe the initial grade and the grade now at time of presentation.
  - Site of food getting stuck: Neck/upper chest/lower chest
- History of loss of weight, loss of appetite

Table 2.1: Definition of significant weight loss
○ Loss of > 10% body weight in 6 months
○ Loss of > 7.5% body weight in 3 months
○ Loss of > 5% body weight in 1 month
○ Loss of > 2% body weight in 1 week

- History to suggest malignant dissemination: abdominal distension, jaundice, respiratory discomfort, hemoptysis, bone and back pain
- Treatment history:
  - Investigation

- o Treatment
- Past history:
  - o Of comorbid illness: DM, HTN, Coronary artery disease (CAD), tuberculosis (TB), chronic obstructive pulmonary disease (COPD), Bronchial asthma (BA)
  - o Surgery
- Personal history:
  - o Smoking history:
    - Type of smoke: Cigarette, cigar or bidi
    - Number of smokes per day; number of years of smoking; calculate pack years
    - Any attempts to quit smoking.
  - o History of alcohol consumption:
    - Type of liquor
    - Frequency of consumption: Per week/per month
    - Quantity
    - Total duration
    - Attempt at abstinence
- Family history: history of cancer in first and second degree family
- Performance history:
  - o Whether he/she is
    - Able to perform all daily routine activity (sedentary and/or strenuous)
    - Able to perform all self care
    - Bed ridden
  - o Whether he/she is able to climb two flight of stairs comfortably or not

Table 2.2: ECOG/ WHO performance scale

0: Fully active; no performance restrictions.

1: Fully ambulatory and able to carry out light work. Strenuous physical activity restricted.

2: Capable of all self-care but unable to carry out any other work activities. Up and about > 50% of waking hours.

3: Capable of only limited self-care; confined to bed or chair > 50% of waking hours.

4: Completely disabled; cannot carry out any self-care; totally confined to bed or chair.

Format for Examination

- What is the appearance of the patient: Young/middle aged/elderly lady/gentleman
- Whether the patient is clinically
  - Poorly/averagely/well built
  - Poorly/averagely/well nourished
  - Height, weight, BMI

Table 2.3: Clinical features suggesting poor nourishment

- Temporal wasting
- Sunken eyes
- Flattened cheeks, Buccal hollow
- Supraclavicular hollow
- Squaring of shoulders
- Prominent scapula
- Prominent intercostal spaces
- Scaphoid abdomen
- Prominent hip bones
- Prominent knee and elbows
- Pedal edema
- Decreased mid arm circumference
- Decreased skin fold thickness

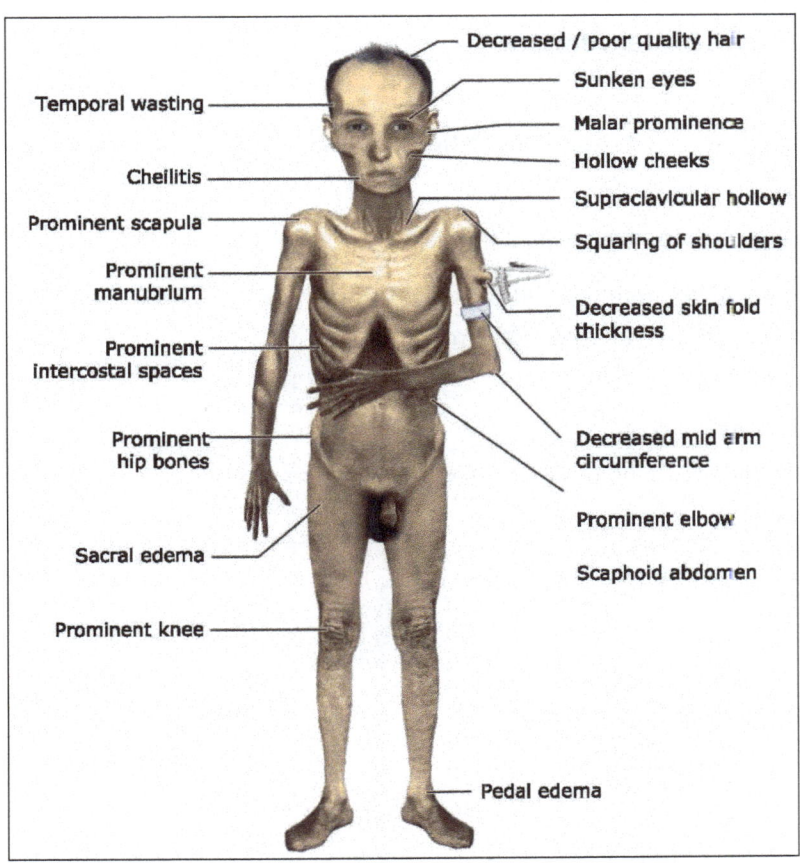

Figure 2.1: Clinical feature suggesting poor nourishment.

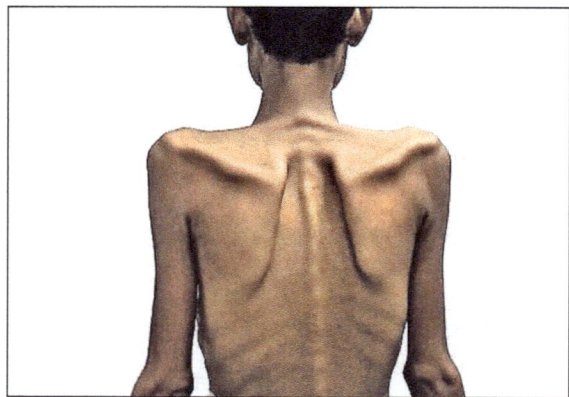

Figure 2.2: Posterior aspect of a poorly nourished patient showing prominent scapula, and spine.

- Whether the patient is clinically
    - Conscious/stuporous
    - Co-operative/un-cooperative
    - Well/poorly oriented to time, place and person
    - Lying comfortably in bed/in discomfort/in pain(rolling in pain)
    - Well hydrated/dehydrated
    - Febrile/Afebrile
- Pulse, BP, Respiratory rate, breath holding time
- Look for
    - Pallor, jaundice, cyanosis, clubbing
    - Generalized or localized lymphadenopathy
    - Palpable left supraclavicular lymph node
    - Pedal or dependent edema
    - Skin lesions
    - Stigmata of chronic liver disease

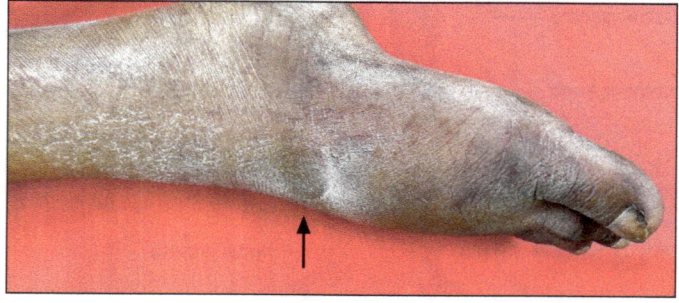

Figure 2.3: Pitting Pedal edema seen in Hypoprotienemia, Cardiac Failure, Renal Failure.

Table 2.4: Stigmata of chronic liver disease (top to bottom)

- Icterus
- Malar erythema
- Fetor hepaticus
- Parotid swelling
- Spider nevi/spider angiomata
- Gynecomastia
- Reduced chest hair
- Reduced axillary hair
- Dupuytren contracture
- Palmar erythema
- Leukonychia
- Flapping tremors/Asterexis
- Abdominal distension
- Caput medusae
- Reduced pubic hair
- Testicular atrophy
- Pedal edema

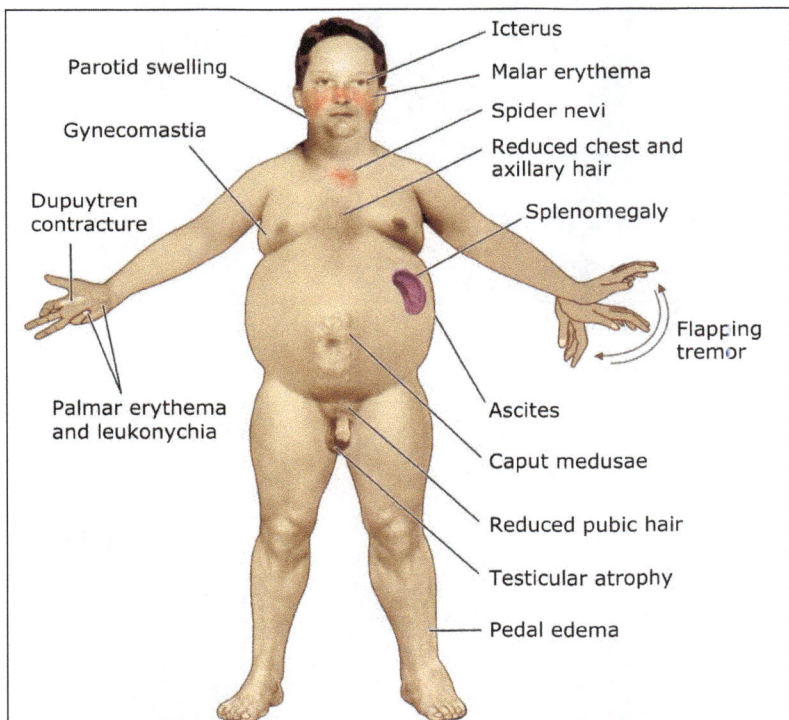

Figure 2.4: Stigmata of chronic liver disease.

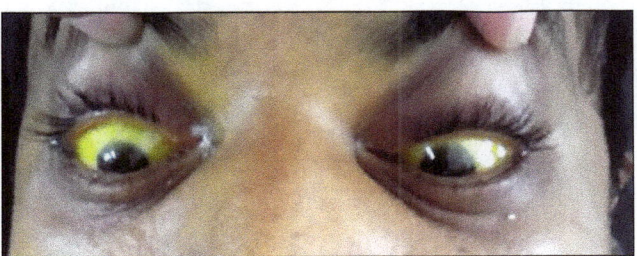

Figure 2.5: Icterus.

- Examination of oral cavity: Look for:
  - Mouth opening: Look for reduced mouth opening or trismus
  - Mucosal lesion: Look for any obvious mucosal lesion like leukoplakia, erythroplakia, ulcers or growth
  - Oral hygiene: Look for dental caries, tobacco stains, foul smell/halitosis
  - Tongue movement: Normal or impaired

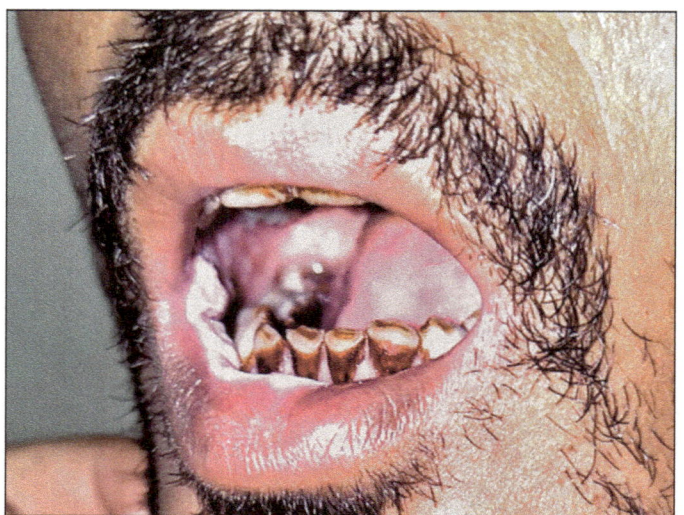

Figure 2.6: Examination of Oral Cavity revealing Leukoplakia, tobacco stain and poor oral hygiene.

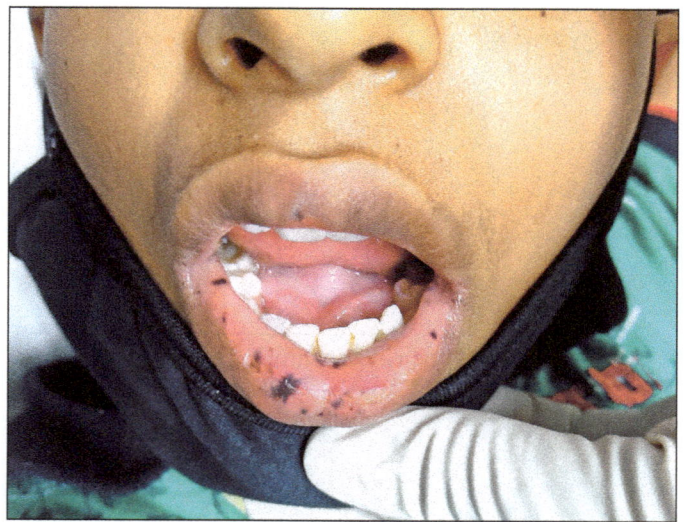

Figure 2.7: Pigmented macules seen on lips and oral mucosa in a patient with Peutz Jeghers syndrome.

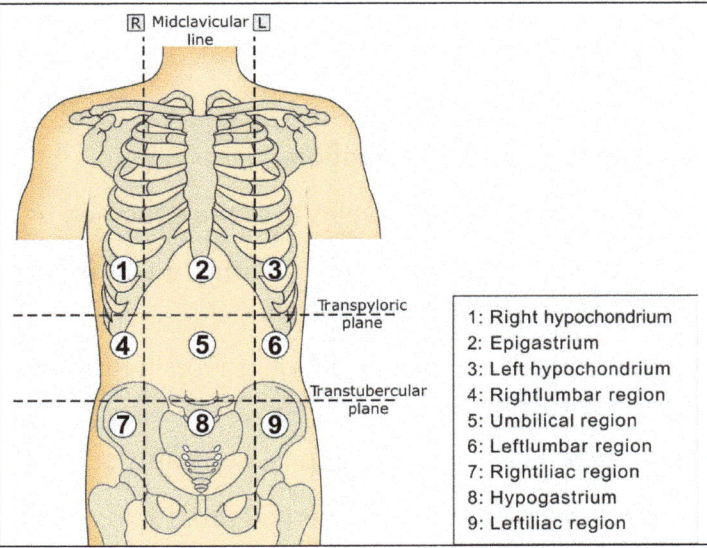

Figure 2.8: Nine quadrants of the abdomen.

- Examination of the abdomen:
  - On Inspection: See if:
    - Abdomen is flat/distended/scaphoid.
    - Umbilicus is central/displaced (upwards/downwards/sideways) inverted/everted/flat.

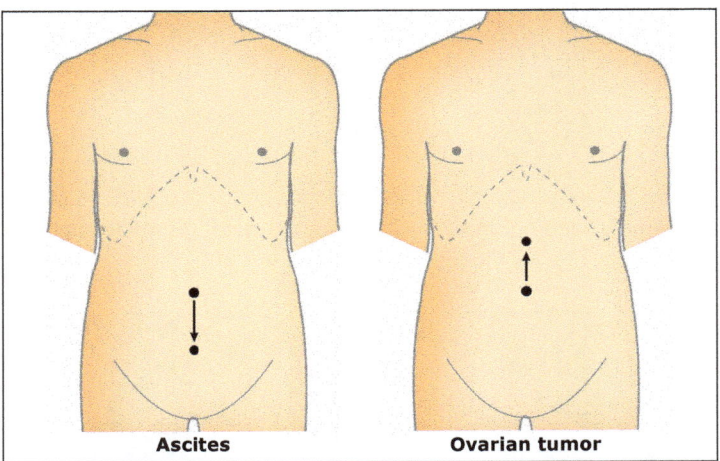

Figure 2.9: Tanyon sign of displacement of umbilicus.

    - All quadrants are moving equally with respiration or not
    - See if there is any visible lump.
      - If visible describe:
        - Size

- Site
- Shape
- Surface and
- Movement with respiration

■ Look for dilated or engorged veins over the abdomen or flank:

– Dilated peri-umbilical veins radiating away from the umbilicus is suggestive of portal hypertension.

– Dilated veins in cranio-caudal orientation in the flanks is suggestive of caval obstruction

■ Look for visible scar, sinus, pulsations, peristalsis or cough impulse.

■ Don't forget to inspect the groin hernial sites (to look for swelling or cough impulse i.e. hernia) and genitalia.

■ Inspection of renal angles to look for fullness

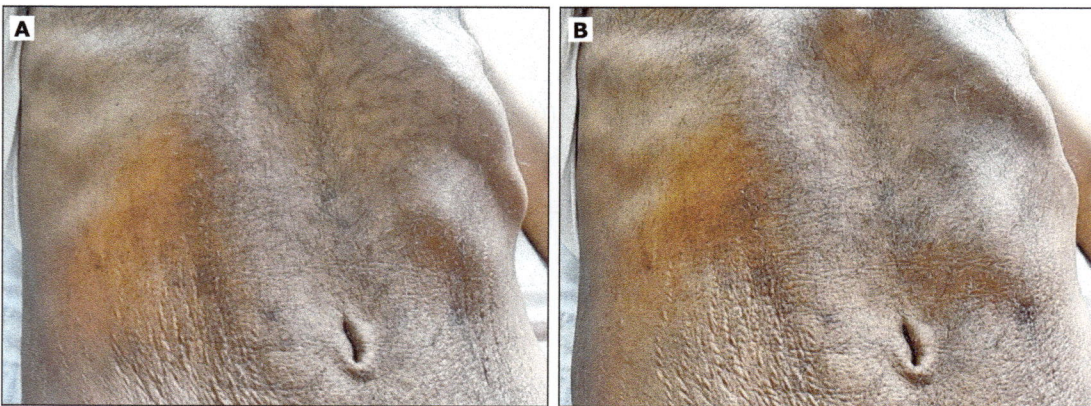

Figure 2.10: Splenomegaly seen on abdominal inspection; note the medial and caudal movement of the spleen with inspiration.

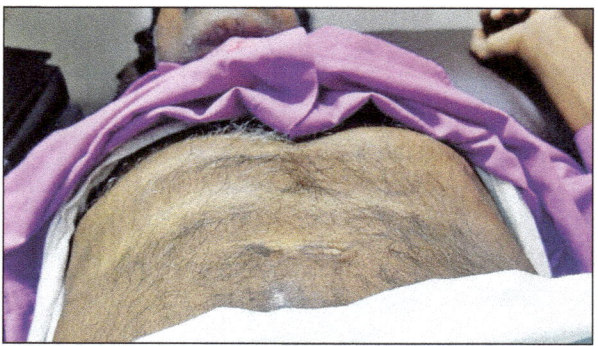

Figure 2.11: Tangential inspection of the abdomen from the leg end revealing a Right upper quadrant bulge which on palpation was confirmed to be Gall Bladder.

CHAPTER 2: GENERAL FORMAT FOR HISTORY TAKING, EXAMINATION AND WORK-UP IN A GI CASE

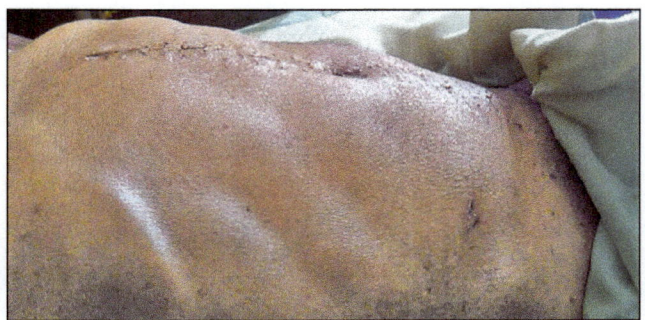

Figure 2.12: Inspection of abdomen showing 'step-ladder' pattern of peristalsis in a patient with intestinal obstruction.

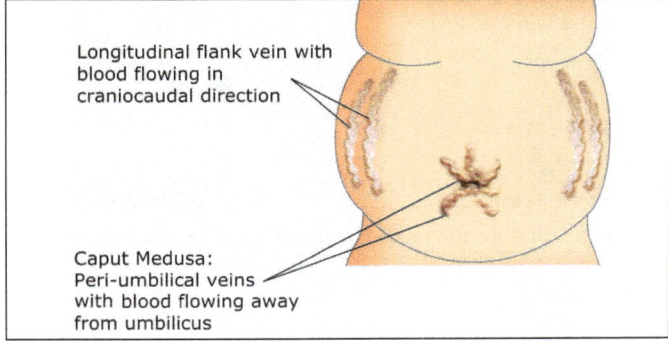

Figure 2.13: Abdominal veins.

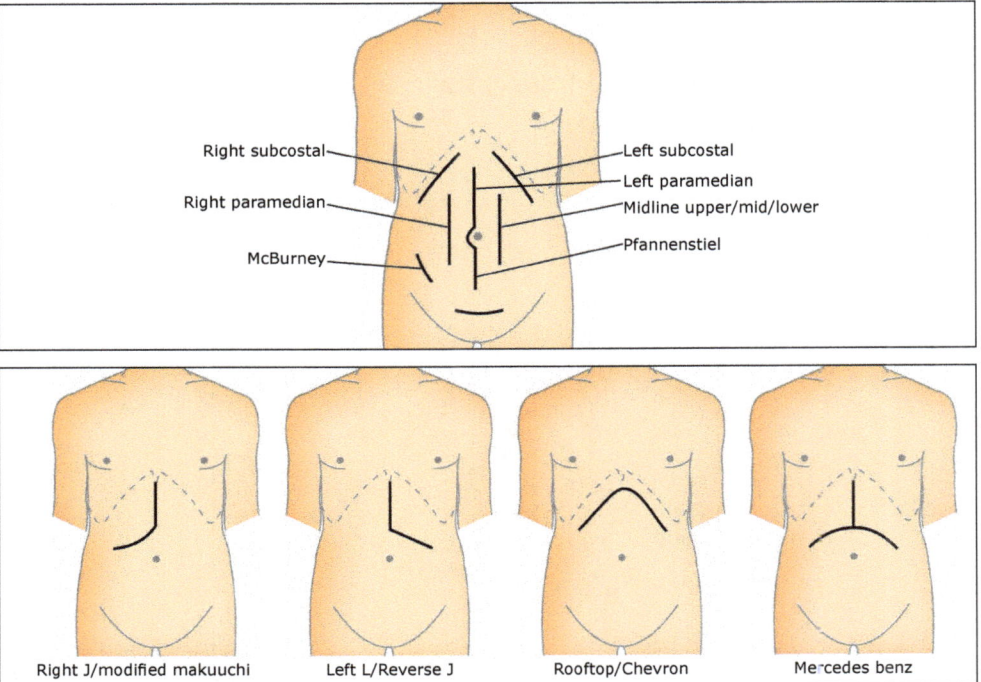

Figure 2.14: Scars of previous abdominal incisions.

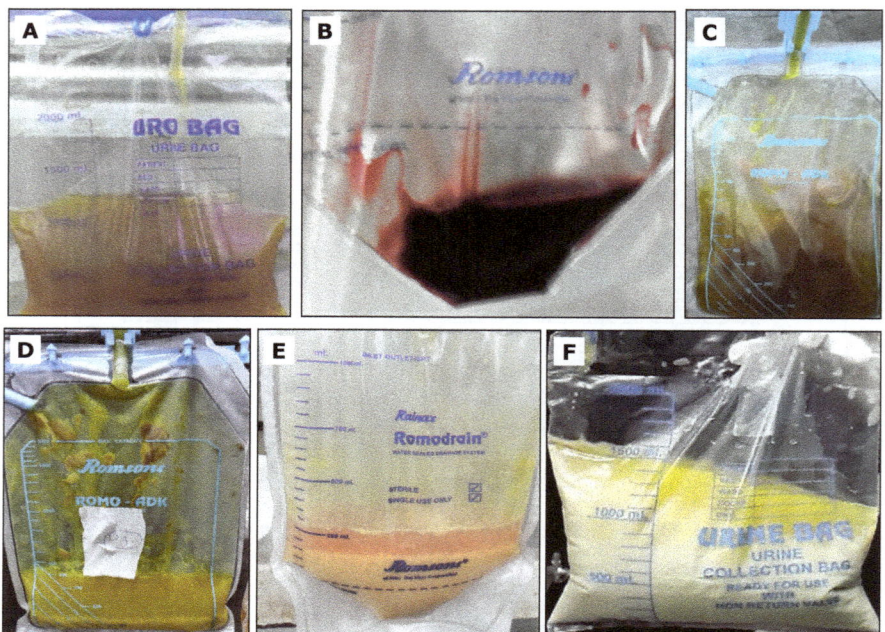

Figure 2.15: If a drain is in-situ note the type of drain effluent. A. Serous; B. Sanguinous; C. Bilious; D. Enteric; E. Purulent; F. Chylus.

- On Palpation: See if:
  - Abdomen is soft and non-tender (Alternatively abdomen could be rigid and/or tender)
  - Liver is palpable or not
    - If yes, measure size from costal margin in midclavicular line in unit of cm or number of fingers

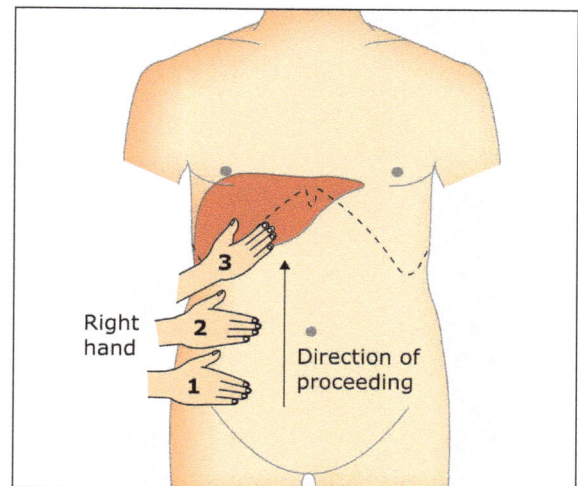

Figure 2.16: Technique of palpation of liver.

- See if:
  - It is tender/nontender
  - Surface is smooth/nodular
  - Borders are round/sharp, regular/irregular
  - Consistency is soft/firm/hard
  - Moving with respiration or not
- Spleen is enlarged or not
  - If yes, measure size from costal margin along its long axis
  - Note its:
    - Extent: upto mid-clavicular line/umbilicus/beyond umbilicus
    - Surface
    - Margins; look for splenic notch along the anterior margin
    - Consistency
    - Movement with respiration
    - See if it is tender/nontender
  - Grading of splenomegaly:
    - Mild: < 3 cm from costal margin
    - Moderate: 3–5 cm from costal margin
    - Massive: > 7 cm from costal margin

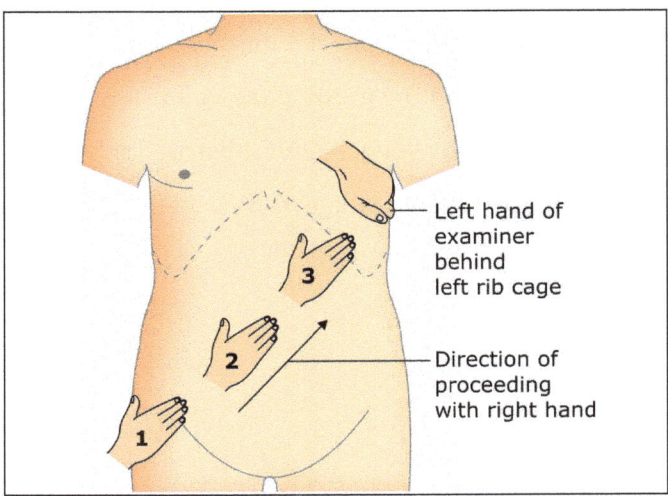

Figure 2.17: Technique of palpation of spleen.

- Any other palpable lump. If present note the following points about the lump
  - Site
  - Size
  - Shape
  - Surface
  - Margins
  - Tenderness
  - Consistency
  - Mobility
  - Movement with respiration
  - Plane
    - Whether the lump is intraperitoneal or not: by performing leg raising test
    - Whether the lump is retroperitoneal or not: by asking the patient to assume lateral decubitus position and palpating if the lump falls forward or not. A retroperitoneal mass won't fall ahead. Knee elbow test is no longer recommended as it would be inhuman to make a patient assume a knee-elbow position.
- If dilated veins are seen over the abdomen then note the direction of blood flow in it:
  - Direction of blood flow in the peri-umbilical veins in patients with portal hypertension is away from the umbilicus.
  - Direction of blood flow in the flank veins:
    - Below upwards suggests IVC obstruction
    - Above downwards suggests SVC obstruction

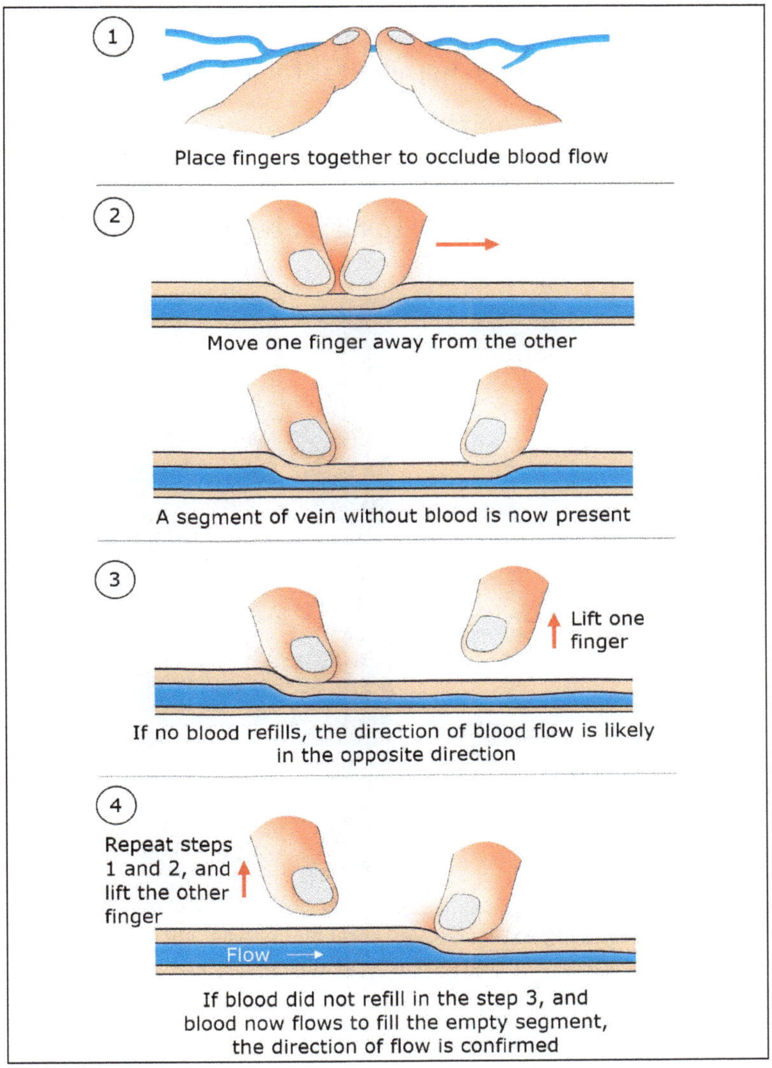

Figure 2.18: Technique to identify direction of Blood Flow in a vein.

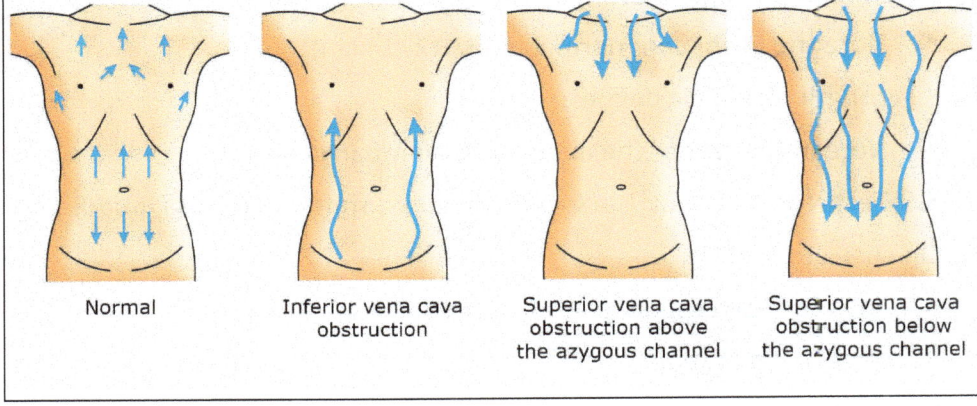

Figure 2.19: Direction of blood flow in Abdomino-Thoracic veins and its significance.

- Do not forget:
  - To palpate the groin hernia sites to look for cough impulse
  - Examination of genitals
  - To look for tenderness in Renal angles
  - Examination of back and spine for tenderness/gibbus.

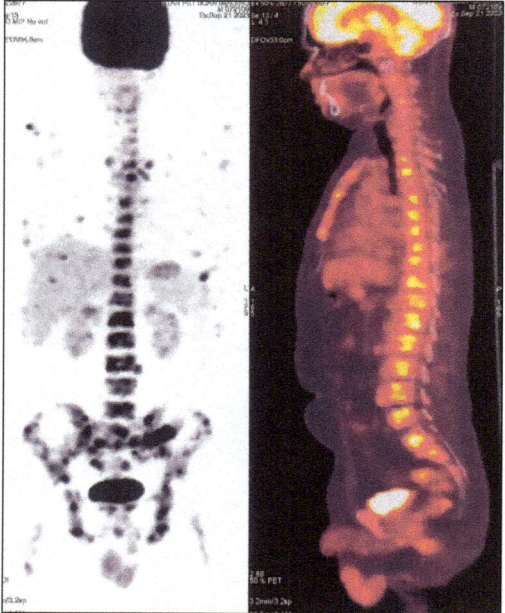

Figure 2.20: FDG-PET-CT revealing extensive Vertebral Metastasis, such metastasis can cause spine tenderness and/or gibbus.

- On Percussion:
  - Look for upper border of liver dullness (generally in the 5th intercostal space) in midclavicular line.
  - Note the liver span (normal being 12–14 cm)
  - Length of splenic dullness
  - Note in the rest of the abdomen: Typmpanic or dull
  - Tests for free fluid: Horseshoe dullness, shifting dullness, puddle sign
- On auscultation:
  - Look for bowel sounds, bruit, hum and rub
- Per rectal examination:
  - Examination of perianal area: Look for fissure, skin tag, external

hemorrhoids, external opening of fistula in ano, perianal abscess, sinus, growth or prolapse, skin excoriation
- Digital rectal examination: with a gloved finger:
  - To note the anal tone and squeeze pressure
  - to palpate for any mucosal lesion. If present, note:
    - The distance of the growth from anal verge.
    - The longitudinal extent in cm
    - Circumferential extent to be mentioned as extending from …'O' clock to …'O' clock
    - Proximal extent of the growth
    - Consistency: soft/firm/hard
    - Form: Ulcerative/proliferative/ulcero-proliferative/polypoidal
    - Fixity: fixed or not
    - Also note what is seen on the gloved finger: normal stool/blood/mucus/pus.
  - Perform proctoscopy if available

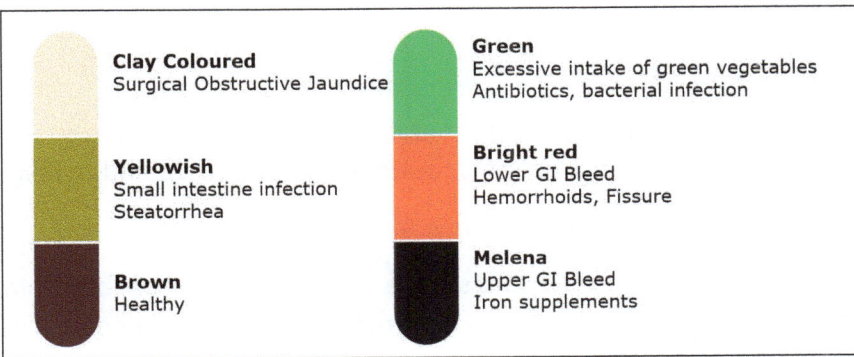

Figure 2.21: Stool color and its significance.

- Respiratory examination:
  - Inspection:
    - Whether the trachea is in midline or is deviated
    - Bilateral chest movement: equal or not
  - Palpation:
    - Trachea: central or deviated
    - Chest: look for warmth and tenderness

- Bilateral chest movement: equal or not
- Tactile vocal fremitus:
  - It is increased in case of pleural effusion and consolidation.
- Auscultation: most important part of respiratory examination:
  - Breath sounds:
    - Bilaterally equal or not
    - Reduced in any lung field: right/left; upper/mid/lower zone. Reduced breath sounds would suggest either pleural effusion or consolidation.
  - Adventitious sounds:
    - Crepts: coarse crepts would suggest aspiration pneumonitis, whereas fine crepts would suggest pulmonary edema.
    - Ronchi/wheeze
- Percussion:
  - Normal percussion note is resonant.
  - Dull note suggests consolidation or pleural effusion.
- Rest systemic examination

How to Work-Up a GI Case

- Review previous clinical records, including previously recorded history and examination findings, investigations, treatment provided up and follow up
- Correction of acute disturbances if any:
  - Respiratory distress: Check and secure airway (A); facilitate breathing with via provision of O_2 via mask, prongs or ventilator as deemed necessary (B)
  - Hypotension: Initiate fluid resuscitation (C)
  - Dehydration: Initiate hydration with crystalloids and/or colloids.
  - Dyselectrolytemia: Correction of electrolyte imbalances such as
    - Hypokalemia: Potassium levels < 3.5 mEq/L
    - Hyperkalemia: Potassium levels > 5 mEq/L
    - Hyponatremia: Sodium levels < 135 mEq/L
    - Hypernatremia: Sodium levels > 145 mEq/L

- Hypocalcemia: Calcium levels < 8.5 mg/dl
- Hypercalcemia: Calcium levels > 10.5 mg/dl
- Others: Hypo/Hyper-Magnesemia, Hypo/Hyper-Phosphatemia
  - Correction of anemia: With blood transfusion
  - Correction of coagulopathy: With transfusion of blood products like fresh frozen plasma (FFP), cryoprecipitate; administration of Vitamin K.
  - Correction of blood sugar levels:
    - In case of hypoglycemia: administer glucose solution orally or intravenously (10%, 25% or 50%)
    - In hyperglycemia: check for ketoacidosis (ABG) and ketones in urine. Then start insulin drip
  - Hypertension: start anti-hypertensive
- Once patient has been stabilized, investigations are performed: Investigations can broadly be divided into four types:
  - Routine investigations: including routine blood tests, X-ray chest and ECG (electro-cardiogram)
  - Investigation for Diagnosis
  - Investigation for Staging
  - Investigation for assessing fitness for surgery
- Routine blood investigations
  - Hemogram
  - LFT: Liver Function Test
  - RFT: Renal Function Test
  - SE: Serum Electrolyte
  - INR
  - Blood sugar levels
- Additional/special laboratory investigation as deemed necessary. E.g.:
  - ABG: arterial blood gas
  - Lactate levels

- o CRP: C-Reactive protein
- o ESR: erythrocyte sedimentation rate
- o Blood grouping and Cross matching
- o Viral markers: HIV, HBsAg, HCV
- o Serum calcium, magnesium, phosphorus levels
- o Lipid profile
- o HBa1c levels
- o Thrombophilic work-up
- o Pancreatic exocrine function testing: Fecal fat estimation, fecal elastase levels
- o Stool testing
- o Urine testing
- o Ascitic fluid testing
- o Sputum testing
- X-ray chest is performed as a routine for all patients. Significance:
  - o Look for consolidation, pulmonary infiltrates, pleural effusion etc.
  - o To look for lung metastasis in suspected cases of malignancy
- X-ray abdomen: In case intestinal obstruction (multiple air-fluid level) or perforation (free gas under diaphragm) is suspected

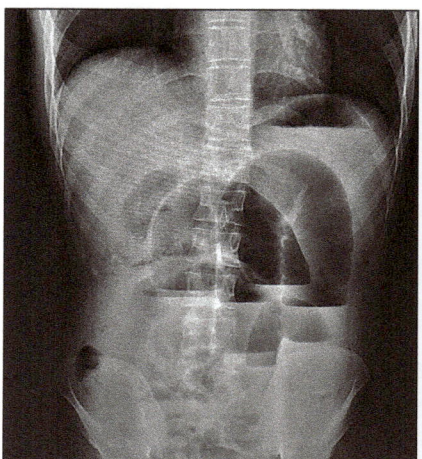
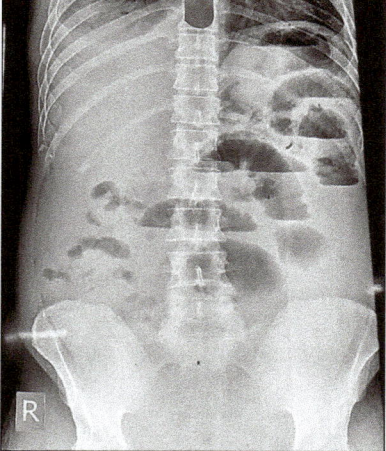

Figure 2.22: X-ray abdomen showing multiple air fluid levels suggesting intestinal obstruction. Note the step ladder pattern of air-fluid level on the right.

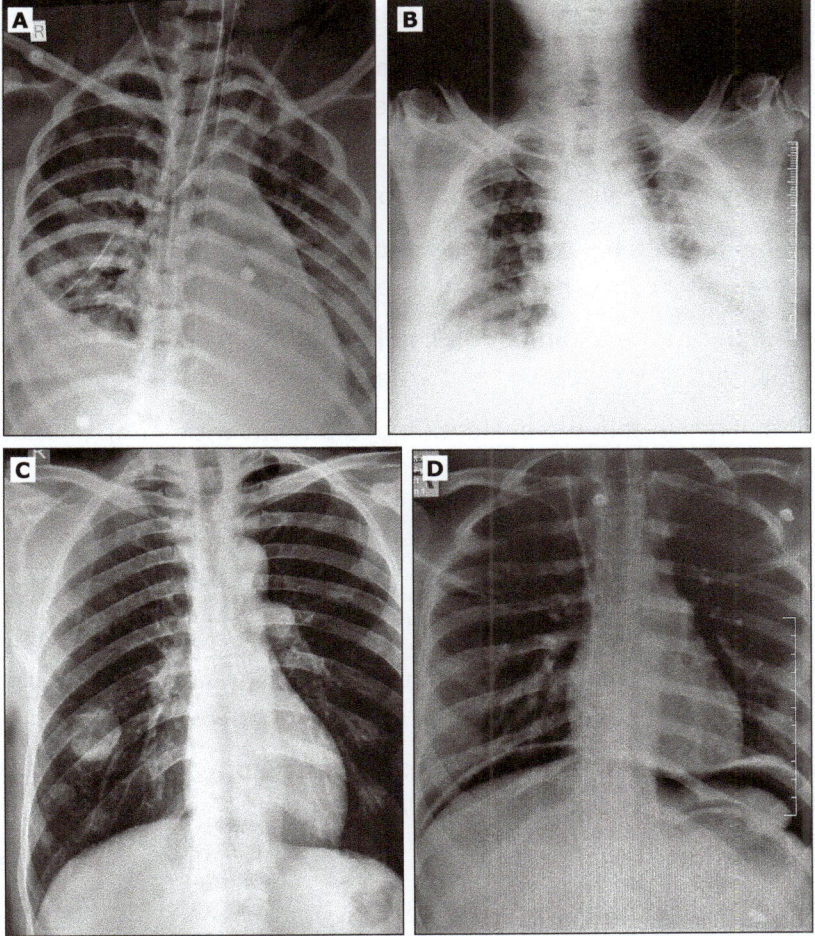

Figure 2.23: X-ray chest showing: A. Pleural effusion; B. Pneumonitis; C. Cannon ball metastasis; D. Free gas under diaphragm.

- Investigations for Diagnosis and Staging. Modalities used:
    - Upper GI endoscopy with or without biopsy: in patients with upper GI symptoms such as dysphagia, dyspepsia, gastric outlet obstruction, upper GI bleed
    - Colonoscopy with or without biopsy: In patients with lower GI symptoms such as per rectal bleed, altered bowel habits (constipation, diarrhea)
    - USG Abdomen and Pelvis:
        - It is an extension of bed side clinical evaluation, it's cheap, noninvasive and easily available
        - It's an excellent tool for evaluation of Hepato-Biliary system. It helps in:
            - Diagnosis and evaluation of liver diseases such as cirrhosis
            - Diagnosis and characterization of space occupying lesion (SOL) in liver

- Diagnosis and evaluation of biliary diseases such as gall stones
- Evaluation of patient with obstructive jaundice (OJ). It can confirm OJ by looking for IHBRD (intra-hepatic biliary radical dilatation). It can also be used to look for the cause of OJ: stone, stricture or mass
- Pancreas may be examined, if not obscured by bowel gas
- It can be used for the evaluation of spleen and bowel, and to look for intra-abdominal lymph nodes and free fluid
- Doppler mode examination can help in evaluation of mesenteric, splenic and hepatic vasculature and great vessels (aorta and IVC)
- It can be used in the evaluation of a patient with Lump in abdomen to:
  - See the site of origin
  - Characterize the lump: its size, shape, extent, margin
- To look for liver metastasis, ascites, omental/peritoneal metastasis, Krukenberg tumor in case of malignancy.
- It can be used for the evaluation of kidney, adrenals, ureter, urinary bladder, prostate, uterus and tubo-ovarian structures
- CECT (contrast enhanced computerized tomography) of the abdomen and pelvis with or without CT of the neck and/or chest:
  - To diagnose the disease and in case of malignancy to stage the disease:
    - To evaluate the site, size, extent of growth
    - Involvement of adjacent organs/vessels
    - To look for regional and distant lymph nodes
    - To look for liver metastasis, omental/peritoneal metastasis, Krukenberg tumor, ascites, lung metastasis, pleural effusion.
  - To look for abdominal complication like:
    - Intestinal obstruction
    - Intestinal Perforation
    - Abscess, phlegmon, fistula formation
    - Vascular complication: thrombosis, pseudoaneurysm
  - To examine chest for:
    - Pneumonia
    - Pleural effusion

- Aspiration
  - Type of CECT:
    - Triple phase CECT: generally performed CT
    - 4 phase CECT: for evaluation of liver disorders
    - Pancreatic protocol CT: for evaluation of pancreatic cancer
    - CT Enterography: for evaluation of bowel related conditions
- MRI abdomen and pelvis:
  - Largely role is similar to CT
  - Advantage over CT:
    - No ionizing radiation
    - May be performed in patients with deranged renal functions
  - Disadvantage:
    - Long acquisition time
    - Expensive
    - Not easily available
    - Risk of contrast associated nephrogenic systemic fibrosis
  - Generally, CT is preferred over MRI
  - However, it has special importance in the evaluation of:
    - Hepato-Pancreatico-Biliary disorders: mainly as it can provide cholangiogram and pancreatogram. Conditions where MRI has a definite role
      - Hilar cholangiocarcinoma
      - Benign biliary stricture due to bile duct injury
      - Liver SOL
      - Chronic pancreatitis
      - Cystic neoplasm of pancreas
    - Rectal cancer: MRI rectal protocol is performed
    - Ano-rectal disorders: Fistula in ano, peri-anal abscess
- FDG-PET-CT: PET is done in cases of malignancy to rule out distant metastasis
- Staging laparoscopy: Done in cases of malignancy to look for peritoneal

metastasis/occult liver metastasis missed on imaging. Main role is to avoid nontherapeutic laparotomy
- Additional investigation as indicated:
  - Tumor markers:
    - AFP (alfa feto proteins) and DCP (des-gamma carboxy prothrombin): (also known as PIVKA- Protein Induced by Vitamin K Absence): For hepatocellular carcinoma
    - CEA (Carcino-embryonic antigen): for colo-rectal carcinoma
    - CA-19-9: for pancreatico-biliary carcinoma
  - CEUS: Contrast enhanced ultrasound for evaluation of liver SOL
  - Contrast study: Upper GI contrast study, barium meal follow through, enteroclysis, rectal contrast study
  - EUS: endoscopic ultrasound with or without fine needle aspiration (FNA) and/or core biopsy
  - EMR: endoscopic mucosal resection
  - ESD: endoscopic submucosal dissection
  - SVE: Side viewing endoscopy
  - Capsule endoscopy, enteroscopy
  - ERCP: endoscopic retrograde cholangio-pancreaticography
  - Cholangioscopy
  - PTC: percutaneous transhepatic cholangiography
  - Liver volumetry
  - ICG (indocyanine green) clearance test
  - Fibroscan, transient elastography
  - Interventional radiology
  - Esophageal manometry, 24 hour pH study
  - Bone scan
- Treatment planning:
  - Following diagnosis and staging (for malignancy), treatment planning is done. Treatment of complex GI diseases generally includes both surgical and non-surgical modalities. Management is best planned in the setting of MDT (multi-disciplinary team) meeting consisting of:

- Surgeon: Surgical gastroenterologists/oncologist, transplant surgeon, general surgeon
- Radiologist: Diagnostic and interventional
- Medical gastroenterologist
- Medical oncologist
- Radiation oncologist
- Pathologist

- Pre-operative Preparation:
  - Baseline investigations
  - PAC: Pre-anesthesia checkup. It is always good to ask your OT anesthetist to evaluate the patient right at the outset once surgery is planned. A thorough evaluation by a good anesthetist may bring out certain correctable/uncorrectable points which may have implications on the surgical outcomes. These can then be accordingly acted upon
  - Investigation for assessing fitness for surgery
    - Assessment of cardio-vascular system:
      - ECG
      - 2-D Echocardiography
      - Tread-mill stress test
      - Dobutamine stress test
      - Cardiac angiography
      - Carotid doppler to look for atherosclerosis
    - Assessment of respiratory system:
      - X-ray chest
      - PFT: pulmonary function test
      - Baseline ABG
  - Correction of underlying coexisting co-morbidities and consultations:
    - Respiratory co-morbidity such as bronchial asthma (BA), chronic obstructive pulmonary disease (COPD): consider pulmonology consultation, bronchodilator, steroids, antibiotics, nebulization and chest physiotherapy
    - Cardiac comorbidity: Hypertension, ischemic heart disease: consider cardiology consultation, antihypertensives, anti-platelets, anti-coagulants,

exercise, SOS angioplasty, CABG (coronary artery bypass grafting)
- Diabetes: Pre-operative control of BSL is important to prevent post-operative morbidity and mortality. Consider endocrinology consultation, diet control and exercise, oral hypoglycemic agents and insulin
- Anemia: administration of oral hematinic, IV iron, blood transfusion
- Coagulopathy: Administration of IV vitamin K, FFP, cryoprecipitates
- Addiction to Smoking and Alcohol: Advise strict abstinence from smoking and alcohol. May consider psychiatry consultation.

- Nutritional assessment and optimization:
  - Assess nutritional status using SGA (subjective global assessment). Consider referral to a dietician for calculation of calorie and protein requirement
  - Patients awaiting major surgery are generally advised high calorie, high protein diet
  - Nutritional therapy may be total or supplemental and may be provided enterally or parenterally
- Chest Physiotherapy: It is a must prior to any major abdominal surgery. It consists of deep breathing exercises, incentive spirometry
- Immediate pre-operative preparation
  - Consent: Patient and a responsible relative should be thoroughly counselled regarding his/her disease, treatment options, planned surgery, expected surgical complications, morbidity and mortality. this is followed by a written informed consent
  - Arrange for blood and blood products
  - Tetanus toxoid (TT) injection
  - Advise regarding Diet: Explain regarding dietary restrictions if any and duration of fasting expected prior to surgery. Generally, patients are advised to be nil per oral from midnight. However, protocols may vary depending on whether or not ERAS (enhanced recovery after surgery) is followed
  - Advice regarding drugs patient is already consuming:
    – Anti-hypertensives: Given on day of surgery
    – Steroid: Given on day of surgery
    – Oral hypoglycemic: Morning dose skipped on day of surgery
    – Aspirin: Continued till day before surgery

- Clopidogrel: Stopped atleast 5 days before surgery
- Warfarin: Change over to UFH (unfractionated heparin) or LMWH (low molecular weight heparin) a week before surgery and continue it till 6 hours and 12 hours prior to surgery respectively
- Skin preparation: Clear the surgical site of hair using either trimming/clipping (preferred), shaving or depilatory cream. Advise the patient to take bath on the day of surgery with an anti-septic solution
- Pre-operative antibiotics at time of induction to prevent surgical site infection
  - Generally, Cephalosporin (Cefazolin or Cefuroxime) is used.
  - In case anaerobic contamination is expected as in esophageal or colorectal surgery then metronidazole needs to be added
- DVT prophylaxis: it generally consists of:
  - Pharmacological prophylaxis: LMWH, UFH
  - Mechanical prophylaxis: DVT stockings, pneumatic compression stockings, crepe bandage application
- Special preparation:
  - In case of GOO (gastric outlet obstruction):
    - Correction of dehydration and dyselectrolytemia (hypokalemic hypochloremic metabolic alkalosis)
    - Gastric lavage with the help of naso-gastric tube for at least 2-3 days prior to surgery
  - In case of Colo-Rectal cancers:
    - Bowel preparation may or may not be performed depending on unit protocol. It consists of:
      - Dietary restriction: Low residue diet for few days prior to planned surgery. Only clear liquids on the day before surgery
      - Bowel wash with polyethylene glycol on the day before surgery
      - Antibiotics: Oral neomycin, erythromycin on the day before surgery
  - In case of obstructive jaundice:
    - Correction of Coagulopathy: administration of IV vitamin K, FFP, cryoprecipitates
    - Pre-operative IV hydration

- In case of planned splenectomy:
  - Vaccination is advised 14 day before or after surgery. Vaccines to be administered:
    - Meningococcal vaccine
    - Pneumococcal vaccine
    - Hemophilus influenza type B vaccine

3 Case of Dysphagia due to Carcinoma Esophagus, Achalasia Cardia

Introduction
- The purpose of history taking and examination in these cases is to confirm the presence of dysphagia and know the probable diagnosis
- Differentials that will be discussed in this chapter:
  - Carcinoma Esophagus
  - Achalasia Cardia

Format for History Taking
- History of dysphagia/difficulty in swallowing: Describe the dysphagia in detail
  - Duration
  - Onset: insidious or sudden
  - Nature: whether it is intermittent, stable or progressive
  - The grade of dysphagia
  - If progressive, describe the initial grade and the grade now at time of presentation
- Site of food getting stuck: neck/upper chest/lower chest
- History of odynophagia, neck pain, neck swelling
- History of halitosis, neck swelling or gurgling sound while swallowing
- History of difficulty initiating swallowing, nasal regurgitation, nasal twang, dysarthria
- History of associated chest pain
- History of regurgitation
- History of relation of the dysphagia to the temperature of food i.e. precipitation or relief of dysphagia with hot or cold beverages
- History of postural modulation to facilitate swallowing
- History of corrosive intake
- History of long standing gastro-esophageal reflux disease: heartburn, regurgitation
- History of hematemesis, melena
- History of cough with expectoration, recurrent upper respiratory tract infection, recurrent fever with or without chills

- History of backache, choking or coughing after swallowing food, hoarseness of voice
- History of abdominal pain, distension, nausea, vomiting, altered bowel habits
- History of loss of weight, loss of appetite
- History of abdominal distension, jaundice, respiratory discomfort, hemoptysis, bone and back pain
- Treatment history: Evaluation with cross-sectional imaging (this includes USG, CT, MRI), upper GI endoscopy with/without biopsy
- Whether chemotherapy and/or radiotherapy was initiated
  - Its intent: Neoadjuvant, Definitive, Palliative
  - When was it initiated, duration of therapy received, time of completion, time since completion
  - History of adverse events during chemo-radiotherapy, Post CRT course
- Past history:
  - Of comorbid illness: DM, HTN, Coronary artery disease (CAD), tuberculosis (TB), chronic obstructive pulmonary disease (COPD), Bronchial asthma (BA)
  - Surgery
  - Oral malignancy
- Personal history:
  - Smoking history in detail including:
    - Type of smoke: cigarette, cigar or biddi
    - Number of smokes per day; number of years of smoking; calculate pack years
    - Any attempts to quit smoking
  - History of alcohol consumption
- Family history: history of cancer in first and second degree family
- Performance history:
  - Whether he/she is
    - Able to perform all daily routine activity (sedentary and/or strenuous)
    - Able to perform all self care
    - Bed ridden
  - Whether he/she is able to climb two flight of stairs comfortably or not

Justification for Each Component in History

- History of dysphagia:
    - Dysphagia refers to difficulty in swallowing.
    - Depending on the site of the pathology it may be classified as either transfer/oropharyngeal dysphagia or esophageal dysphagia.
    - Transfer dysphagia means patient has difficulty transferring food from oral cavity into the esophagus via the pharynx; most common cause being neurological disorders such as stroke.
    - Esophageal dysphagia occurs due to pathology in esophagus, most common causes being malignancy and motility disorder. Most likely cause of dysphagia in an exam setting (especially in an elderly patient) are carcinoma esophagus and achalasia cardia.
- Onset of dysphagia:
    - Insidious onset: dysphagia in carcinoma esophagus and achalasia cardia is usually insidious in onset.
    - Sudden onset: Sudden onset dysphagia is seen in other types of esophageal motility disorders like diffuse esophageal spasm and jackhammer esophagus.
    - Sudden onset aphagia is seen in patient with Schatzki ring.
- Nature of dysphagia: whether it is intermittent, stable or progressive:
    - Intermittent dysphagia would suggest esophageal motility disorder.
    - Progressive dysphagia would suggest carcinoma esophagus, achalasia cardia.
    - Stable dysphagia would suggest chronic benign stricture like peptic stricture.
- The grade of dysphagia

Table 3.1: Grades of dysphagia (as described by Suguhara et al)
▪ 1: Able to swallow solid meals with some difficulty
▪ 2: Able to swallow solid meals but requires liquids along with it
▪ 3: Able to swallow only semisolid meals
▪ 4: Able to swallow only liquids
▪ 5: Able to swallow only saliva
▪ 6: Unable to swallow anything including saliva

-
    - It is important while taking history to note the grade of dysphagia. If dysphagia is progressive in nature then note the grade of dysphagia at the onset of symptoms and what is the grade at presentation.

- Site of food getting stuck: neck/upper chest/lower chest: it is usually said that the actual site of obstruction is below the site of obstruction as perceived by the patient. So for example, if patient says that the site of dysphagia is in the neck, then the site of obstruction will be somewhere below i.e. any where in the thoracic esophagus or esophago-gastric junction.

- History of Odynophagia: Odynophagia refers to pain while swallowing. Its presence suggests a painful oro-pharyngeal pathology such as tonsillitis, quinsy, pharyngitis or acute corrosive injury.

- History of neck pain: it suggests an inflammatory or infective pathology in the neck such as retro pharyngeal abscess.

- History of neck swelling: it could suggest goiter of any cause (especially malignant cause) compressing the esophagus resulting in dysphagia. Alternatively, a zenker's diverticulum could also occasionally cause neck swelling.

- History of halitosis, neck swelling, gurgling sound while swallowing: these symptoms suggest Zenker's diverticulum.

- History of difficulty initiating swallowing, nasal regurgitation, nasal twang, dysarthria: all would suggest oropharyngeal/transfer dysphagia most commonly due to neurological cause such as stroke.

- History of associated chest pain: presence of gripping type of chest pain suggests motility disorder.

- History of regurgitation: it would suggest either motility disorder or gastro esophageal reflux disease with resultant peptic stricture/Adenocarcinoma GE junction.

- History of relation of the dysphagia to the temperature of food i.e. precipitation or relief of dysphagia with hot or cold beverages: it would suggest motility disorder.

- History of postural modulation to facilitate swallowing: some patient extend their neck and/or straighten their spine to facilitate the act of swallowing. It is usually seen in long standing dysphagia of benign etiology as in motility disorder.

- History of corrosive intake: it is important to rule out previous history of either accidental or intentional corrosive (acid or alkali) consumption. In such case the dysphagia would be due to caustic esophageal stricture. At times there may be accidental consumption of corrosive without the patient's knowledge and he may present with dysphagia at a later date due to corrosive stricture.

- History of long-standing gastro- esophageal reflux disease: heartburn, regurgitation: Long standing GERD may result in peptic stricture. Long standing GERD is also an etiological factor for adenocarcinoma of the GE junction. So, if present suspect an adenocarcinoma of the GEJ or peptic stricture.

- History of hematemesis, melena: it may have many implications. GI bleed may be seen in carcinoma or in acute corrosive esophageal injury. Hematemesis may also occur as a complication of dilatation therapy for corrosive esophageal stricture. Alternatively, patient might have dysphagia as a sequelae of sclerotherapy done for variceal GI bleed.

- History of cough with expectoration, recurrent upper respiratory tract infection, recurrent fever +/- chills: patients with progressive esophageal obstruction (as in achalasia cardia, malignancy) develop gradually increasing proximal esophageal dilatation in which food gets accumulated. The patient may aspirate the esophageal content when supine leading to respiratory tract infection, manifesting as cough with expectoration, fever with chills.

- History of backache: History of backache in an elderly patient with dysphagia points towards advanced esophageal malignancy infiltrating the posterior mediastinal nerves and vertebra.

- History of choking or coughing after swallowing food: this is a grave symptom which would suggest tracheo- esophageal fistula. This should point towards advanced unresectable esophageal malignancy with tracheal involvement leading to tracheo-esophageal fistula. Alternatively choking or coughing within first few seconds after swallowing food may be seen in transfer/oropharyngeal dysphagia due to neurological cause (stroke).

- History of hoarseness of voice: this again is a grave symptom suggesting recurrent laryngeal nerve involvement in a patient with advanced unresectable esophageal malignancy.

- History of loss of weight, loss of appetite: these are alarming symptoms pointing towards malignancy. However, one has to remember that any patient with dysphagia of more than a few weeks duration is bound to develop weight loss even if the etiology is benign. So be aware before labelling the patient to have dysphagia of malignant origin just based on the fact that patient gives history of loss of weight.

Table 3.2: Definition of significant weight loss
▪ Loss of > 10% body weight in 6 months
▪ Loss of > 7.5% body weight in 3 months
▪ Loss of > 5% body weight in 1 month
▪ Loss of > 2% body weight in 1 week

- History of abdominal distension; respiratory discomfort; hemoptysis; Bony pain; back pain; blackout; seizures: all these symptoms are suggestive of metastatic disease.
    - Abdominal distension: Due to malignant ascites
    - Respiratory discomfort: Due to pleural effusion and lung metastasis
    - Hemoptysis: Due to lung metastasis
    - Bony pain: Due to bony metastasis
    - Back pain: Due to vertebral metastasis
    - Blackout, Seizures: due to brain metastasis
- Treatment history of evaluation with upper GI endoscopy and a biopsy, administration of chemotherapy, radiotherapy would hint the candidate towards diagnosis of malignant dysphagia.
- Whether chemotherapy and/or radiotherapy was initiated, when was it initiated, duration of therapy received, time of completion, time since completion, history of adverse events during chemo-radiotherapy, post CRT course: Although such history helps confirm the clinical diagnosis of malignant dysphagia, it is best to mention this part of history briefly, and not elaborate on the same. Some examiners may not like it.
- History of comorbid illness: It is very important to know about the patient's co-morbidities, especially pulmonary diseases like bronchial asthma and chronic obstructive pulmonary disease. One cannot plan surgery in a patient with disabling respiratory co morbidity/depleted respiratory reserve as they won't tolerate surgery well.
- Past history of oral or upper digestive tract cancer: Patient with such history are at higher risk for esophageal cancer due to field cancerisation
- Smoking history: It is very important to know in detail about patient's smoking habit. Smoking tobacco is an etiological factor for esophageal malignancy. Additionally patients who smoke usually do not tolerate surgery well.
- Performance history: To assess whether patient can withstand required treatment including chemotherapy, radiotherapy and surgery. Patients with poor effort tolerance, as in those who cannot climb two flights of stairs usually do not tolerate aggressive treatment well. Performance status of the patient is determined as per ECOG (Eastern Cooperative Oncology Group) classification for malignant diseases and WHO (world health organization) classification for benign diseases.

> **Table 3.3: ECOG/WHO performance scale**
> - 0: Fully active; no performance restrictions.
> - 1: Fully ambulatory and able to carry out light work. Strenuous physical activity restricted
> - 2: Capable of all self-care but unable to carry out any other work activities. Up and about > 50% of waking hours.
> - 3: Capable of only limited self-care; confined to bed or chair > 50% of waking hours.
> - 4: Completely disabled; cannot carry out any self-care; totally confined to bed or chair.

- Patients with performance status (PS) ECOG 0 and 1 usually tolerate major surgery well, whereas those with PS ECOG 3 and 4 usually do not tolerate any kind of aggressive treatment. Patients with PS ECOG 2 are borderline.

Format for Examination
- Remember:
  - In a case of dysphagia it is very unlikely to find positive findings on abdominal examination
  - It is important to mention findings of oral, neck and chest examination
- What is the appearance of the patient: young/middle-aged/elderly, lady/gentleman
- Whether the patient is clinically
  - Poorly/averagely/well built
  - Poorly/averagely/well nourished
  - Clinical features suggesting poor nourishment
    - Temporal wasting
    - Sunken eyes
    - Flattened cheeks, Buccal hollow
    - Supraclavicular hollow
    - Squaring of shoulders
    - Prominent scapula
    - Prominent intercostal spaces
    - Scaphoid abdomen
    - Prominent hip bones
    - Prominent knee and elbows

- Pedal edema
- Decreased mid arm circumference
- Decreased skin fold thickness

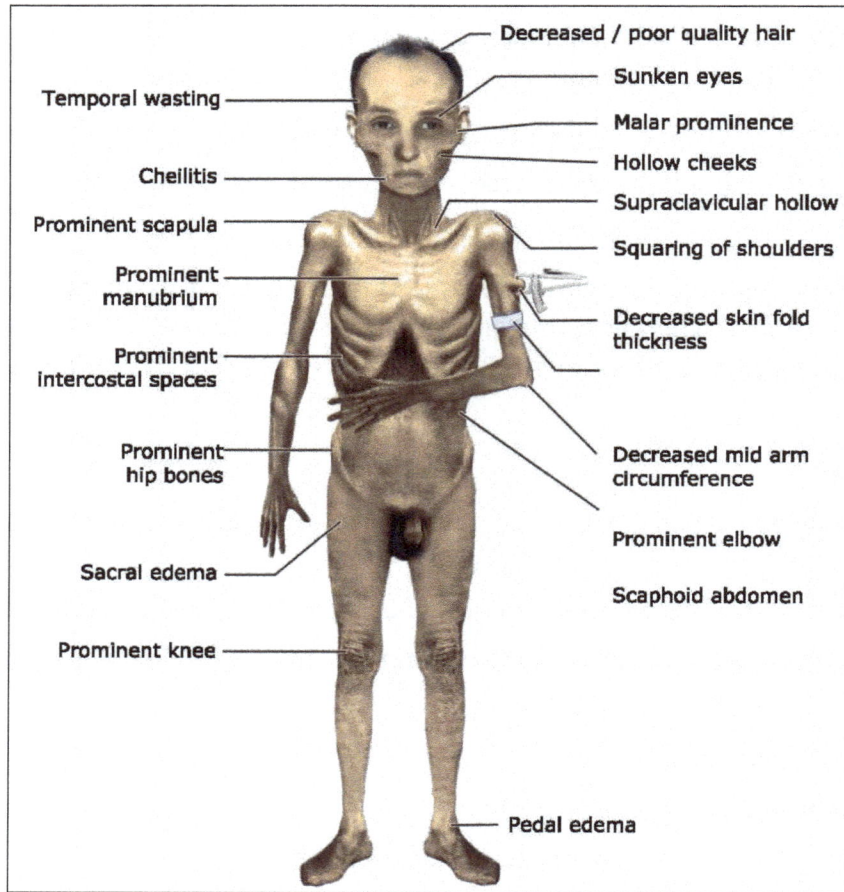

Figure 3.1: Clinical features suggesting poor nourishment.

- Measure height, weight, BMI
- It is very important to clinically assess the patient's nutritional status. Many a times even though a patient may have radiologically resectable esophageal cancer, patient's poor nutritional status may not permit surgical resection.
• Whether the patient is clinically
  - Conscious/stuporous
  - Cooperative/un-cooperative
  - Well/poorly oriented to time, place and person;

- o Well hydrated/dehydrated
- o Lying comfortably in bed/in discomfort/in pain
- o Preferred decubitus: whether patient prefers sitting position or he/she can comfortably lie in supine position
- o Febrile/Afebrile.
- Mention Pulse, BP, respiratory rate.
- Breath holding time: Along with vitals it would be good to mention the breath holding time (normal being > 22 seconds) in a patient with dysphagia suspected to be due to malignancy. Apart from nutritional status assessment, this is another clinical method of assessing fitness for surgery.
- Look for
  - o Pallor, jaundice, cyanosis, clubbing
  - o Generalized or localized lymphadenopathy
  - o Palpable cervical and left supraclavicular lymph node
  - o Pedal or dependent edema
  - o Skin lesions, if any
- Examination of oral cavity: it is an important component of examination in case of dysphagia. Look for:
  - o Mouth opening: look for reduced mouth opening or trismus. It could be present in patients with submucosal fibrosis or oral malignancy. Submucosal fibrosis itself is an etiological factor for squamous cell carcinoma of the upper digestive tract.
  - o Mucosal lesion: look for any obvious mucosal lesion like leukoplakia, erythroplakia, ulcers or growth. Leukoplakia and erythroplakia are precursors to oral malignancy. At times there may be co-existing oral and esophageal malignancy. At times, patient may have previously undergone surgery for oral cancer and later patient develop dysphagia due to esophageal malignancy (concept of field cancerization).
  - o Oral hygiene: look for dental caries, tobacco stains, foul smell/halitosis.
  - o Tongue movement: Normal or impaired: impaired tongue movement would suggest either tumor infiltration or neurological disease as in stroke.

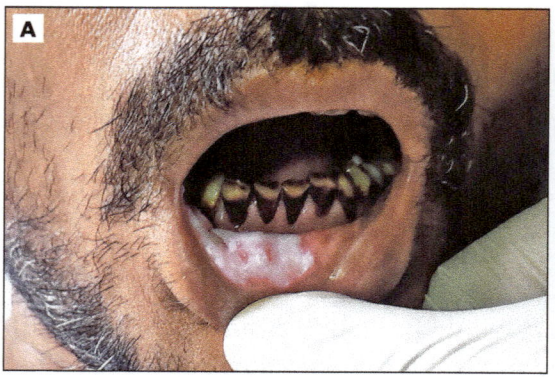 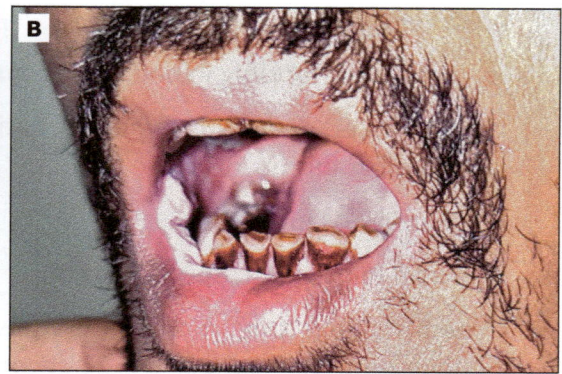

Figure 3.2: Oral examination showing (A) Leukoplakia; (B) poor oral hygiene and tobacco stains.

- Examination of the abdomen: (in a case of dysphagia it is usually unremarkable)
  - On Inspection: See if:
    - Abdomen is flat/distended/scaphoid
    - Umbilicus is central/displaced (upwards/downwards/sideways); inverted/everted/flat.
    - All quadrants are moving equally with respiration or not
    - See if there is any visible lump
    - Look for visible scar, sinus, engorged veins, pulsations, peristalsis or cough impulse.
    - Don't forget to inspect the groin hernial sites (to look for swelling or cough impulse i.e. hernia) and examine genitalia.
    - Inspection of renal angles to look for fullness
  - On Palpation: See if:
    - Abdomen is soft, non-tender
    - Liver is palpable or not; hepatomegaly may be present in case of liver metastasis
      - If yes, measure its extent from costal margin in midclavicular line in units of centimeter or number of fingers below costal margin
      - See if:
        - It is tender/nontender;
        - Surface is smooth/nodular;
        - Borders are round/sharp, regular/irregular,
        - Consistency is soft/firm/hard

- Spleen is enlarged or not (unlikely to find splenomegaly)
- Any other palpable lump. Do not forget to look for umbilical nodule/Sister Mary Joseph nodule which would suggest metastatic disease.
- Do not forget to:
  - Palpate groin hernia sites to look for cough impulse
  - Examine genitals
  - Look for tenderness in Renal angles
  - Examine back and spine for tenderness/gibbus.
- On Percussion:
  - Look for upper border of liver dullness (generally in the 5th intercostal space) in midclavicular line.
  - Note the liver span (normal being 12–14 cm)
  - Percussion note in the rest of the abdomen (generally tympanic)
  - Tests for free fluid
- On auscultation:
  - Auscultate for bowel sounds.
  - Bruit, hum and rub
- Per rectal examination
- Respiratory examination:
  - Inspection:
    - Whether the trachea is in midline or is deviated
    - Bilateral chest movement: equal or not
  - Palpation:
    - Trachea: central or deviated
    - Chest: look for warmth and tenderness
    - Bilateral chest movement: equal or not
    - Tactile vocal fremitus:
      - It is increased in case of pleural effusion and consolidation.
  - Auscultation: most important part of respiratory examination:
    - Breath sounds:
      - Bilaterally equal or not

- Reduced in any lung field: right/left; upper/mid/lower zone. Reduced breath sounds would suggest either pleural effusion or consolidation.
    - Adventitious sounds:
        - Crepts: coarse crepts would suggest aspiration pneumonitis, whereas fine crepts would suggest pulmonary edema.
        - Ronchi/wheeze
  - Percussion:
    - Normal percussion note is resonant.
    - Dull note suggests consolidation or pleural effusion.
- Rest systemic examination

EXAMPLE CASE

History

- My patient Mrs XYZ, is a 64-year-old lady hailing from Mumbai, is a homemaker.
- She presented with chief complaints of difficulty in swallowing since 2 months.
- She was apparently alright 2 months back, when she developed difficulty in swallowing solid food, which was insidious in onset with the sensation of food being stuck in lower chest. She required water along with solid foods to facilitate the act of swallowing
- Gradually the dysphagia has progressed such that she is now able to consume only liquids
- She gives history of having lost 10 kg over last 2 months with an associated history of decreased appetite
- She gives no history of:
  - Odynophagia
  - Chest pain, regurgitation, relation of dysphagia to temperature of food or posture.
  - Difficulty initiating swallowing, nasal regurgitation, nasal twang, dysarthria or choking sensation
  - Halitosis, neck swelling, gurgling sound while swallowing
  - Cough with expectoration, upper respiratory tract infection, recurrent fever with chills
  - Coughing/choking after swallowing, hoarseness of voice, pain in back

- o Hematemesis, melena
- o Abdominal pain, nausea, vomiting, altered bowel habits
- o Corrosive intake or long standing symptoms of GERD
- o Jaundice, respiratory distress, bony or back pain
- She seeked medical care for these symptoms for which she was evaluated with upper GI endoscopy and biopsy and CT abdomen.
- There is no previous history of bronchial asthma, COPD, TB, diabetes, hypertension, ischemic heart disease.
- She has not undergone any major surgery in the past.
- There is no history of alcohol consumption or smoking
- She is post menopausal,
- Family history is not contributory
- She is able to perform all her daily routine activity without any difficulty and is able to climb two flight of stairs without difficulty

Examination

- My patient is an elderly lady, who is averagely built, poorly nourished, with a height of 160 cm, weight of 45 kg and BMI being 17.6 kg/m^2
- She is conscious, cooperative, well oriented to time, place and person; Lying comfortably in bed; well hydrated and afebrile.
- Pulse is 72/min, BP is 110/70 mm Hg, respiratory rate is 14 per min and breath holding time is 24 seconds.
- There is no pallor, jaundice, cyanosis, clubbing, generalized or localized lymphadenopathy. There is no palpable cervical or left supraclavicular lymph node; pedal or dependent edema or skin lesions
- Examination of oral cavity reveals adequate mouth opening, tongue movement and oral hygiene with no obvious mucosal lesions.
- Examination of the abdomen:
  - o On inspection: Abdomen is flat, umbilicus is central, inverted. All quadrants are moving equally with respiration. There is no visible lump, scar, sinus, engorged veins, pulsations, peristalsis or cough impulse.
  - o Inspection of groin hernial sites reveals no swelling or cough impulse and Inspection of genitalia is unremarkable. Inspection of renal angles reveals no fullness

- On Palpation: Abdomen is soft and non-tender. Liver and spleen are not palpable. There isn't any other palpable lump.
- There is no palpable cough impulse over groin hernia sites and examination of genitals is unremarkable. There is no tenderness in renal angles. Examination of back and spine is essentially normal.
- On Percussion, upper border of liver dullness is in the 5th intercostal space in midclavicular line with liver span being 14 cm. Rest of the abdomen is tympanitic with no evidence of free fluid.
- On auscultation normal bowel sounds are heard. There is no bruit, hum or rub
- Per rectal examination is unremarkable.
- Examination of respiratory system:
    - Trachea is central
    - Bilateral chest movement is equal
    - On percussion there is resonant note in bilateral lung fields.
    - On auscultation air entry is bilaterally equal, with normal vesicular breath sounds heard and there is no crepts or wheeze.
- Rest systemic examination is essentially normal

To Summarize

- My patient is a 64-year-old female with no co-morbid illness with ECOG 1 performance status, presents with 2 months history of gradually progressive dysphagia, first to solids and now to liquids with associated history of loss of weight and appetite
- On examination she is poorly nourished with BMI being 17.6 kg/m^2. Examination of neck, chest and abdomen is unremarkable

The Most Probable Diagnosis in my patient is malignant dysphagia due to carcinoma esophagus

How to Proceed: (Sequence and Justification)

- Review available medical records
- Routine blood investigations (Hemogram, Liver Function Test, Renal Function Test, Serum Electrolyte, INR)
- Upper GI endoscopy: to confirm the diagnosis/to confirm the presence of a neoplastic growth in the esophagus/GE junction; if present note:

- The site and size
- The extent: Longitudinal and circumferential extent. Relation to cricopharynx and GE junction
- Morphology: Proliferative/ulcerative/ulcero-proliferative/infiltrative
- Whether passable or not
- Presence of synchronous lesions: Malignancy elsewhere in the upper GI tract, Barrett's esophagus, concomitant gastric pathology
- Presence of bleed
- Siewert Stein type in case of GEJ malignancy
  - Type I: Epicentre of tumor between 1 and 5 cm above GEJ
  - Type II: Epicentre of tumor between 1 above GEJ and 2 cm below GEJ
  - Type III: Epicentre of tumor between 2 and 5 cm below GEJ
- Biopsy: 6-8 in number

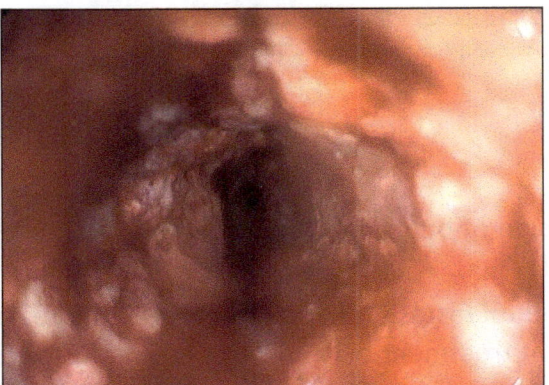

Figure 3.3: Upper GI endoscopy showing stricturing growth in mid esophagus.

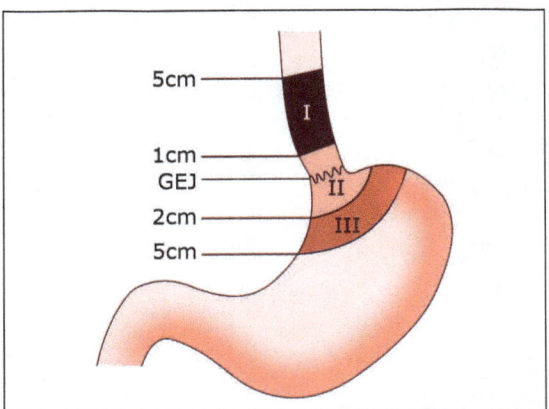

Figure 3.4: Siewert-Stein classification of GEJ adenocarcinoma.

- X-ray chest: to look for lung metastasis. If present it deems the patient in-operable and palliative intent treatment may be initiated. Further investigation may not be warranted

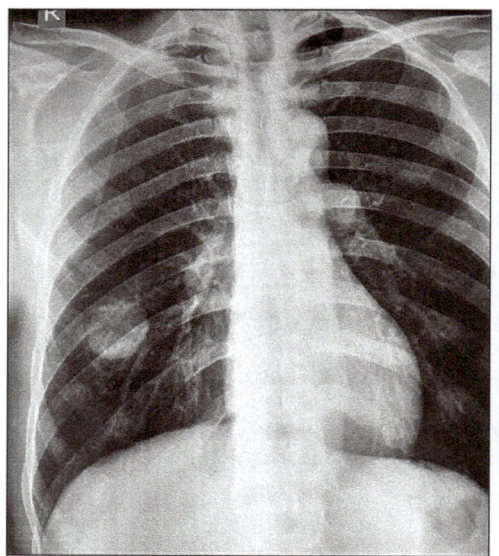

Figure 3.5: X-ray chest showing cannon ball metastasis.

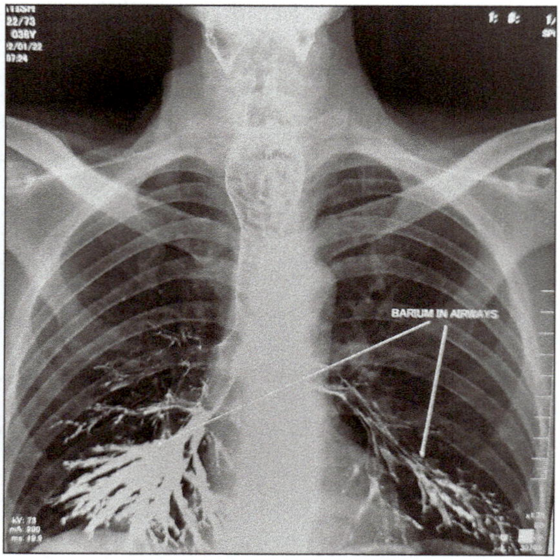

Figure 3.6: Upper GI Contrast Study revealing a Tracheo-Esophageal Fistula.

- USG (A+P):
  - It is an extension of bed side clinical evaluation, it's cheap, non invasive and easily available
  - To look for liver metastasis, ascites, omental/peritoneal metastasis. If present, palliative intent treatment may be initiated and further investigation may not be warranted

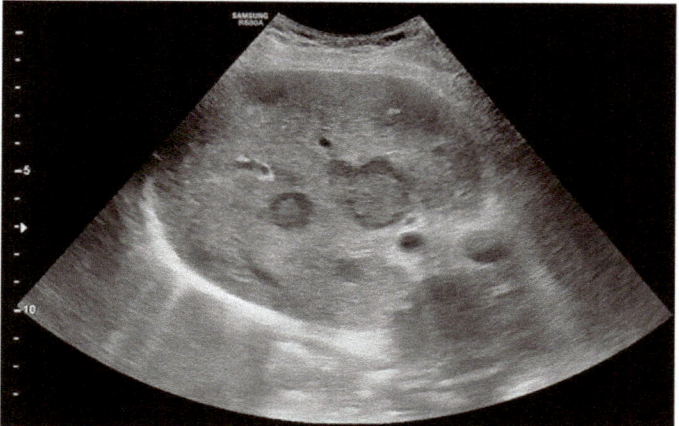

Figure 3.7: USG abdomen showing liver metastasis.

- CECT of the neck, chest, abdomen and pelvis: to stage the disease:
  - To evaluate the site, size, extent of growth
  - Involvement of adjacent organs/vessels: pericardium, heart, trachea, bronchi, lung, aorta, vertebra, liver, spleen, pancreas, diaphragmatic crus, celiac artery. In case of aortic involvement note the Picus angle.

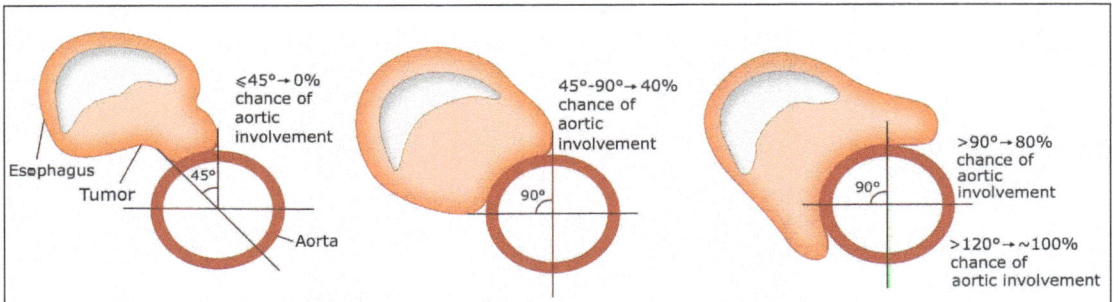

Figure 3.8: Angle of contact between esophageal cancer and aorta: Picus angle.

  - To look for lymph nodes: cervical, mediastinal, paratracheal, tracheo-bronchial, lung hilar, para-aortic, aorto-pulmonary, diaphragmatic, perigastric, left gastric, celiac, hepatic, splenic artery
  - To look for liver metastasis, omental/peritoneal metastasis, Krukenberg tumor, ascites, lung metastasis, pleural effusion.

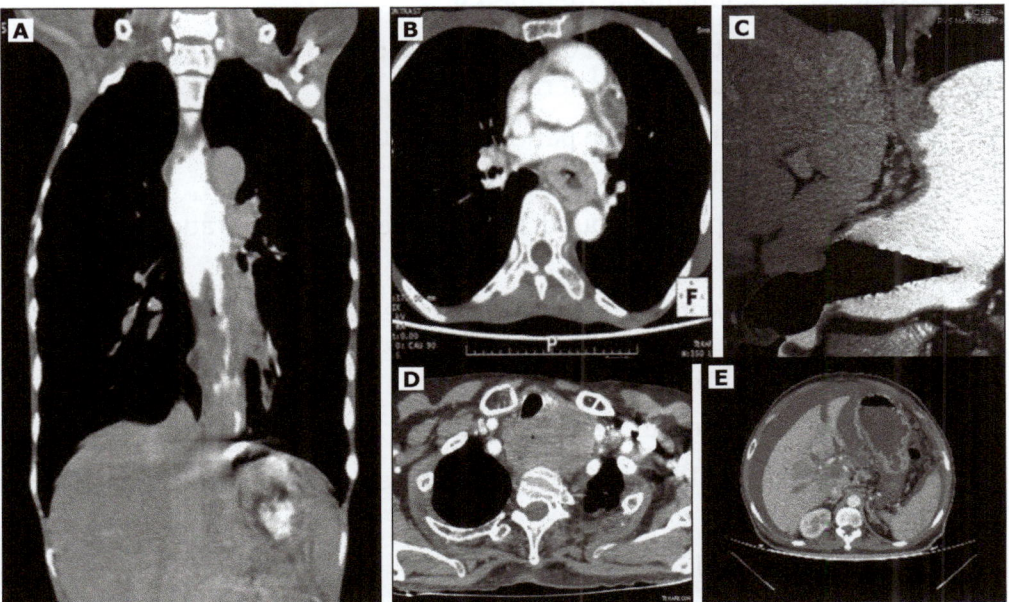

Figure 3.9: CT showing: apple core like malignancy with shouldering in mid-lower esophagus (A); esophageal wall thickening due to malignancy in mid esophagus (B); GEJ tumor (C); cervical- proximal esophageal tumor (D); malignant ascites (E)

- FDG-PET-CT: PET is done primarily to rule out distant metastasis. It is less efficacious for local staging. Note that, poorly differentiated adenocarcinoma/signet ring adenocarcinoma are less FDG avid
- Staging laparoscopy with or without peritoneal cytology: performed in cases of GEJ adenocarcinoma. Done to look for peritoneal metastasis/occult liver metastasis. Main role is to avoid nontherapeutic laparotomy

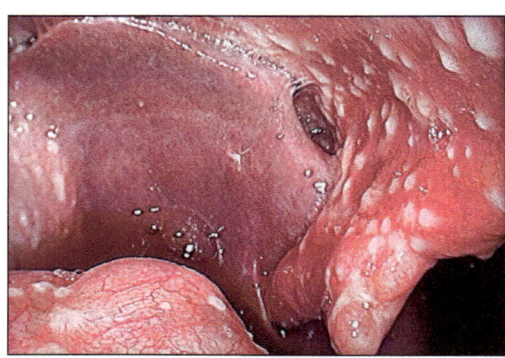

Figure 3.10: Staging laparoscopy (and not diagnostic laparoscopy) revealing peritoneal metastasis.

- Optional staging investigation:
  - EUS: endoscopic ultrasound: useful modality for T and N staging. Guided fine needle aspiration (FNA) and/or core biopsy is possible with EUS
  - EMR: endoscopic mucosal resection: It is considered for clinically early stage T1 cancers. It is potentially therapeutic.
  - ESD: endoscopic submucosal dissection: It is considered for clinically early stage T1 cancers. It is potentially therapeutic.
  - Bronchoscopy: performed in patients with tumors above the carina to rule out tracheal involvement
  - Endo-bronchoscopic ultrasound: Guided fine needle aspiration is possible with EBUS
  - At the end of the work up, the tumor is staged as per AJCC-TNM staging system
- Management principles:
  - In esophageal squamous cell carcinoma:
    - Treatment would generally include Neoadjuvant chemoradiation followed by surgery
    - Alternative options:
      - Upfront surgery followed by adjuvant chemoradiation
      - Definitive chemoradiation

Table 3.4: AJCC-TNM staging system for esophageal carcinoma

- T stage:
  - T1: Tumor invades submucosa
  - T2: Tumor invades muscularis propria
  - T3: Tumor invades adventitia
  - T4: Tumor invades adjacent structures
- N stage:
  - N1: Metastasis to 1–2 lymph nodes (LN)
  - N2: Metastasis to 3–6 LN
  - N3: Metastasis to 7 or more LN
- M stage:
  - M0: No distant metastasis
  - M1: Distant metastasis present

- In esophageal/GEJ adenocarcinoma:
    - Treatment would generally include pre-operative chemotherapy followed by surgery followed by post-operative chemotherapy (i.e. peri-operative chemotherapy)
    - Alternative options:
        - Neoadjuvant chemoradiation followed by surgery
        - Upfront surgery followed by adjuvant chemoradiation
        - Upfront surgery followed by adjuvant chemotherapy
- Enteral nutrition:
  - Modalities:
    - Naso-gastric tube insertion
    - Naso-jejunal tube insertion
    - Feeding jejunostomy
    - SEMS (self-expansile metallic stent) insertion.
  - This needs to be achieved before initiating any kind of neo-adjuvant therapy or definitive CRT
- Neoadjuvant therapy
  - Advantage:
    - To downstage/downsize the tumor

- To evaluate tumor biology i.e.
  - if the cancer progresses on therapy then it suggests aggressive tumor biology and such patients would not benefit from any kind of aggressive therapy.
  - On the contrary good response to therapy suggests good tumor biology and hence better prognosis.
- Therapy is given to tissues with intact vascularity and which are well oxygenated
- Radiated tissues will be removed at surgery
- Systemic micro-metastasis is dealt with by the systemic chemotherapy
- Higher proportion of patients will receive chemotherapy and/or radiation
    - Disadvantage:
        - Loss of window of opportunity in case the disease progresses. That is if a resectable cancer becomes unresectable during the course of neoadjuvant therapy then the window of opportunity to resect the tumor is lost
    - Indication: tumors with clinical TNM stage >/= T2, >/= N1, M0
- Neo-adjuvant chemoradiation:
    - CROSS regimen is commonly used. It consists of carboplatin + paclitaxel + 41.4 gray radiation.
    - Primarily preferred for squamous cell carcinoma
- Peri-op chemotherapy:
    - Primarily preferred for adenocarcinoma
    - Options are:
        - ECF: MAGIC regimen: epirubicin, cisplatin and 5-Fluorouracil. 3 cycles pre and post surgery
        - DCF: Docetaxel, cisplatin and 5-Fluorouracil. 3 cycles pre and post surgery
        - FLOT: 5-FU, leucovorine, oxalilatin and docetaxel. 4 cycles pre and post surgery
- Response assessment:
    - Modalities used:
        - CT

- PET-CT
- Upper GI endoscopy
- Surgery:
  - Options are:
    - Orringers trans-hiatal esophagectomy: laparotomy and cervical exploration with cervical anastomosis
    - Trans-thoracic Ivor-Lewis (two hole) esophagectomy: laparotomy and thoracotomy with intrathoracic anastomosis
    - Trans-thoracic Mc Evans (three hole) esophagectomy: thoracotomy, laparotomy and cervical exploration with cervical anastomosis
    - Minimally invasive esophagectomy
    - Hybrid esophagectomy: combination of minimally invasive and open surgical modality
    - Radical total D2 gastrectomy for Siewerts type 3 GE junction adenocarcinomas
    - Proximal Gastrectomy for Siewerts type 3 GE junction adenocarcinomas (less preferred option)

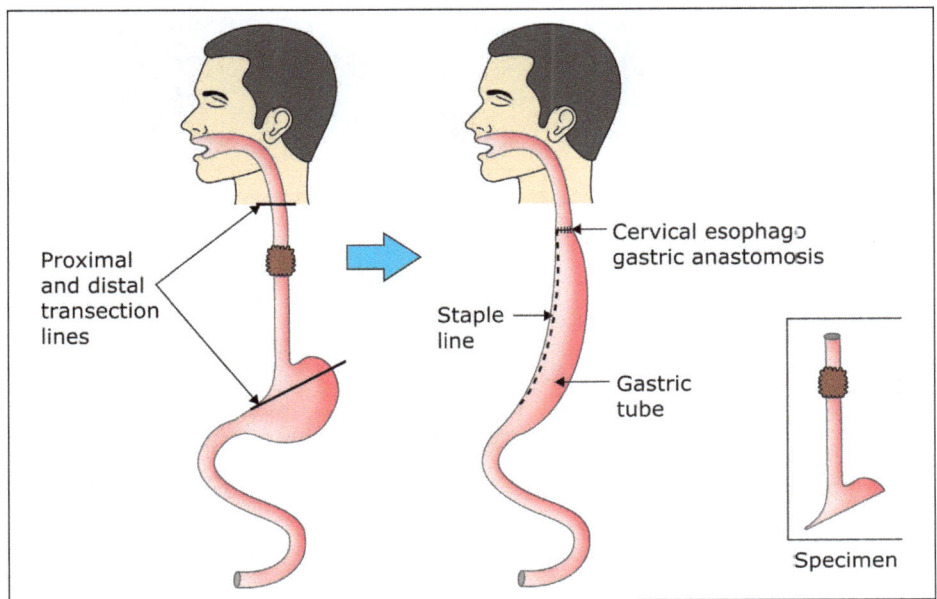

Figure 3.11: Esophagectomy with cervical anastomosis.

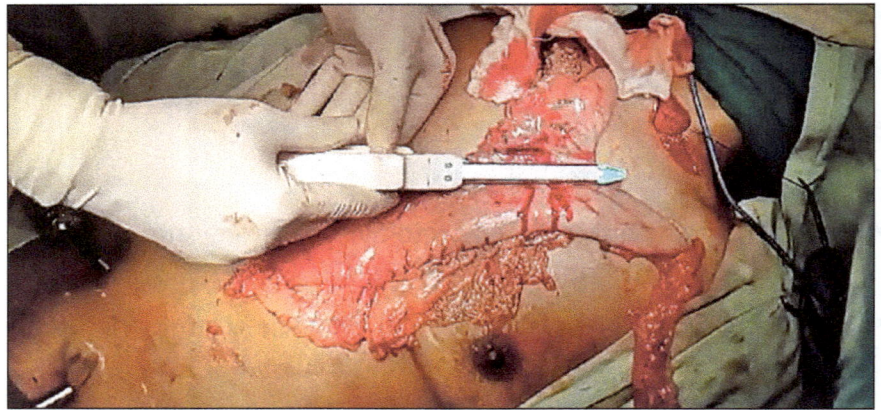

Figure 3.12: Intra-operative picture showing creation of a Tubularized Gastric Conduit.

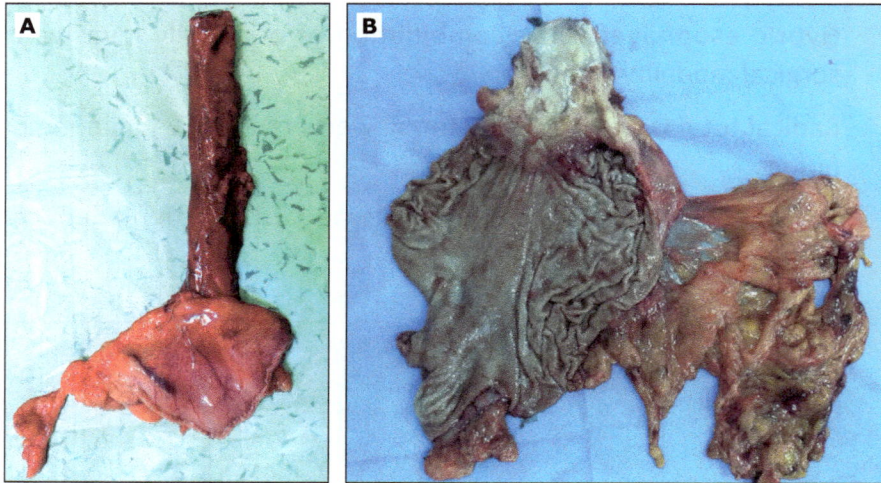

Figure 3.13: Total esophagectomy specimen (A); distal esophagectomy with proximal gastrectomy specimen revealing GEJ tumor (B).

- Adjuvant therapy:
  - Indication:
    - In case neoadjuvant radiation was not given and if a margin positive resection was performed (R1, R2)
      - Resection margin or R:
        - R0: no cancer at resection margin
        - R1: microscopic disease at resection margin
        - R2: gross disease at resection margin

- o Options:
  - ▪ Adjuvant Chemoradiation: Fluoropyrimidine based chemoradiation
  - ▪ Adjuvant chemotherapy: Cape-Ox: capecitabine and oxaliplatin
- o In GEJ/Gastric cancer:
  - ▪ If a D2 gastrectomy is performed then adjuvant chemotherapy suffices.
  - ▪ However, if a surgery amounting to less than D2 resection is performed then adjuvant chemoradiation would be preferred
- Definitive chemo-radiation:
  - o Indication:
    - ▪ For cervical and proximal esophageal squamous cell carcinomas
    - ▪ Non surgical candidates

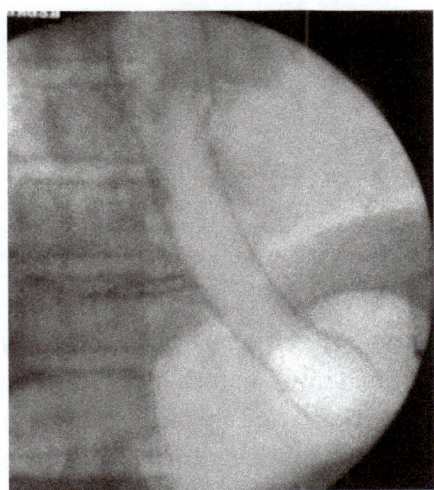

Figure 3.14: Insertion of SEMS to palliate dysphagia in a case of stage 4 esophageal malignancy.

- Surveillance
  - o Modality used:
    - ▪ History and examination
    - ▪ Biochemistry: CBC, LFT
    - ▪ USG
    - ▪ CT
    - ▪ Endoscopy
- **Go through chapter 13 for literature on the subject.**

How to Proceed in a Suspected case of Achalasia Cardia: (Sequence and Justification for Each in Brief)

- Routine blood tests and X ray chest
- Upper GI contrast study: look for esophageal dilatation with 'bird beak' like narrowing in the lower esophagus. In long standing cases, patients may develop megaesophagus (dilated esophagus) or sigmoid esophagus (dilated esophagus with axis deviation) which is best evaluated on a contrast swallow study.

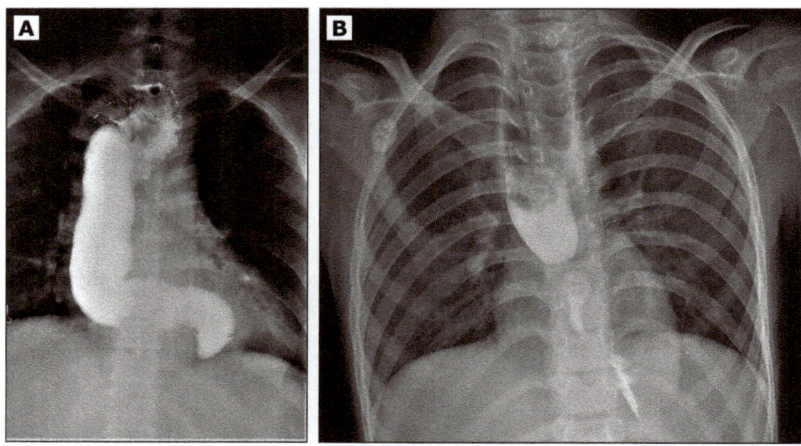

Figure 3.15: Upper GI contrast study on the left shows dilated esophagus with axis deviation (sigmoid esophagus) and bird beak sign suggestive of Achalasia cardia. On the right it reveals dilated esophagus with rat tail sign more suggestive of carcinoma.

- Upper GI endoscopy: look for dilated esophagus with residual food in the esophagus and stasis ulcers. Lower esophageal sphincter is spastic with a certain give away felt while passing the scope through it. J maneuver should be performed to rule out gastric fundus malignancy which may present with pseudoachalasia.
- Esophageal Manometry:
  - Findings include:
    - Elevated lower esophageal sphincter pressure
    - Absent peristalsis
    - Pan esophageal pressurization
  - Using high resolution manometry one may diagnose achalasia cardia (integrated relaxation pressure [IRP] >/= upper limit of normal and 100% failed peristalsis or spasm) and also classify it as per Chicago classification
    - Type 1: Classical achalasia: absent peristalsis
    - Type 2: Pan esophageal pressurization
    - Type 3: Spastic achalasia

- Treatment: Therapeutic options include:
  - Pharmacological therapy: nitrates, calcium channel blocker
  - Endoscopic Botox therapy
  - Pneumatic dilatation therapy
  - Laparoscopic Hellers cardiomyotomy
  - POEM: Per oral endoscopic myotomy

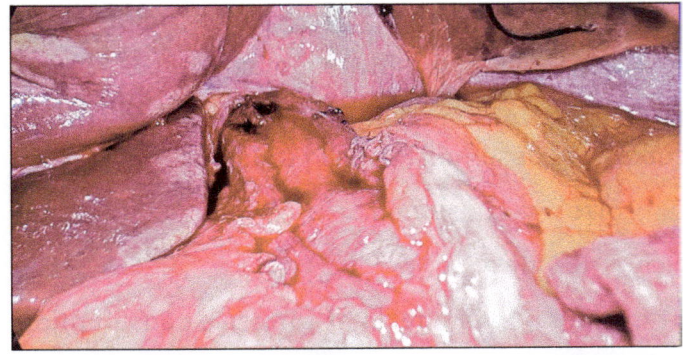

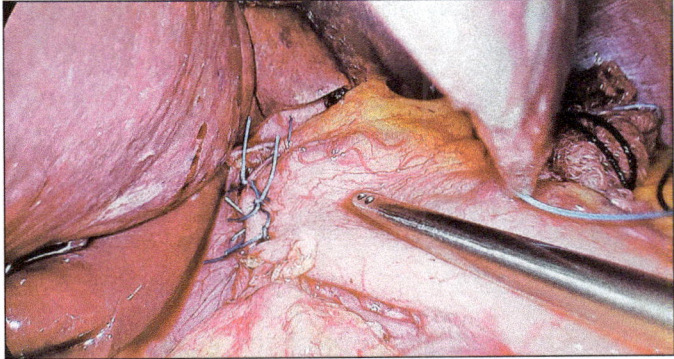

Figure 3.16: Intra-operative picture of Laparoscopic Heller's Cardiomyotomy with Dor's Fundoplication which is the Gold Standard treatment for Achalasia Cardia.

- **Go through chapter 13 for literature on the subject.**

4 Case of Dysphagia due to Corrosive Esophageal Injury

Format for History Taking

- Alleged history of corrosive intake:
    - Day and time of consumption
    - The intent of consumption, i.e. whether suicidal or accidental
    - Whether patient was under influence of any substance, e.g. alcohol, drugs
    - Nature of corrosive consumed i.e. acidic or alkaline, strong or weak; physical form of corrosive consumed i.e. solid or liquid
    - Quantity of corrosive consumed
- History of psychiatric illness
- Enquire about the immediate effects of corrosive consumption:
    - In mild disease patient may either be asymptomatic or have throat pain
    - Alternatively in moderate to severe disease patient may have:
        - Odynophagia, dysphagia
        - Drooling of saliva
        - Hematemesis
        - Chest pain, epigastric pain
        - Stridor, hoarseness of voice, coughing, respiratory distress
- History of treatment immediately given:
    - Was patient admitted in ward or ICU
    - Did the patient require emergency intubation or tracheostomy and ventilatory support
    - Was endoscopy performed; if yes at what time point from corrosive consumption was it performed
    - Was naso-gastric or naso-jejunal tube inserted
    - What imaging was performed: X-ray, CT
    - Was feeding jejunostomy tube insertion performed

- Later disease course:
  - Is the patient able to swallow or not. If patient has dysphagia/difficulty in swallowing then describe the dysphagia in detail:
    - Duration
    - Onset (usually insidious)
    - Progress (usually progressive)
    - The grade of dysphagia: initially and now at presentation.
    - Site of food getting stuck: neck/upper chest/lower chest
  - Current diet: what does he/she eat or drink, and the time taken for the patient to eat a portion of meal
  - History of odynophagia/painful swallowing
  - History of post prandial nausea, vomiting
  - History of early satiety
  - History of colicky abdominal pain, abdominal distension, nausea, vomiting, ball rolling sensation, borborygmi
  - History of hematemesis, melena
- Quality of life
- Performance status
- Treatment history for dysphagia:
  - History of contrast studies, CT, endoscopy
  - History of dilatation procedure: number of dilatation sessions and the interval between each session
  - History of relief of dysphagia with dilatation, duration of relief, and recurrence of dysphagia after dilatation therapy
  - History of any endoscopy related complication
  - Compliance to treatment
- Past history of comorbidities, surgery, psychiatric illness and previous suicidal tendency
- Personal history of alcohol consumption, smoking and any other substance abuse
- Family history

Justification for Each Component in History

- It is better to mention the term **Alleged:** Because we don't know what actually happened on day of corrosive consumption. Therefore it is good to mention 'alleged history of corrosive intake'
- Day and time of consumption: It is important to know when corrosive was consumed to know about the total duration of the disease.
- The intent of consumption, i.e. whether suicidal or accidental:
  - Patient with suicidal intent corrosive consumption usually tend to consume small quantity of corrosive hesitantly and slowly with multiple attempts at consumption, very much similar to hesitant cuts in suicidal wrist or throat cut.
  - Where as in case of accidental corrosive consumption, patient is unaware that he is consuming a corrosive. He/she mistakes corrosive for water (most likely when corrosive is stored in a water bottle). So thinking it to be water the patient may gulp down large quantity of corrosive hastily.
  - The result is that, in suicidal consumption, oral cavity, oropharynx, pharyngesophageal junction and proximal esophagus are more likely to be injured, where as in accidental consumption distal esophagus and stomach are more likely to be involved.
- Whether patient was under influence of any substance, e.g. alcohol: again, patient with history of corrosive consumption under influence of alcohol is likely to consume large quantity of corrosive hastily leading to lower esophageal and/or stomach injury.
- Nature of corrosive consumed i.e. acidic or alkaline:
  - 'Acid licks the esophagus and bites the stomach', i.e. gastric injury is more severe compared to esophageal injury in case of acid consumption. This is because acid causes coagulative necrosis with eschar formation. This prevents deeper penetration of acid into the esophageal wall. Whereas in stomach it causes pyloric spasm delaying gastric emptying, leading to longer contact times and hence more severe gastric injury.
  - The opposite is true for alkaline consumption (i.e. esophageal injury is more severe compared to gastric injury). This is because alkali causes liquefactive necrosis, hence penetrating through the layers of esophageal wall as it passes through it with higher risk of perforation.
  - This point is important in India where acid (which is freely available and cheap) consumption is much more common than alkaline consumption (which is more expensive and less freely available).

- Nature of corrosive consumed i.e. strong or weak: more concentrated/stronger the corrosive consumed, more severe the expected injury.
- Physical form of corrosive consumed i.e. solid or liquid:
  - Gastric emptying time for solid is more as compared to liquids
  - Hence solid corrosive consumption will lead to more contact time in stomach leading to more severe gastric injury.
  - Alternatively, liquid alkali may cause small bowel injury.
- Quantity of corrosive consumed: higher the quantity, more severe the expected injury and vice versa.
- Immediate effects following corrosive consumption: it is important to note the immediate symptoms following corrosive consumption to clinically grade the severity of the injury:
  - Patients who are asymptomatic or have just some mild throat pain usually have only mild disease
  - Alternatively, patients with moderate to severe disease present with odynophagia, dysphagia, drooling of saliva, hematemesis, chest pain, epigastric pain, stridor, hoarseness of voice, coughing, respiratory distress,
    - Odynophagia, Drooling of saliva: suggests moderate to severe involvement of oral cavity.
    - Dysphagia is due to esophageal inflammation
    - Hematemesis is usually a significant event suggesting severe disease
    - with poor overall prognosis.
    - History of chest pain should hint towards thoracic esophageal perforation
    - History of severe epigastric pain should hint towards gastric perforation
    - Stridor, hoarseness of voice, coughing, respiratory distress: would suggest laryngeal or tracheal involvement. Additionally, it could be due to aspiration
- Immediate treatment given:
  - Admitted in ward or ICU: admission to ICU suggests severe disease or occurrence of disease related complication (like perforation, hemorrhage). History of treatment on OPD basis suggests mild disease.
  - History of intubation and/or tracheostomy: it suggests severe injury and/or respiratory involvement.

- Details regarding endoscopic evaluation: It is important to know if endoscopy was performed or not; and at what time point from consumption was it performed. It is usually done within first 2–3 days of consumption and is generally contraindicated after 96 hours. It is performed to grade the severity of the injury which will help with prognostication and treatment planning. Zargar classification is used to grade the damage.

Table 4.1: Zargar Classification
- Grade 1: Only erythema and edema
- Grade 2a: Superficial erosions
- Grade 2b: Deep and/or circumferential ulcers
- Grade 3a: Scattered areas of necrosis
- Grade 3b: Extensive necrosis
- Grade 4: Perforation

- Naso-gastric or naso-jejunal tube is usually inserted after completion of endoscopic evaluation for two reasons: to facilitate enteral nutrition (immediate) and dilatation therapy (later).
- If naso-gastric or naso-jejunal tube is not inserted a feeding jejunostomy is usually performed to facilitate enteral nutrition. Note when was it performed.

Table 4.2: Phases of Caustic Injury
- Acute Necrotic Phase: < 72 Hours
- Ulcerative Granular Phase: 3 days to three weeks
  - Esophagus is the weakest in this phase, hence any intervention is to be avoided during this period
- Cicatrization & Stricturing Phase: 3 weeks to 3 months
  - It's in this phase that the patient starts developing stricture resulting in dysphagia

- Later disease course:
  - It is important to note patients diet pattern and his current diet. Patients with mild disease may be able to consume both solid and liquids without any difficulty. On the other hand patients with moderate to severe injury will gradually develop corrosive esophageal stricture. Such patients will develop dysphagia. So inquire if patient is able to swallow solids, liquids or just saliva.

Also note the quantity of food patient is able to eat and the time taken for him/her to consume it. Patients may be able to consume one portion of food; but if he/she takes more than usual time to consume it should hint towards presence of dysphagia.

- o History of dysphagia: Dysphagia in corrosive esophageal stricture is usually progressive in nature. see for the grade initially and what is the grade now at presentation.

Table 4.3: Grades of dysphagia (as described by Suguhara et al)
- 1: able to swallow solid meals with some difficulty
- 2: able to swallow solid meals but requires liquids along with it
- 3: able to swallow only semisolid meals
- 4: able to swallow only liquids
- 5: able to swallow only saliva
- 6: Unable to swallow anything including saliva

- o Site of food getting stuck: Neck/upper chest/lower chest: it is usually said that the actual site of obstruction is below the site of obstruction as perceived by the patient. So for example, if patient says that the site of dysphagia is in the neck, then the site of obstruction will be somewhere below i.e. any where in the lower cervical or thoracic esophagus or esophago-gastric junction.
- o Odynophagia: It would suggest presence of painful oral or oropharyngeal ulcers.
- o History of post prandial nausea, vomiting: Would suggest gastric outlet obstruction due to corrosive gastric stricture.
- o History of early satiety: Would suggest extensive gastric cicatrization resulting in linitus plastica like picture (type 4 gastric stricture).
- o History of colicky abdominal pain, abdominal distension, nausea, vomiting, ball rolling sensation, borborygmic: All these symptoms would suggest small bowel involvement with stricture formation.
- o History of hematemesis, melena: Could be due to esophageal/gastric ulcers/ erosions.
- Treatment history for dysphagia:
  - o History of contrast studies/cross sectional imaging/endoscopy: Patients with corrosive esophageal stricture are usually evaluated by barium esophagogram and/or endoscopy to get a road map for endoscopic dilatation therapy. This help with further treatment planning (endoscopic dilatation therapy/surgery).

The sequence: Barium esophagogram followed by endoscopy or endoscopy followed by barium is controversial.

- History of dilatation therapy: Endoscopic dilatation therapy is initiated after 4–6 weeks once the inflammation subsides and before the process of scarring completely obliterates the lumen. It is usually done with Savary Gillard dilators at 2–3 week interval. Target is to achieve an esophageal lumen size of 14 mm (40 fr) for complete relief of dysphagia. It is important to note the compliance to treatment.
    - Indications for surgery:
        - Refractory stricture: Inability to accomplish a luminal diameter of 14 mm over 5 sessions done at 2 week intervals
        - Recurrent stricture: Inability to maintain satisfactory luminal diameter for 4 weeks once target diameter(14 mm) is achieved
        - Failure to pass guidewire across stricture
        - Long stricture > 10 cm
        - Multiple strictures (> 3)
        - Dilatation related complication
        - Stricture with pseudodiverticulae

- History of psychiatric illness: It is important to inquire regarding previous history of psychiatric illness, history of previous suicidal tendencies. Such patients are less compliant to treatment.
- History of comorbid illness: It is very important to know about the patient's co-morbidities, especially pulmonary diseases like bronchial asthma and chronic obstructive pulmonary disease. One cannot plan surgery in a patient with disabling respiratory co-morbidity/depleted respiratory reserve as they won't tolerate surgery well.
- Smoking history: It is very important to know in detail about patient's smoking habit. Patient who smokes usually do not tolerate surgery well.
- Quality of life and performance status: It is very important to inquire regarding patient's quality of life and assess his performance status for treatment planning/modification and to evaluate patient's tolerability for surgery respectively.

Format for Examination

- Remember:
    - Most patients with corrosive esophageal strictures will have some degree of dysphagia, will be dehydrated and malnourished (usually all skin and bones).

Those with absolute dysphagia will usually have a small jug/pan with them, into which they would spit their saliva every few minutes since they are not able to swallow it.
- o Most may have naso gastric/naso-jejunal or feeding jejunostomy tube in situ.
- o Do not forget to look for surgical scars in neck, chest, and abdomen.
- o It is very important to mention findings of oral and chest examination

Now Let's Start
- What is the appearance of the patient: young/middle-aged/elderly, lady/gentleman
- Whether the patient is clinically
  - o Poorly/averagely/well built
  - o Poorly/averagely/well nourished; It is very important to clinically assess patient's nutritional status.
  - o Clinical features suggesting poor nourishment
    - Temporal wasting
    - Sunken eyes
    - Flattened cheeks, Buccal hollow
    - Supraclavicular hollow
    - Squaring of shoulders
    - Prominent scapula
    - Prominent intercostal spaces
    - Scaphoid abdomen
    - Prominent hip bones
    - Prominent knee and elbows
    - Pedal edema
    - Decreased mid arm circumference
    - Decreased skin fold thickness
- Measure height, weight, BMI
- Mention if NG/NJ tube is seen insitu. Also mention if central line/IV line is in situ and whether IV fluids, enteral or parenteral feed is being given

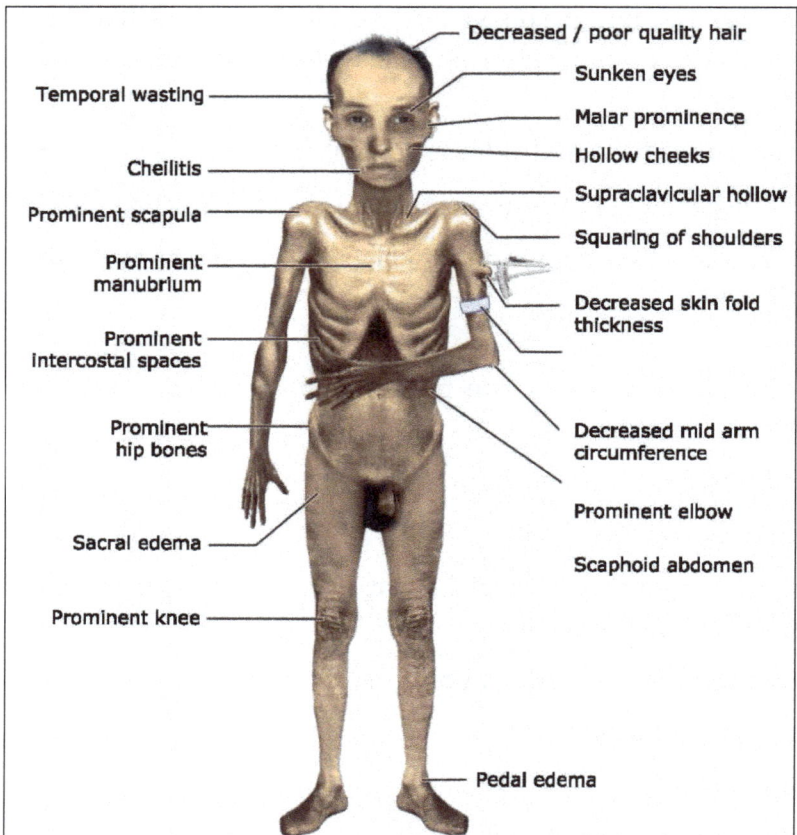

Figure 4.1: Clinical features suggesting poor nourishment.

- Whether the patient is clinically
    - Conscious/stuporous
    - Co-operative/un-cooperative
    - Well/poorly oriented to time, place and person
    - Well hydrated/dehydrated
    - Lying comfortably in bed/in discomfort/in pain
    - Preferred decubitus: Whether patient prefers sitting position or he/she can comfortably lie in supine position
    - Febrile/Afebrile.
- Mention Pulse, BP, respiratory rate.
- Breath holding time: Along with vitals it would be good to mention the breath holding time (normal being > 22 seconds). After assessing nutritional status this is another clinical method of assessing fitness for surgery.

- Look for
    - Pallor, jaundice, cyanosis, clubbing
    - Generalized or localized lymphadenopathy
    - Pedal or dependent edema
    - Previous suicidal cuts. Skin lesions, if any
- Examination of oral cavity: Look for:
    - Mouth opening: Look for reduced mouth opening or trismus. It suggests oral scarring.
    - Mucosal lesion: Look for erythema, edema, discoloration of mucosa, ulcer, slough, eschar or any other obvious mucosal lesion.
    - Oral hygiene: Look for dental caries, tobacco stains, foul smell/halitosis.
    - Tongue movement: Normal or impaired/restricted (due to scarring).

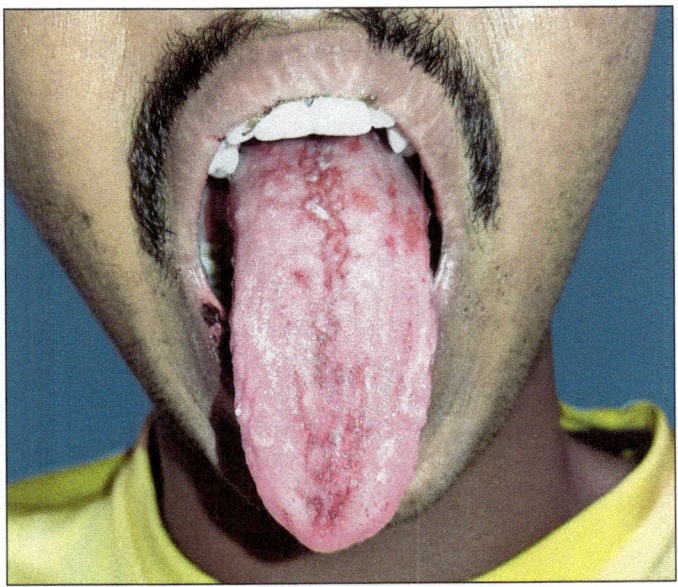

Figure 4.2: Oral examination revealing erythema, ulcer and slough; also note the eschar on the lips.

- Examination of the neck
    - Look for scar of previous cervical exploration, which may have been done for esophageal perforation in which case diversion cervical esophagostomy would have been created.
    - Alternatively cervical exploration may be done for esophageal guidewire insertion to facilitate dilatation.

- Examination of the abdomen:
    - On Inspection: See if:
        - Abdomen is flat/distended/scaphoid;
        - Umbilicus is central/displaced (upwards/downwards/sideways) inverted/everted/flat.
        - All quadrants are moving equally with respiration or not
        - Look for surgical scar of previous laparotomy for corrosive induced perforation. Look for gastrostomy, feeding jejunostomy tube
        - Look for visible gastric peristalsis (from left to right) which will be seen in patients with gastric outlet obstruction.
        - Look for visible lump, sinus, engorged veins, pulsations or cough impulse.
        - Don't forget to inspect the groin hernial sites (to look for swelling or cough impulse i.e. hernia) and genitalia.
        - Inspection of renal angles to look for fullness

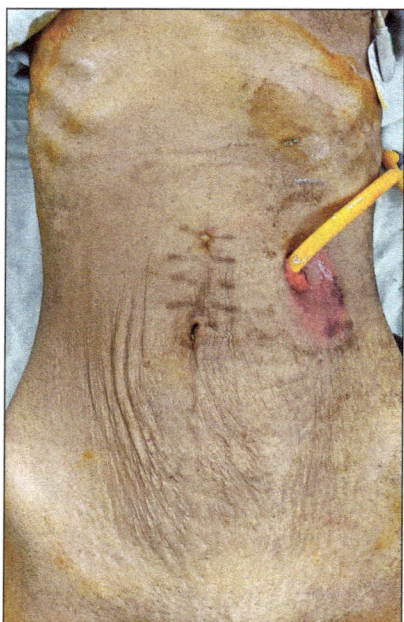

Figure 4.3: Abdominal inspection revealing a Feeding Jejunostomy tube, skin excoriation around it, an upper midline Scar and features of poor nourishment.

    - On Palpation: See if:
        - Abdomen is soft and non-tender
        - Liver is palpable or not

- Spleen is enlarged or not
- Any other palpable lump
- Do not forget to:
  - Palpate groin hernia sites to look for cough impulse
  - Examine genitals
  - Look for tenderness in renal angles
  - Examine back and spine
- On Percussion:
  - Look for upper border of liver dullness (generally in the 5th intercostal space) in midclavicular line.
  - Note the liver span (normal being 12–14 cm)
  - Percussion note in the rest of the abdomen (generally tympanic)
  - Tests for free fluid
- On auscultation:
  - Auscultate for bowel sounds.
  - Bruit, hum and rub
- Per rectal examination
- Respiratory examination:
  - Inspection:
    - Whether the trachea is in midline or is deviated
    - Bilateral chest movement: equal or not
  - Palpation:
    - Trachea: centralized or deviated
    - Look for warmth and tenderness
    - Bilateral chest movement: equal or not
    - Tactile vocal fremitus:
      - It is increased in case of pleural effusion and consolidation.
  - Auscultation: most important part of respiratory examination:
    - Breath sounds:
      - Bilaterally equal or not

- Reduced in any lung field: right/left; upper/mid or lower zone. Reduced breath sounds would suggest either pleural effusion or consolidation.
        - Adventitious sounds:
            - Crepts: coarse crepts would suggest aspiration pneumonitis, whereas fine crepts would suggest pulmonary edema.
            - Ronchi/wheeze
    - Percussion:
        - Normal percussion note is resonant.
        - Dull note suggests consolidation or pleural effusion.
- Rest systemic examination

EXAMPLE CASE

History

- My patient Mrs XYZ, is a 22-year-old lady hailing from Mumbai, is a homemaker.
- She presented with chief complaints of difficulty in swallowing since 1.5 months and loss of weight since 2 months.
- Her history dates back to 3 months back when she gives alleged history of consuming 100 ml of liquid toilet cleaner on __/__/____(date) at __.__ am/pm (time) with suicidal intent.
- Immediately following consumption of corrosive she developed throat pain and odynophagia; however she did not have chest pain, abdominal pain, hoarseness of voice, stridor, respiratory distress or hematemesis
- For this, she was immediately taken to the hospital where she was admitted in ICU. An endoscopy was performed after 12 hours of corrosive consumption, at the end of which a nasal tube was inserted.
    - She did not require intubation and/or tracheostomy
    - An abdominal tube was surgically placed within the first week of admission, most probably feeding jejunostomy, through which feeds were initiated.
- She was discharged after 4 weeks at which point of time she was receiving around 2.5 litre of FJ feeds daily. She was able to swallow saliva and liquids orally
- Following discharge she continued tube feeding, apart from which was consuming liquids and occasionally semisolids.

- Now since last 1.5 month patient is having difficulty in swallowing semisolids. The dysphagia has gradually progressed such that now she is able to swallow only saliva and small quantity of liquids. She has sensation of food getting stuck at level of mid chest
- She has been gradually losing weight over last 2 months, and has lost around 12 kg.
- At present there is no:
    - History of odynophagia/painful swallowing
    - History of post prandial nausea, vomiting
    - History of early satiety
    - History of colicky abdominal pain, abdominal distension, nausea, vomiting, ball rolling sensation, borborygmi
    - History of hematemesis, melena
- One month back she was evaluated for these symptoms with contrast study, following which she supposedly underwent 2 sessions of endoscopic dilatation therapy. She is able to swallow liquids but not semisolid or solid food since the last session
- There is no previous history of any co morbid or psychiatric illness or history of previous suicidal tendency
- There is no history of alcohol consumption, smoking or any other substance abuse
- Family history is not contributory
- She is able to perform all self-care but not strenuous physical activity.

Examination

- My patient is a young lady, who is averagely built, poorly nourished, with a height of 160 cm, weight of 45 kg and BMI being 17.6 kg/m^2
- She is conscious, co-operative, well oriented to time, place and person; Lying comfortably in bed; well hydrated and afebrile.
- Pulse is 72/min, BP is 110/70 mm Hg, respiratory rate is 14 per min and breath holding time is 24 seconds.
- Naso gastric tube is seen insitu
- There is no pallor, jaundice, cyanosis, clubbing, generalized or localized lymphadenopathy, pedal or dependent edema or skin lesions

- Examination of oral cavity reveals adequate mouth opening and oral hygiene, normal tongue movement and no obvious mucosal lesions.
- Examination of the neck is unremarkable
- Examination of the abdomen:
  - On inspection: Abdomen is flat, umbilicus is central, inverted. All quadrants are moving equally with respiration.
  - Feeding jejunostomy tube is seen insitu in the left lumbar region through which feed is being given. There is a 5 cm mid midline laparotomy scar which has healed well.
  - There is no visible lump, sinus, engorged veins, pulsations, peristalsis or cough impulse.
  - Inspection of groin hernial sites reveals no swelling or cough impulse and Inspection of genitalia is unremarkable. Inspection of renal angles reveals no fullness
  - On Palpation: Abdomen is soft and non-tender. Liver and spleen is not palpable. There isn't any other palpable lump. There is no cough impulse over the midline scar.
  - There is no palpable cough impulse over groin hernia sites and examination of genitals is unremarkable. There is no tenderness in renal angles. Examination of back and spine is essentially normal.
  - On Percussion, upper border of liver dullness is in the 5th intercostal space in midclavicular line with liver span being 14 cm. Rest of the abdomen is tympanitic with no evidence of free fluid.
  - On auscultation normal bowel sounds are heard. There is no bruit, hum or rub,
  - Per rectal examination is unremarkable.
- Examination of respiratory system:
  - Trachea is central.
  - Bilateral chest movement is equal.
  - On percussion there is resonant note in bilateral lung fields.
  - On auscultation air entry is bilaterally equal, with normal vesicular breath sounds heard and there is no crepts or wheeze.
- Rest systemic examination is essentially normal.

To Summarize

- My patient is a 22 year old female with no co-morbid or psychiatric illness with WHO 1 performance status, presents with alleged history of consuming 100 ml of liquid toilet cleaner 3 month back following which she immediately developed throat pain and odynophagia for which she required hospital admission and underwent upper GI endoscopy and feeding jejunostomy. Following discharge at 4 weeks from admission she was consuming liquids and occasionally semisolid. However since last 1.5 months she has developed gradually progressive dysphagia, associated with history of loss of weight. She received 2 session of dilatation therapy for the same following which there is some relief in the dysphagia
- On examination she is poorly nourished with BMI being 17.6 kg/m² with naso-gastric tube in situ.
- Examination of abdomen reveals healthy midline laparotomy scar and feeding jejunostomy tube in situ. Examination of oral cavity, neck and chest is otherwise unremarkable

The Most Probable Diagnosis in my patient is corrosive esophageal stricture

How to Proceed: (Sequence and Justification)

- Review available medical records
- Routine blood investigations (Hemogram, Liver Function Test, Renal Function Test, Serum Electrolyte, INR)
- X-ray chest: to look for features of aspiration pneumonitits (e.g.: patchy infiltrates)
- Upper GI contrast study: to diagnose and further evaluate the stricture. To note:
    - Number, location and length of strictures
    - To see caliber of lumen

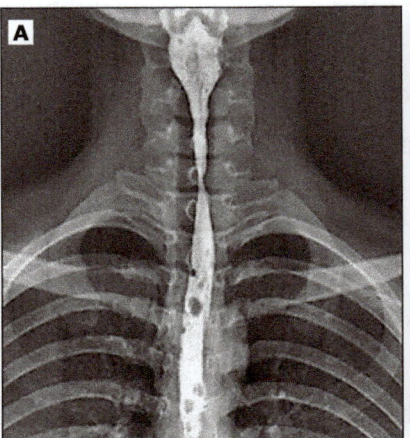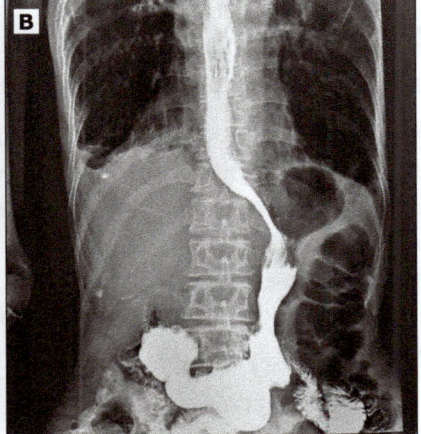

Figure 4.4: Upper GI contrast study on the left reveals esophageal stricture (A) and on the right shows gastric stricture (B).

- o To get a roadmap for dilatation therapy
- o To look for treatment related complication
- Upper GI endoscopy: to evaluate the stricture and facilitate guidewire guided dilatation therapy

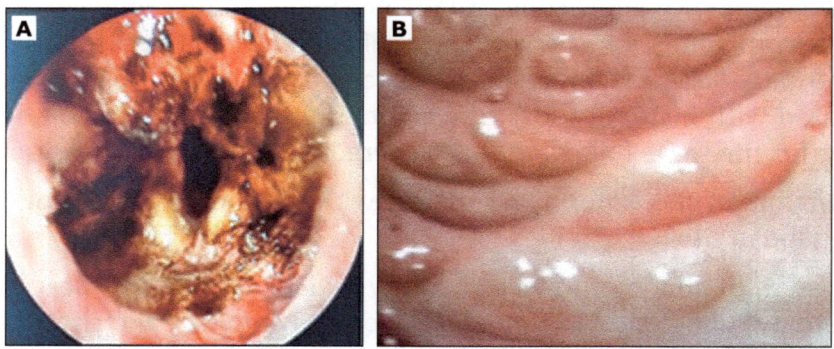

Figure 4.5: Upper GI endoscopy on the left reveals esophageal stricture (A) and on the right shows gastric cicatrization (B).

- CECT with oral contrast:
  - o To understand esophageal and gastric anatomy and evaluate the stricture
  - o To evaluate treatment related complications and disease related complication such as perforation, tracheo-esophageal fistula
  - o To evaluate pleural cavity and lungs for pleural effusion and consolidation respectively
  - o Additionally, in case coloplasty is planned, CT may be performed to evaluate the patency of inferior mesenteric vessels and rule out colonic pathology
- Indirect laryngoscopy and hypopharyngoscopy: to examine the epiglottis, vocal cords, posterior pharyngeal wall and pyriform sinus. It is invaluable in planning management of pharyngeal strictures.
- Psychiatry consultation in case of suicidal intent corrosive consumption.
- Endoscopy-Fluoroscopy guided dilatation therapy: To non surgically relieve the dysphagia. The dilatation programme is generally initiated after 4-6 weeks. It consists of passage of a Savary Gilard dilator over an endoscopically placed guide wire with dilatation done under fluoroscopy guidance. It is performed at an interval of 2 weeks over 6 sessions. Aim is to achieve a target lumen diameter of 14 mm at completion of dilatation programme, which is maintained for atleast 4 weeks.
  - o Rule of 3: in each session no more than 3 bougie dilators of sequentially larger size should be passed starting with the size with which moderate resistance was felt in the previous session.

- Colonoscopy: to rule out colonic pathology in case you are considering coloplasty.
- Surgery:
    o Esophageal replacement for esophageal stricture

Table 4.4: Indication for surgery in Corrosive Esophageal Stricture
▪ Refractory stricture: unable to achieve a luminal diameter of 14 mm over 5 session
▪ Recurrent stricture: unable to maintain a luminal diameter of 14 mm over 4 weeks or recurrence of dysphagia within 4 weeks of achieving diameter of 14 mm
▪ Long stricture (> 10 cm), multiple strictures (> 3)
▪ Failure to pass guidewire across stricture
▪ Stricture with pseudodiverticulae
▪ Dilatation related complication

   o Surgical options:
      ▪ Esophago-coloplasty: colon is the preferred conduit
         – Right colon Esophago-coloplasty: based on middle colic pedicle

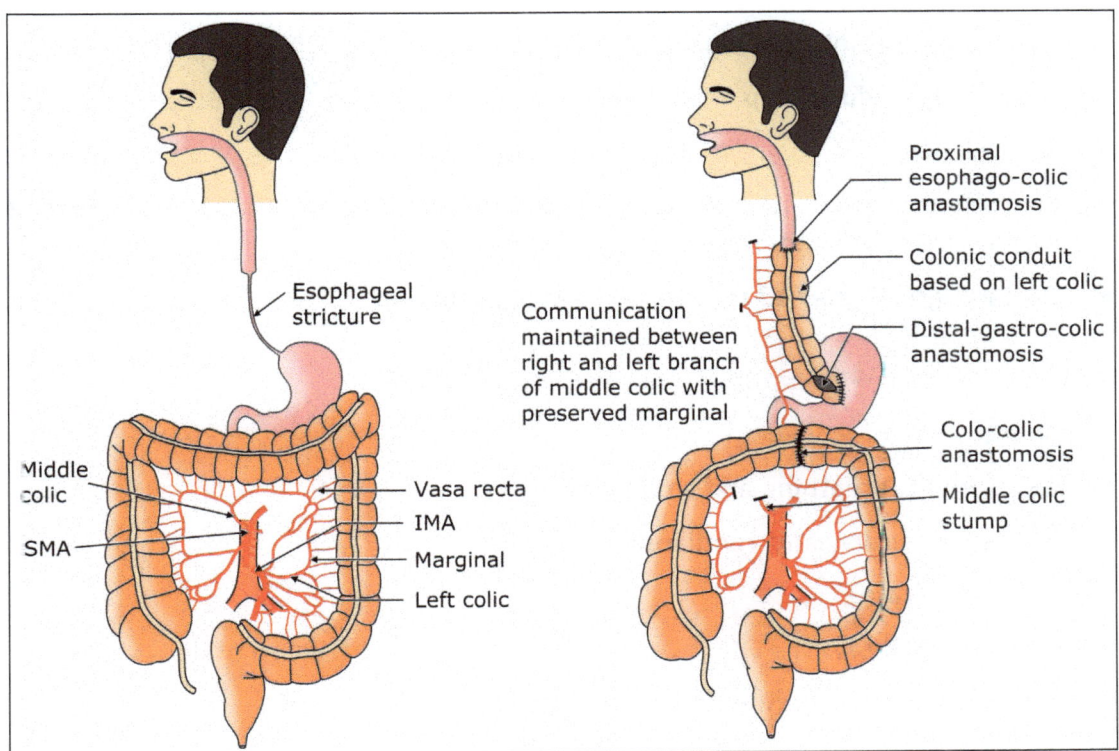

Figure 4.6: Esophagocoloplasty.

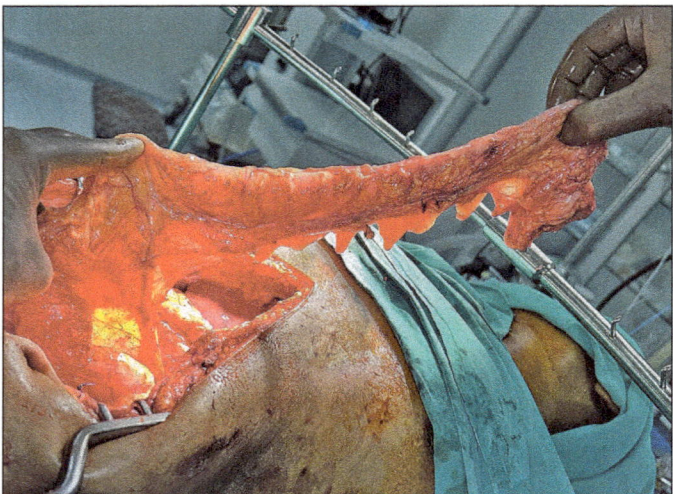

Figure 4.7: Intra-operative picture showing the colonic conduit ready to be transposed. Image courtesy Dr. K. Sutariya.

- Left colon Esophago-coloplasty: based on left colic pedicle
- Mid colon Esophago-coloplasty: based on left colic pedicle
- Stomach is less preferred as a conduit as it may also be damaged by the corrosive
- Jejunal interposition
- Free jejunal flap
- Surveillance
- Remember: at super specialty level you are in addition expected to know regarding management of pharyngo-esophageal strictures
- **Go through chapter 13 for literature on the subject.**

Principles of Management in the Acute Setting: In Brief

- Admit
- ABC: airway, breathing and circulation
  - Secure airway and ventilation
  - Resuscitate
- Blood tests, X-rays
- Endoscopy within 72 hours to note Zargar grade and extent

Table 4.5: Zargar Classification

- Grade 1: Only erythema and edema
- Grade 2a: Superficial erosions
- Grade 2b: Deep and/or circumferential ulcers
- Grade 3a: Scattered areas of necrosis
- Grade 3b: Extensive necrosis
- Grade 4: Perforation

- Further management is decided by the Zargar grade:
  - Grade 1, 2a: observe for 24–48 hours; once he can swallow saliva > start liquids and discharge once he/she tolerates it
  - Grade 2b, 3a: these patients are prone for stricture formation
    - Place NG/NJ tube; plan FJ tube insertion during index admission
    - Provide enteral nutrition via NG/NJ/FJ tube
    - May consider starting liquids once he is able to swallow saliva and gradually proceed to more solid diet as and when he tolerates it
    - To plan Dilatation therapy
  - Grade 3b, 4: these patients generally require emergency surgery as these patients tend to develop perforation.
- **Go through chapter 13 for literature on the subject.**

5 Case of Gastric Outlet Obstruction due to Carcinoma Stomach

Introduction

In this chapter the main focus of discussion will be on Carcinoma of body or distal stomach which presents predominantly with features of gastric outlet obstruction. Carcinoma of the gastro-esophageal junction predominantly presents with dysphagia which has already been discussed in chapter 3.

Format for History Taking

- History of vomiting:
    - Onset
    - Duration
    - Frequency
    - Quantity: Small or large volume, alternatively one could describe quantity in form of cup
    - Contents:
        - Bilious or not
        - Contains food previously eaten or not: If yes then describe if it is undigested/partially digested/completely digested (Chyme)
    - Projectile or not
    - Related to meals or not i.e. post prandial or not
    - Is there a sense of relief after vomiting
- History of sensation of postprandial fullness
- History of early satiety
- History of hematemesis or Melena: If yes then ask for history of postural dizziness, syncope, fatigue, shortness of breath, need for blood transfusion.
- History of dyspepsia: Epigastric pain, burning, fullness, bloating
- History of pain:
    - Site
    - Onset: Insidious or sudden

- o Duration
- o Nature: Intermittent/continuous
- o Character of pain: Dull aching or colicky
- o Intensity: Mild/moderate/severe
- o Radiation of pain
- o Precipitated by meals or not
- o Precipitated by fasting or not
- o Relation with posture
- o Inquire whether there is any recent change in character of pain.
- o Relieving factor: Spontaneous/oral analgesic/intra venous analgesic
- History of loss of weight, loss of appetite
- History of abdominal distension; respiratory discomfort; hemoptysis; bony pain; back pain; blackout; seizures
- Treatment history: Evaluation with cross-sectional imaging, upper GI endoscopy with/without biopsy.
- Past history of comorbid illness: DM, HTN, TB; past history of surgery.
- Personal history: Smoking history; History of alcohol consumption.
- Family history: History of cancer in first and second degree family
- Performance history

Justification for Each Component in History

- History of vomiting: Antrum is most common site of gastric carcinoma. Distal gastric growths cause gastric outlet obstruction, main feature of which is vomiting. In GOO vomiting occurs within a few hours of eating, it is large in volume, non bilious and contains partially digested food particles. Bilious vomiting rules out obstruction proximal to the second part of the duodenum.
- History of sensation of postprandial fullness: Post prandial epigastric fullness, bloating or distension could suggest gastric outlet obstruction, and it occurs due to gastric distension. At times patient may even feel the gastric peristalsis, going from left to right in the upper abdomen.
- History of early satiety: Early satiety suggests reduced gastric distensibility which may be seen in linitus plastica and extensive gastric cicatrization due to corrosive intake.

- History of hematemesis or Melena: Patients with gastric carcinoma may have GI bleed. It is usually low volume painless bleed leading to anemia rather than manifesting as hematemesis or/and melena. GIST on the contrary are highly vascular tumors which may cause frank GI bleed.
- History of postural dizziness, syncope, fatigue, shortness of breath, need for blood transfusion should be inquired for in case patient gives history of GI bleed. It is suggestive of anemia and helps quantify the blood loss
- History of dyspepsia: Gastric adenocarcinoma and lymphoma may both present with dyspepsia. Patients in whom there was malignant transformation of gastric peptic ulcer, may also give history of dyspepsia. New onset dyspepsia after age of forty should raise the suspicion of gastric malignancy.
- History of pain: patients in whom there is malignant transformation of gastric peptic ulcer, may give history of pain. Pain is in the epigastrium, dull in nature, precipitated by meals. Pain in duodenal ulcer on the contrary is precipitated by fasting and hence usually occurs in the middle of the night. It is relieved on consuming meals. There may be radiation of pain to the back in case of penetrating posterior duodenal ulcer.
- History of loss of weight, loss of appetite: These are pointers towards malignancy.
- History of abdominal distension; respiratory discomfort; hemoptysis; Bony pain; back pain; blackout; seizures: these symptoms suggest dissemination of malignancy
    - Abdominal distension: Due to malignant ascites
    - Respiratory discomfort: Due to pleural effusion and lung metastasis
    - Hemoptysis: Due to lung metastasis
    - Bony pain: Due to bony metastasis
    - Back pain: Due to vertebral metastasis
    - Blackout, Seizures: Due to brain metastasis
- Treatment history of evaluation with upper GI endoscopy with biopsy, administration of chemotherapy would hint the candidate towards diagnosis of malignant GOO.
- History of comorbid illness: To assess patient's tolerability for surgery.
- Smoking history: Patient who smokes usually do not tolerate surgery well.
- Family history: it is important to inquire about family history of gastric cancer as it may suggest Hereditary Diffuse gastric cancer due to CDH-1 gene mutation

Table 5.1: Laurens Classification of Gastric Cancer

Intestinal Type Adenocarcinoma	Diffuse type Adenocarcinoma
• Environmental	• Familial
• Affects elderly (M > F)	• Affects younger population (F > M)
• Associated with H. Pylori Infection, Chronic Atrophic Gastritis, Intestinal Metaplasia & Diet high in Nitrosamines	• Associated with CDH 1 Gene Mutation
• Arises from Mucosa	• Arises from Lamina Propria
• Gland forming	• Non Gland forming
• Involves Distal Stomach	• Involves Proximal Stomach
• Hematogenous spread	• Spreads through Sub-Mucosa; Lymphatic metastasis is common; tendency for Transmural spread with Peritoneal metastasis.
	• Linitus Plastica is a rare form of Diffuse Gastric Cancer

- Performance history: To assess patient's tolerability for surgery.

Format for Examination

- What is the appearance of the patient: Young/middle-aged/elderly, lady/gentleman
- Whether the patient is clinically
    - Poorly/averagely/well built
    - Poorly/averagely/well nourished
- Measure height, weight, BMI
- Whether the patient is clinically
    - Conscious/stuporous
    - Co-operative/un-cooperative
    - Well/poorly oriented to time, place and person
    - Lying comfortably in bed/in discomfort/in pain (rolling in pain). Also note patient's posture.

- o Well hydrated/dehydrated
- o Febrile/Afebrile.
- Mention Pulse, BP
- Look for:
  - o Pallor, jaundice, cyanosis, clubbing
  - o Generalized or localized lymphadenopathy
  - o Palpable left supraclavicular lymph node: Virchow node
  - o Palpable left anterior axillary Lymph node: Irish node
  - o Pedal or dependent edema
  - o Skin lesions

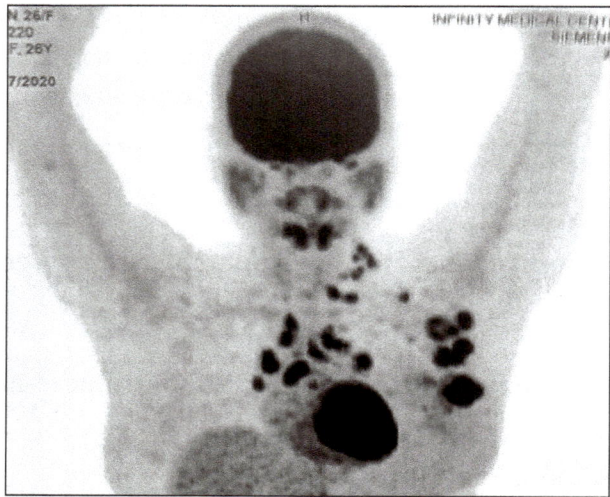

Figure 5.1: PET CT showing Left Supra-Clavicular, Left Axillary and mediastinal Lymph Nodes, this should not be missed out on examination, in cases of GI cancer.

- Examination of oral cavity: Look for oral hygiene and any obvious mucosal lesions
- Examination of the abdomen:
  - o On Inspection: See if:
    - Abdomen is flat/distended/scaphoid;
    - Umbilicus is central/displaced (upwards/downwards/sideways), inverted/everted/flat.
    - All quadrants are moving equally with respiration or not

- Look for upper abdominal fullness (due to distended stomach)
- Look for any visible lump in the upper abdomen.
    - If visible describe:
        - Size
        - Site
        - Shape
        - Surface
        - Movement with respiration.
- Look for umbilical nodule: Sister Mary Joseph nodule. It is suggestive of metastatic disease similar to Virchows node (palpable supra-clavicular node).
- Look for visible gastric peristalsis: Waves moving from left to right in the upper abdomen
- Look for visible scars, sinus, engorged veins, pulsations, or cough impulse.
- Don't forget to inspect the groin hernial sites (to look for swelling or cough impulse i.e. hernia) and genitalia.
- Inspection of renal angles to look for fullness

o On Palpation: See if:
- Abdomen is soft and non-tender (Alternatively abdomen could be rigid and/or tender)
- Liver and/or spleen is palpable or not
- There is any other palpable lump:
    - Gastric tumors are less likely to be palpable. If it's palpable consider possibility of GIST or advanced adenocarcinoma.
    - One is more likely to palpate the over-distended stomach in the form of a water-filled bag in the upper abdomen.
    - Also look for lump in lower abdomen in females which could be due to Krukenberg tumor (metastatic spread of gastric cancer to the ovary)
    - If present describe:
        - Site
        - Size
        - Shape

- Surface
- Margins
- Tenderness
- Consistency
- Mobility
- Movement with respiration
- Plane:
  - ☐ Whether the lump is intraperitoneal or not: by performing leg raising test
  - ☐ Whether the lump is retroperitoneal or not: by asking the patient to assume lateral decubitus position and palpating if the lump falls forward or not. A retroperitoneal mass won't fall ahead.

- Do not forget to:
  - Palpate groin hernia sites to look for cough impulse
  - Examine genitals
  - Look for tenderness in renal angles
  - Examine back and spine for tenderness/gibbus.

○ On Percussion:
  - Look for upper border of liver dullness (generally in the 5th intercostal space) in midclavicular line.
  - Note the liver span (normal being 12–14 cm)
  - Perform ausculto-percussion test to delineate the outline of greater curvature of the distended stomach and mark it to demonstrate it to the examiner, if asked for.
  - Note the percussion note over rest of the abdomen (it is generally tympanic)
  - Tests for free fluid. Presence of free fluid or ascites in a patient with gastric carcinoma could be due to either metastasis or hypoalbuminemia.

○ On auscultation:
  - Auscultate for bowel sounds.
  - Look for succussion splash. Prior to performing the test, the examiner

has to confirm that the patient has been nil per oral for adequate duration of time (atleast 2 hours for liquids and 4 hours for solids). Also, succussion splash may not be checked for in case the stomach has been decompressed with a nasogastric tube.
     - Auscultate for Bruit, hum and rub
   o Per rectal examination: to look for Blumer shelf or metastatic deposit in the Pouch of Douglas
- Rest systemic examination:
   o Respiratory examination in form of auscultation
   o Assessment of breath holding time is important for clinically evaluating patient's fitness for surgery.
- Important points to remember: do not forget to look for and mention
   o Hydration status
   o Naso-gastric tube

EXAMPLE CASE

History

- My patient Mr ABC, is a 64-year-old gentleman hailing from Nagpur, is a farmer by occupation.
- He presented with chief complaints of dyspepsia since 2 months and vomiting since 1 month.
- My patient was apparently alright 2 months back when he developed upper abdominal burning discomfort. Present almost throughout the day, aggravated by meals.
- It was associated with sensation of upper abdominal fullness since 1.5 months, aggravated by meals.
- Since last one month he began to vomit large volume of non bilious vomitus within one hour of his meal. It contained partially digested food which he had previously consumed. There was a slight sensation of relief in the fullness following vomiting.
- He has lost around 2 kg weight in two months and appetite has also decreased
- There is no history of:
   o Early satiety

- o Hematemesis or Melena; postural dizziness, syncope, fatigue, shortness of breath, need for blood transfusion.
- o Abdominal pain
- o Altered bowel habits
- o Abdominal distension; respiratory discomfort; hemoptysis; Bony pain; back pain; blackout; seizures
- For these symptoms an upper GI endoscopic evaluation was attempted 3 days back. It was however told to be incomplete due to excessive food residue, following which a tube was inserted through the nose, which got accidentally removed yesterday
- There is no history of DM, hypertension, TB, or any previous abdominal surgery
- He smokes around 10 bidis per day but denies consuming alcohol.
- He is able to perform all daily routine activities.

Examination

- My patient is an elderly gentleman, who is averagely built, poorly nourished, with a height of 160 cm, weight of 45 kg and BMI being 17.6 kg/m^2
- He is conscious, cooperative, well oriented to time, place and person; Lying comfortably in bed; well hydrated and afebrile.
- Pulse is 72/min, BP is 110/70 mm Hg
- There is no pallor, icterus, cyanosis, clubbing, generalized or localized lymphadenopathy. There is no palpable left supraclavicular or left anterior axillary lymph node; pedal or dependent edema.

    (Note: in case the examiner asks you "is it routine to examine for left axillary node?", the answer you can say is that: following complete history and examination since one of my differential diagnosis is Gastric carcinoma I retrospectively looked for it)

- Examination of oral cavity reveals adequate oral hygiene with no obvious mucosal lesions
- Examination of the abdomen:
  - o On inspection:
    - Abdomen is flat, umbilicus is central, inverted. All quadrants are moving equally with respiration. There is no visible fullness, lump, umbilical

nodule, scar, sinus, engorged veins, pulsations, peristalsis or cough impulse.
- Inspection of groin hernial sites reveals no swelling or cough impulse and Inspection of genitalia is unremarkable. Inspection of renal angles reveals no fullness

o On Palpation:
- Abdomen is soft and non-tender. Liver and spleen are not palpable. There isn't any other palpable lump.
- There is no palpable cough impulse over groin hernia sites and examination of genitals is unremarkable. There is no tenderness in Renal angles. Examination of back and spine is essentially normal.

o On Percussion, upper border of liver dullness is in the 5th intercostal space in midclavicular line with liver span being 14 cm. Ausculto-percussion test was performed which revealed the distended stomach. Rest of the abdomen is tympanitic with no evidence of free fluid.

o On auscultation succussion splash is present. Normal bowel sounds are heard. There is no bruit, hum or rub

- Per rectal examination is unremarkable.
- Examination of the respiratory system:
    o On auscultation, air entry is bilaterally equal with normal breath sounds
    o The breath holding time is 25 seconds.
- Rest systemic examination is essentially normal

To Summarize

- My patient is a 64-year-old male with no co-morbid illness with ECOG 1 performance status, is a smoker but does not consume alcohol, presents with new onset dyspepsia of 2 months duration and history suggestive of gastric outlet obstruction since 1 month, with associated history of loss of weight.
- On examination he is poorly nourished with BMI being 17.6 kg/m^2. Succussion splash is present and ausculto-percussion test reveals distended stomach

The Most Probable Diagnosis in my patient is malignant gastric outlet obstruction due to gastric carcinoma

How to Proceed: (Sequence and justification)

- Review available medical records

- Routine blood investigations (Hemogram, Liver Function Test, Renal Function Test, Serum Electrolyte, INR)

- Upper GI endoscopy: to confirm the diagnosis/to confirm the presence of a neoplastic growth in the stomach; if present note:

    o The site, size and extent

    o Relation to GE junction, pylorus greater and lesser curve

    o Morphology: described as per Borman classification which is based on the gross endoscopic appearance

        - Type I: Protruding/proliferative

        - Type II: Fungating/ulcero-proliferative

        - Type III: Ulcerative

        - Type IV: Infiltrative

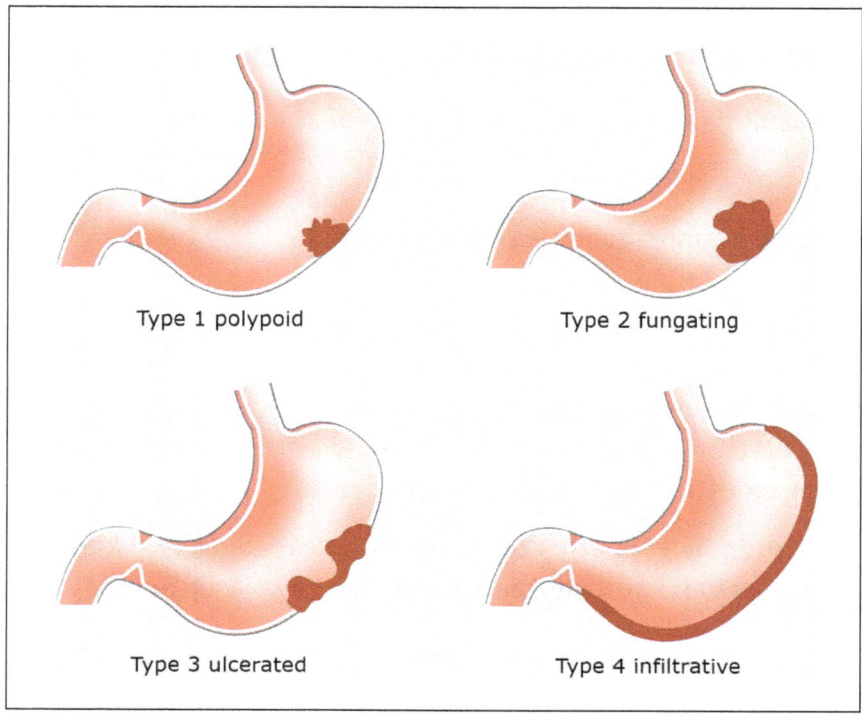

Figure 5.2: Clinical features suggesting poor nourishment.

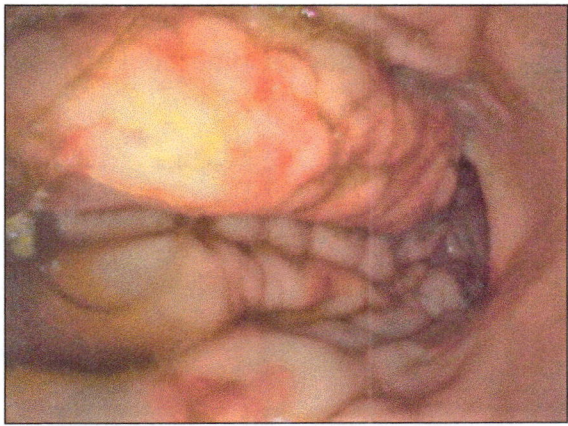

Figure 5.3: Gastroscopy showing proliferative growth in the body of stomach.

- o Passable or not
- o Distensibility of stomach with insufflation (loss of distensibility should suggest linitus plastica)
- o Presence of bleed
- o Presence of features of gastric outlet obstruction: distended stomach and food residue
- o Presence of any other synchronous lesions
- o Siewert Stein type in case of GEJ malignancy
    - Type I: epicenter of tumor between 1 and 5 cm above GEJ
    - Type II: epicenter of tumor between 1 above GEJ and 2 cm below GEJ
    - Type III: epicenter of tumor between 2 and 5 cm below GEJ
- o Biopsy: 6–8 in number

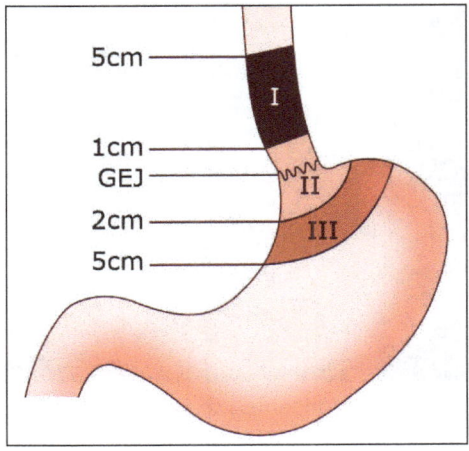

Figure 5.4: Siewert-Stein classification of GEJ adenocarcinoma.

- X-ray chest: to look for lung metastasis. If present it deems the patient in-operable and palliative intent treatment may be initiated. Further investigation may not be warranted

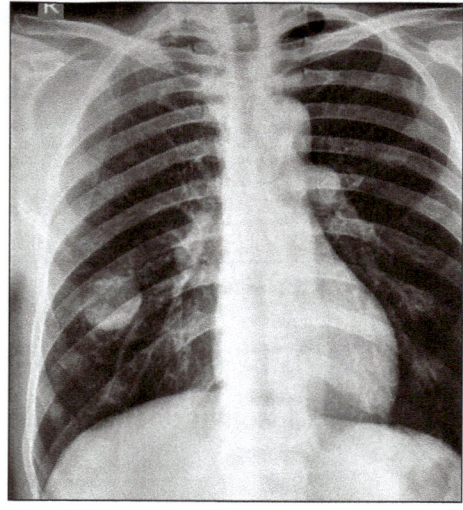

Figure 5.5: X-ray chest showing cannon ball metastasis.

- USG (A+P):
  - It is an extension of bed side clinical evaluation, it's cheap, non invasive and easily available
  - To look for liver metastasis, ascites, omental/peritoneal metastasis. If present, palliative intent treatment may be initiated and further investigation may not be warranted

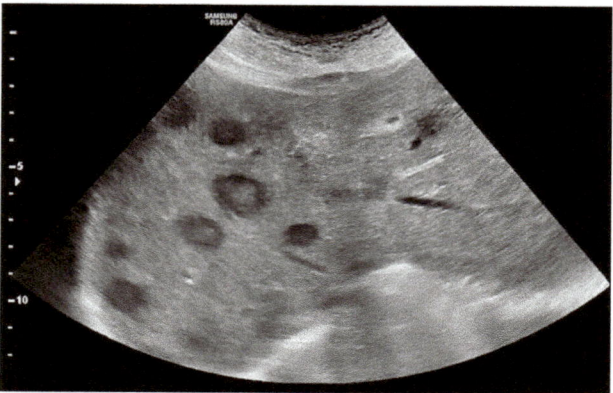

Figure 5.6: USG abdomen showing liver metastasis.

- CECT of the chest, abdomen and pelvis: to stage the disease:
  - To evaluate the site, size, extent of growth
  - Involvement of adjacent organs/vessels: liver, spleen, pancreas, diaphragmatic crus, aorta, celiac artery
  - To look for lymph nodes: perigastric, left gastric, celiac, hepatic, splenic artery
  - To look for liver metastasis, omental/peritoneal metastasis, Krukenberg tumor, ascites, lung metastasis, pleural effusion.

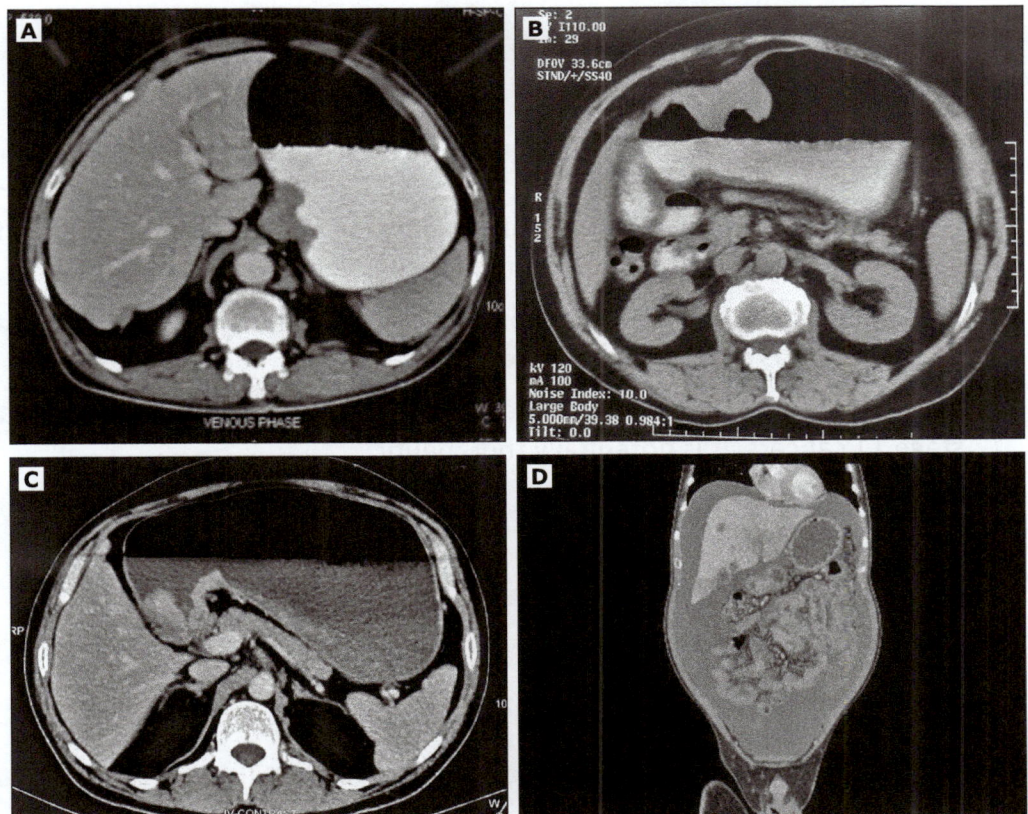

Figure 5.7: CECT showing malignancy in the cardia (A), body (B) and antrum (C) of stomach. CECT labelled (D) reveals malignant ascites..

- FDG-PET-CT: PET is done primarily to rule out distant metastasis. It is less efficacious for local staging. However, poorly differentiated adenocarcinoma/signet ring tumors are less FDG avid
- Staging laparoscopy with or without peritoneal cytology: Done to look for peritoneal metastasis/occult liver metastasis. Main role is to avoid nontherapeutic laparotomy

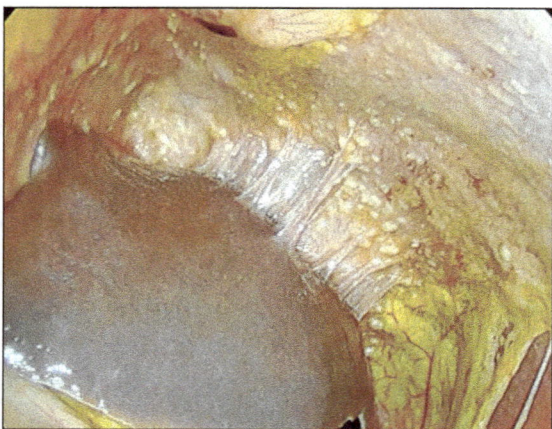

Figure 5.8: Staging Laparoscopy revealing peritoneal metastasis.

- Optional staging investigation:
  - EUS: endoscopic ultrasound: useful modality for T and N staging. Guided fine needle aspiration (FNA) and/or core biopsy is possible with EUS
  - EMR: endoscopic mucosal resection: It is considered for clinically early stage T1 cancers. It is potentially therapeutic.
  - ESD: endoscopic submucosal dissection: It is considered for clinically early stage T1 cancers. It is potentially therapeutic.

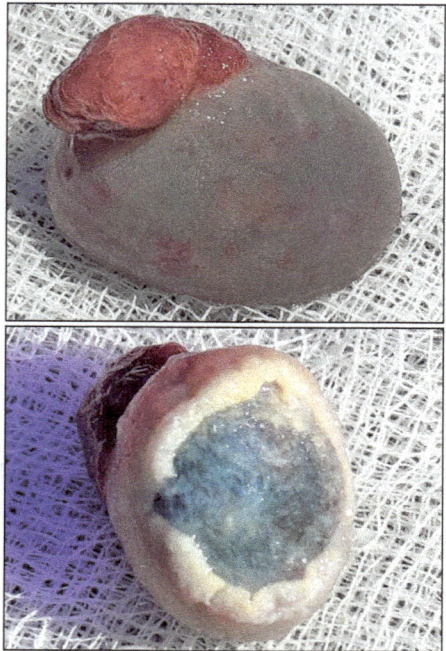

Figure 5.9: ESD specimen. The sub-mucosa will be stained blue due to sub-mucosal methylene blue injection.

- At the end of the work up, the tumor is staged as per AJCC-TNM staging system

Table 5.2: AJCC-TNM staging system for Gastric carcinoma

- T stage:
  - T1: Tumor invades submucosa
  - T2: Tumor invades muscularis propria
  - T3: Tumor invades subserosal connective tissue without penetrating through serosa or invading adjacent structures
  - T4: Tumor invades serosa or adjacent structures.
- N stage:
  - N1: Metastasis to 1–2 lymph nodes (LN)
  - N2: Metastasis to 3–6 LN
  - N3: Metastasis to 7 or more LN
- M stage:
  - M0: No distant metastasis
  - M1: Distant metastasis present

- Management principles:
  - Treatment would generally include pre-operative chemotherapy followed by surgery followed by post-operative chemotherapy (i.e. peri-operative chemotherapy)
  - Alternative options:
    - Upfront surgery followed by adjuvant chemoradiation, in case D0/D1/D1+ dissection is performed (concept of 'D' has been described later)
    - Upfront surgery followed by adjuvant chemotherapy, in case D2 dissection is performed
    - Neoadjuvant chemoradiation followed by surgery in case of GEJ adenocarcinoma
- Enteral nutrition:
  - Modalities:
    - Naso-jejunal tube insertion
    - Feeding jejunostomy
    - SEMS (self-expansile metallic stent) insertion.
  - This needs to be achieved before initiating any kind of neo-adjuvant therapy
- Neoadjuvant therapy
  - Advantage:

- To downstage/downsize the tumor
- To evaluate tumor biology i.e.
  - If the cancer progresses on therapy then it suggests aggressive tumor biology and such patients would not benefit from any kind of aggressive therapy.
  - On the contrary good response to therapy suggests good tumor biology and hence better prognosis.
- Therapy is given to tissues with intact vascularity and which are well oxygenated
- Radiated tissues will be removed at surgery
- Systemic micro-metastasis is dealt with by the systemic chemotherapy
- Higher proportion of patients will receive chemotherapy and/or radiation
  - Disadvantage:
    - Loss of window of opportunity in case the disease progresses. That is if a resectable cancer becomes unresectable during the course of neoadjuvant therapy then the window of opportunity to resect the tumor is lost
  - Indication: Tumors with clinical TNM stage >/= T2, >/= N1, M0
- Peri-op chemotherapy:
  - Options are:
    - ECF: MAGIC regimen: Epirubicin, cisplatin and 5-Fluorouracil. 3 cycles pre and post surgery
    - DCF: Docetaxel, cisplatin and 5-Fluorouracil. 3 cycles pre and post surgery
    - FLOT: 5-FU, leucovorine, oxalilatin and docetaxel. 4 cycles pre and post surgery
- Response assessment:
  - Modalities used:
    - CT
    - PET-CT
    - Upper GI endoscopy
- Surgery:
  - Prior to understanding surgeries for carcinoma stomach, you need to first remember the 16 lymph node stations related to stomach as described by Japanese classification system
    - Station 1, 3, 5: Lymph nodes along lesser curve
    - Station 2, 4, 6: Lymph nodes along greater curve

- Station 7: Lymph nodes along left gastric artery
- Station 8: Lymph nodes along common hepatic artery
- Station 9: Lymph nodes along celiac trifurcation
- Station 10: Lymph nodes in splenic hilum
- Station 11: Lymph nodes along spenic artery
- Station 12: Lymph nodes in hepato-duodenal ligament
- Station 13: Retro-pancreatic lymph nodes
- Station 14: Lymph nodes along Superior Mesenteric vessels
- Station 15: Lymph nodes along Middle Colic vessels
- Station 16: Para-aortic lymph nodes

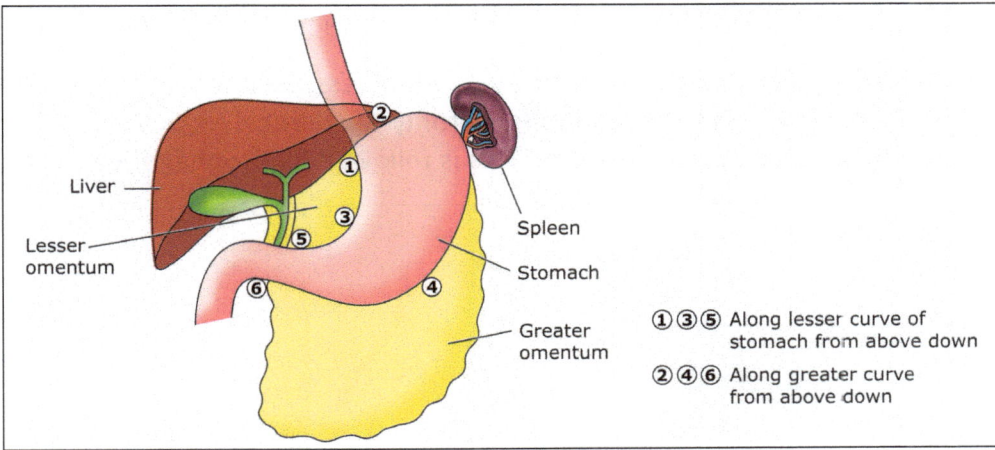

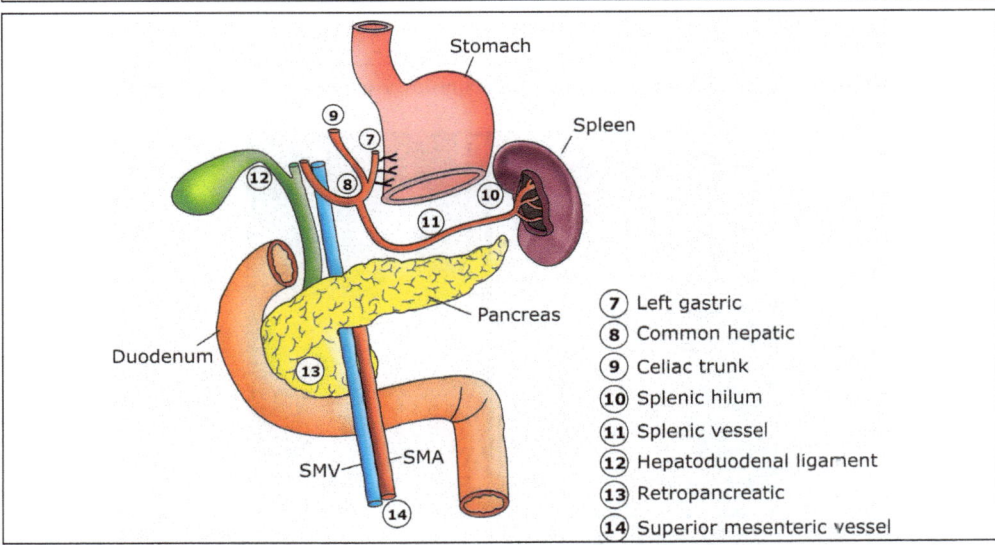

Figure 5.10: Lymph node stations in gastric cancer.

○ Surgeries performed include:
- Radical D2 Subtotal Gastrectomy: It involves resection of atleast 2/3 of the stomach along with lymphadenectomy of station 1, 3, 5, 4, 6, 7, 8, 9, 11, 12 [i.e. station 1–12 except 2 & 10]. This is followed by gastrojejunostomy.

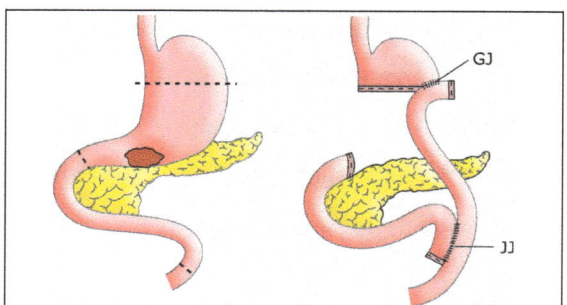

Figure 5.11: Sub-total gastrectomy and Roux-en-y gastrojejunostomy.

- Radical D2 Total Gastrectomy: It involves resection of whole of the stomach along with lymphadenectomy of station 1, 3, 5, 2, 4, 6, 7, 8, 9, 10, 11, 12 [i.e. station 1–12]. This is followed by esophago-jejunostomy

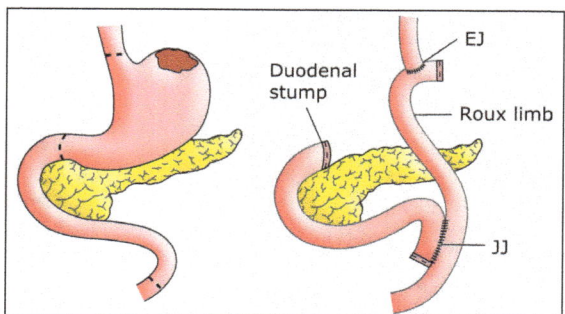

Figure 5.12: Total gastrectomy and Roux-en-y esophagojejunostomy.

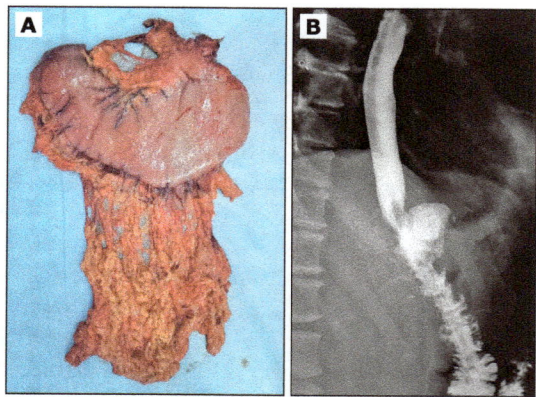

Figure 5.13: Total gastrectomy specimen (A). Upper GI contrast study (B) done on POD 5 reveals intact esophago-jejunal anastomosis. Such dye study is usually performed prior to initiating diet.

- D1 Subtotal Gastrectomy: It involves resection of 2/3 of the stomach along with lymphadenectomy of station 1, 3, 5, 4, 6, 7 [i.e. station 1–7 except 2]. This is followed by gastro-jejunostomy.
- D1 Total Gastrectomy: It involves resection of whole of the stomach along with lymphadenectomy of station 1, 3, 5, 2, 4, 6, 7 [i.e. station 1–7]. This is followed by esophago-jejunostomy
- D1 + (plus) Subtotal Gastrectomy: It involves resection of 2/3 of the stomach along with lymphadenectomy of station 1, 3, 5, 4, 6, 7, 8 and 9 [i.e. station 1–9 except 2]. This is followed by gastro-jejunostomy.
- D1 + Total Gastrectomy: It involves resection of whole of the stomach along with lymphadenectomy of station 1, 3, 5, 2, 4, 6, 7, 8, 9 and 11 [i.e. station 1–11 except 10]. This is followed by esophago-jejunostomy
- D0 Gastrectomy: Resection of a part of stomach without formal lymph node dissection.
- Proximal gastrectomy followed by esophago-gastrostomy: it is performed for proximal gastric tumors. However it is less preferred.
- D2 Gastrectomy is the preferred surgery in the curative setting. Whereas, D0 and D1 are performed in the palliative setting.
- Options for reconstruction:
  - Roux-en-y: Preferred
  - Loop GJ/EJ with Brauns jejuno-jejunostomy
  - Uncut Roux-en-y
  - Loop GJ/EJ: Least preferred

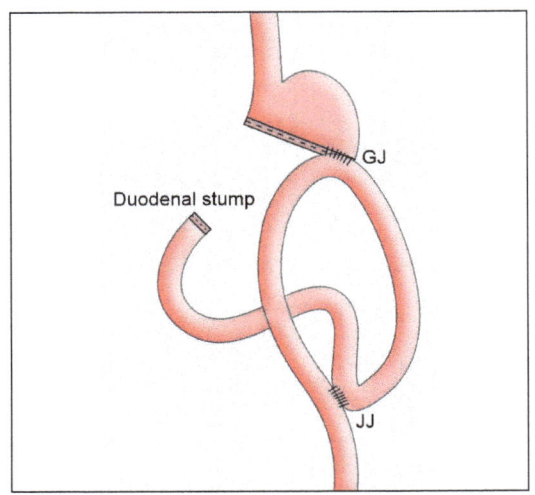

Figure 5.14: Loop Gastro-Jejunostomy with Brauns jejuno-jejunostomy.

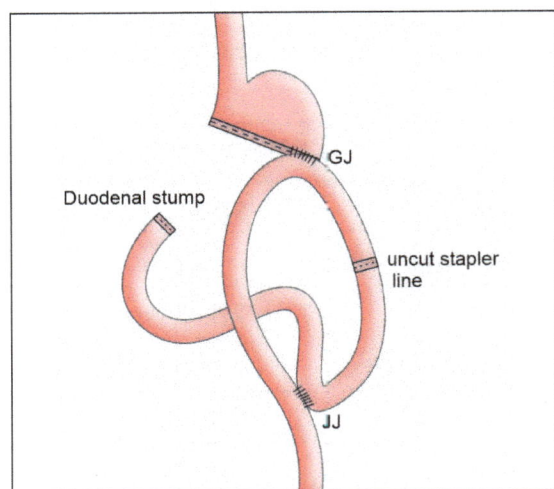

Figure 5.15: Uncut Roux-en-y Gastro-Jejunostomy.

- Adjuvant therapy:
  - Options:
    - Adjuvant Chemoradiation: Fluoropyrimidine based chemoradiation
    - Adjuvant chemotherapy: Cape-Ox: capecitabine and oxaliplatin
  - If a D2 gastrectomy is performed then adjuvant chemotherapy suffices.
  - However if a surgery amounting to less than D2 resection is performed then chemoradiation would be preferred.
- Surveillance
  - Modality used:
    - History and examination
    - Biochemistry: CBC, LFT
    - USG
    - CT
    - Endoscopy
- **Go through chapter 13 for literature on the subject.**

Management of Gastric Gastro-intestinal stromal tumor (GIST)

- Diagnosis of GIST needs to be considered when apart from GOO patient gives history of GI bleed and/or there is a firm to hard lump palpable in the upper abdomen on examination
- Immuno-histochemical analysis is required for diagnosis: CD117, PDGFRA, DOG1
- The malignant potential is estimated based on Joensuu modification of Fletcher criteria

Table 5.3: Joensuu Criteria for Gastric GIST		
Risk	Size	Mitotic index
Very low	< 2 cm	< 6/50 High power field (HPF)
Low	2.1–5 cm	< 6/50 HPF
Intermediate	2.1–5 cm	> 5/50 HPF
	5.1–10 cm	< 6/50 HPF
High	> 5 cm	AND > 5/50 HPF
	Tumor rupture in itself is a high-risk factor	

Table 5.4: Joensuu Criteria for Non-gastric GIST

Risk	Size	Mitotic index
Very low	< 2 cm	< 6/50 High power field (HPF)
Low	2.1–5 cm	< 6/50 HPF
High	> 5 cm	OR > 5/50 HPF
	Tumor rupture in itself is a high-risk factor	

- Treatment:
  - Surgery:
    - Principles of surgery:
      - Complete resection with 1–2 cm gross margin
      - Maximal organ preservation
      - Avoiding violation of tumor pseudo-capsule to avoid tumor rupture.
      - Lymphadenectomy is not required.
  - Targeted therapy:
    - Imatinib Mesylate (Gleevac):
      - It may be given as Adjuvant therapy, neo-adjuvant therapy and palliative therapy
      - Imatinib is indicated in the adjuvant setting for high risk tumors at a dose of 400 mg OD for 3 years
      - If facility is available genotyping should be performed:
        - Tumor with exon 9 c-kit mutation: may consider double dose imatinib therapy
        - Wild type tumors which are c-kit mutation and PDGFRA mutation negative are not sensitive to imatinib
        - Exon 11 c-kit mutation: these tumors have high risk of recurrence, hence there may be role for prolonged therapy in them
    - Sunitinib is second line therapy and Regorafenib is third line therapy in case of imatinib resistance
- Go through chapter 13 for literature on the subject.

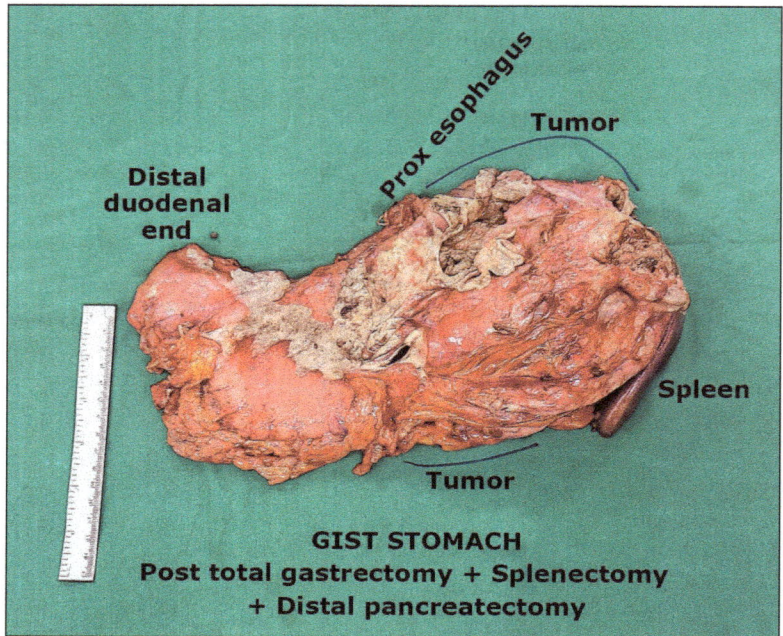

Figure 5.16: Surgical specimen of Total Gastrectomy with Distal Pancreatico-Splenectomy for a large gastric GIST; do remember that palpable gastric masses are usually GIST

Management of Gastric Lymphoma

- GI NHL (Non-Hodgkin lymphoma) is classified as per WHO classification

Table 5.5: WHO Classification of NHL
o   Diffuse Large B cell Lymphoma (DLBC): Most common
o   Extra nodal marginal Lymphoma (MALToma): 2nd most common
o   Follicular cell Lymphoma
o   Mantle cell Lymphoma
o   Burkitt's Lymphoma

- PET-CT and bone marrow examination is additionally required to stage the disease
- Staging of GI NHL is done as per Lugano classification or Ann Arbor classification

Table 5.6: Lugano classification for staging		
Stage	Sub-stage	Description
Stage I		Confined to GI tract
	Stage I1	Confined to mucosa
	Stage I2	Infiltration of sub-mucosa and deeper layers
Stage II		Spread to abdominal lymph nodes (LN)
	Stage II1	Involvement of regional LN
	Stage II2	Involvement of distant abdominal LN
	Stage II E	Infiltration of adjacent organs
Stage IV		Spread to extra-abdominal LN

- Treatment of DLBC:
  o Primary treatment modality is chemotherapy +/- radiotherapy
  o Regimen most commonly used: CHOP-R
    - C: Cyclophosphamide
    - H: Doxorubicin
    - O: Vincristin
    - P: Prednisolone
    - R: Rituximab
- Treatment of MALToma:
  o Treatment depends on stage, H. Pylori status and whether t(11:18) translocation is present or not (on molecular analysis by PCR or FISH)

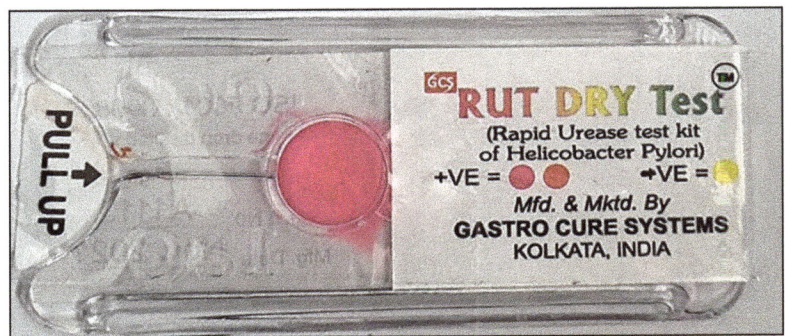

Figure 5.17: H. Pylori status is identified using Rapid Urease Test (RUT) kit on an endoscopic biopsy sample; alternatively, Urea Breath Test may be performed

- Stage I, II
  - H. pylori positive and t(11:18) negative: H. Pylori eradication and re-assess
    - If remitting: Follow-up
    - If progressing: ISRT (involved site radiotherapy)
  - H. pylori positive and t(11:18) positive: H. Pylori eradication and ISRT/rituximab
  - H. pylori negative and t(11:18) positive: ISRT/rituximab
- Stage IV: CHOP-R chemotherapy
- Indications for surgery:
  - Perforation
  - Bleeding
  - In case of diagnostic dilemma

6 Case of Surgical Obstructive Jaundice

Introduction

Differentials to be discussed in this chapter:
- Carcinoma Head of Pancreas
- Carcinoma Gall Bladder
- Peri-Ampullary Cancer
- Hilar Cholangiocarcinoma
- Choledocholithiasis, Choledochal Cyst

Format for History Taking

- History of yellowish discoloration of sclera and high colored urine:
    - Duration
    - Onset: insidious or sudden
    - Nature: intermittent or persistent or progressive or waxing and waning
    - Painless or painful: associated with abdominal pain or not
    - Preceded by prodromal symptoms or not.
    - Identified by self or relative
- History of pruritus (itching):
    - Generalized to whole body or localized to a certain body part
    - Present throughout the day or at certain point of the day (as in, more towards the night)
    - Disturbing lifestyle or not; disturbing sleep or not
- Color of stools:
    - Cholic or acholic, i.e. note whether stool is normal brown colored (cholic) or clay/white colored (acholic) stool
    - Additionally, also ask if patient passes silver paint stools or Melena.
- History of pain:
    - Site

- Onset: insidious or sudden
- Duration: total duration. If intermittent in nature, inquire regarding the frequency and the interval between each episode of pain
- Character of pain: Dull aching or colicky
- Nature: intermittent/persistent/progressive
- Intensity: mild/moderate/severe
- Radiation of pain: whether there is radiation of pain to mid back or right infrascapular region
- Related to meals or not
- Relation to posture: Relieved on bending forward or not
- Relief of pain: whether the pain gets relieved spontaneously or with medications (oral or injectable analgesic). Also note if patient's pain was initially getting relieved with oral medication and now he/she requires injectable analgesics and whether the analgesic requirement is increasing.
- Natural history: Is there any change in the nature, intensity or frequency of pain over course of the disease, i.e. whether there is any increase or decrease in intensity or frequency of pain or change in nature of pain from intermittent to persistent. Inquire whether there is any recent change in character of pain, especially in a patient with chronic pancreatitis.
- History of fever:
    - Duration
    - Onset: insidious or sudden
    - Grade: low or high
    - Nature: intermittent/fluctuating/continuous
    - Associated chills or not.
- History of vomiting:
    - Onset
    - Duration
    - Frequency
    - Quantity: small or large volume, alternatively one could describe quantity in form of cup
    - Bilious or not

- Projectile or not
- Related to meals or not i.e. post prandial or not
- Is there sensation of postprandial fullness or not
- Is there a sense of relief after vomiting or not.
- History of recent onset diabetes or recent change in diabetic pattern
- History of hematemesis or Melena; postural dizziness, syncope, fatigue, shortness of breath, need for blood transfusion.
- History suggestive of fat-soluble vitamin deficiency:
  - Vitamin A deficiency: history of decreased night vision, dryness of eyes
  - Vitamin D deficiency: bone pain, frequent fractures, muscle weakness
  - Vitamin K deficiency: history suggestive of coagulopathy such as ecchymosis, petechiae, easy bruisability
- History suggestive of chronic liver disease:
  - Abdominal distension
  - GI bleed
  - Altered sensorium
  - Features of hypersplenism
    - Anemia: History of shortness of breath, fatigue
    - Leukopenia: History of repeated fever or infection
    - Thrombocytopenia: History of gum bleed, epistaxis, easy bruisability, hematuria, menorrhagia
- History of loss of weight; loss of appetite
- History of abdominal distension; respiratory discomfort; hemoptysis; Bony pain; back pain; blackout; seizures
- Past history:
  - Past history of gallstone disease (in the form of biliary colic)
  - History of previous surgery particularly laparoscopic cholecystectomy.
  - History of co-morbid illness
- Personal history:
  - History of smoking or alcohol consumption.
  - Diet: history of red meat consumption.

- Treatment history:
  - History of any cross sectional imaging
  - History of endoscopic or percutaneous intervention (biopsy, stenting or tube insertion)
- Family history of pancreatitis or cancer
- Performance history:
  - Whether he/she is
    - Able to perform all daily routine activity (sedentary and/or strenuous)
    - Able to perform all self care
    - Bed ridden
  - Whether he/she is able to climb two flight of stairs comfortably or not

Justification for Each Component in History

- History of jaundice:
  - History of yellowish discoloration of sclera and high colored urine: History of yellowish discoloration of sclera suggests jaundice and high colored urine in such patients suggests obstructive jaundice.
  - Duration of jaundice: Duration of jaundice is usually short (few weeks to around 1–2 month) in malignant cases. Longer duration of symptoms (few months to years) is more suggestive of benign cause (choledochal cyst or choledocholithiasis).
  - Onset of jaundice: generally, jaundice due to malignant pathology is insidious in onset; whereas sudden onset jaundice is less likely to be seen in malignant OJ. Sudden onset obstructive jaundice could be due to bile duct obstruction by stone or blood clots (hemobilia)
  - Nature of jaundice:
    - Progressive jaundice means jaundice which is gradually deepening in nature. It is usually seen in carcinoma head of pancreas, carcinoma gall bladder or cholangiocarcinoma.
    - Intermittent jaundice is one in which the bilirubin levels reaches baseline between two episodes of hyperbilirubinemia. It may be seen in choledocholithiasis, hemobilia. Bilirubin level normalizes as the stone or clot passes off.

- Fluctuating jaundice is one in which bilirubin levels does not normalize between two episodes of hyperbilirubinemia; another term for this is waxing and waning. It is seen in peri-ampullary cancers, this is because, initially there would be jaundice as the tumor obstructs the outlet, but then when the tumor sloughs off due to tumor necrosis, the bilirubin levels drop as the obstruction gets partially or fully relieved, causing waning. Also, as the tumor sloughs off, there will be some amount of GI bleed manifesting as Melena or silver paint stools (as described in textbooks).
  - Persistent jaundice is usually seen in jaundice of medical cause as in viral hepatitis or chronic liver disease.
  - Jaundice preceded by prodromal symptoms or not: presence of prodromal symptoms (nausea, vomiting, myalgia, malaise) suggests medical cause for jaundice such as viral hepatitis.
  - Identified by self or relative: this point has no specific significance; may or may not be mentioned.
- History of pruritus:
  - History of pruritus in a jaundiced patient suggests obstructive pathology. The exact reason for pruritus in a patient with obstructive jaundice is controversial. Previously it was thought to be due to deposition of bile salts in skin causing irritation of nerve endings. More recently endogenous opioids, serotonin and lysophosphatidic acid have been implicated. It is important to evaluate the degree to which life has been affected because it has implication on treatment. Severe pruritus affecting quality of life itself is an indication for biliary drainage. (do not underestimate pruritus as a symptom, patients may develop suicidal tendency due to the suffering)
- Color of stools: Cholic or acholic: passage of clay colored stools in a patient with jaundice suggests complete obstruction to flow of bile from bile duct into the intestinal lumen (i.e. obstructive type of jaundice). Where as passage of cholic stools (normal brown colored) suggest that there is no or only a partial obstruction to flow of bile.
- Remember passage of clay colored stools in a jaundiced patient would suggest complete obstruction, whereas pruritus may be present even in case of partial biliary obstruction.
- History of pain:
  - In general, painless progressive obstructive jaundice is said to be due to malignant etiology and painful intermittent jaundice is due to

choledocholithiasis. At super-speciality level however it should be noted that this statement may not be completely true because ½ to ¾ patients with carcinoma head of pancreas will complain of pain; similarly ½ to ¾ patients with carcinoma gall bladder experience pain. Pain is however less common in patients with periampullary cancer and hilar cholangiocarcinoma.

- o Site of pain: common site of pain in hepato-pancreatico-biliary diseases, both benign and malignant is right hypochondrium and epigastrium. Radiation to mid back or right infra-scapular region is common.
- o Onset of pain: pain in choledocholithiasis is usually sudden in onset, whereas pain in malignancy is generally insidious in onset.
- o Duration of pain: pain is usually of short duration in malignant causes (weeks to few months). Whereas long duration of symptoms may be seen in diseases like choledochal cyst and choledocholithiasis.
- o Nature of pain: intermittent/continuous: pain in choledocholithiasis is intermittent; whereas pain in malignant diseases is usually continuous in nature.
- o Character of pain: dull aching type of pain is seen in malignant diseases whereas pain in choledocholithiasis or choledochal cyst is usually colicky in nature.
- o Intensity of pain: mild/moderate/severe: it is important to grade the severity of pain. Also, the degree to which life has been hampered by pain must be inquired for and mentioned.
- o Pain related to meals or not: relation of pain to meals may be seen in diseases of pancreatic or gall bladder origin.
- o Pain relieved on bending forward or not: reduction in pain on bending forwards suggests pancreatic cause for pain.
- o Recent change in character of pain: Recent change in character of pain, especially in a patient with chronic pancreatitis: this is worrisome and could suggest development of malignancy in the setting of long standing chronic pancreatitis.
- History of fever: development of fever in a patient with obstructive jaundice should raise suspicion of cholangitis. Cholangitis is more common in patients with choledocholithiasis vis a vis obstructive jaundice due to malignant cause. In patients with malignant obstructive jaundice, cholangitis usually sets in after some kind of intervention such as ERCP/PTBD.
- History of vomiting is to be inquired for in a patient with obstructive jaundice mainly to rule out gastric outlet obstruction. Post prandial upper abdominal fullness,

voluminous non bilious post prandial vomiting containing previously eaten food suggests gastric outlet obstruction. It may be seen in patients with carcinoma head of pancreas, carcinoma gall bladder and chronic pancreatitis with fibroinflammatory head mass.

- History of recent onset diabetes: recent onset type 2 diabetes mellitus in patients above 50 years of age is a harbinger of pancreatic cancer. It is considered to be a paraneoplastic condition due to adrenomedullin. Similarly, a recent change in diabetic pattern, i.e. worsening of glycemic control, is also worrisome feature hinting towards clinical diagnosis of pancreatic cancer.
- History of hematemesis or Melena: GI bleed may be seen in periampullary cancer
- History of postural dizziness, syncope, fatigue, shortness of breath, need for blood transfusion: these questions need to be asked to grade the severity of blood loss and are to be mentioned only if there is history of GI bleed.
- History suggestive of fat soluble vitamin deficiency: may be found in patient with long standing obstructive jaundice. Vitamin K deficiency is earliest to occur. To be mentioned, only if present.
- History suggestive of chronic liver disease: in a patient with jaundice, one has to always rule out the possibility of chronic liver disease. Clinical features to look out for are:
  - Abdominal distension suggestive of ascites
  - GI bleed suggestive of variceal bleed
  - Altered sensorium suggestive of hepatic encephalopathy
  - Features of hypersplenism
- History of loss of weight; loss of appetite: alarming symptoms, suggestive of malignancy
- History of abdominal distension; respiratory discomfort; hemoptysis; Bony pain; back pain; blackout; seizures: all these symptoms are suggestive of metastatic disease.
  - Abdominal distension: Due to malignant ascites
  - Respiratory discomfort: Due to pleural effusion and lung metastasis
  - Hemoptysis: Due to lung metastasis
  - Bony pain: Due to bony metastasis
  - Back pain: Due to vertebral metastasis
  - Blackout, Seizures: due to brain metastasis

- Past history of gallstone disease (in the form of biliary colic) could suggest that the current symptoms may be due to choledocholithiasis
- Past history of laparoscopic cholecystectomy should raise in mind the possibility of biliary stricture due to bile duct injury.
- History of endoscopic or percutaneous intervention: History of ERCP and endoscopic biliary stenting, or alternatively percutaneous drain tube insertion (PTBD or percutaneous transhepatic biliary drainage) draining greenish fluid (bile) should be asked for. Both would suggest obstructive jaundice. PTBD is more likely to be done for proximal blocks (either hilar cholangiocarcinoma, carcinoma gall bladder) whereas endoscopic biliary stenting is commonly done for distal blocks (carcinoma head of pancreas, periampullary cancer, distal cholangiocarcinoma).
- History of endoscopic biopsy: History of endoscopic biopsy is more likely to suggest periampullary cancer.
- Family history: There are many hereditary pancreatic cancer syndromes:
    - Hereditary pancreatitis (related to mutation in PRSS1 gene)
    - Familial Adenomatosis Polyposis (related to mutation in Adenomatosis Polyposis Coli [APC] gene)
    - Hereditary Non Polyposis Colon Cancer (related to mutation in Mismatch Repair [MMR] gene)
    - Hereditary breast and ovarian cancer (related to mutation in BRCA gene)
    - Familial atypical mole melanoma syndrome (related to mutation in p16 gene)
- Performance history: to clinically assess fitness for surgery. Most of the malignant differential diagnoses discussed in this chapter would necessitate performance of a major surgery like Whipples Pancreaticoduodenectomy (WPD) or hepatectomy in order to achieve cure. Enquiring about performance status in history is a simple way of clinically assessing patient's ability to tolerate such a major surgery.

Characteristic Features Pointing Towards a Particular Diagnosis

- **Carcinoma Head of Pancreas**
    - Painful progressive obstructive jaundice (remember: although textbooks classically describe carcinoma head of pancreas to present with "painless progressive jaundice"; one has to remember that in clinical practice (and at super-specialty level) this is not completely true and pain is seen in ½ to ¾ of the patients)

- Pain is dull aching in nature and radiates to back
- Pain is slightly relieved on bending forwards
- Lump in abdomen (due to distended gall bladder)
- Post prandial fullness, post prandial vomiting (due to gastric outlet obstruction)
- Recent onset diabetes or change in diabetic pattern
- Patient from south India.

- **Carcinoma Gall Bladder**
    - Painful progressive obstructive jaundice
    - Dull aching pain radiating to right infra scapular region
    - Lump in abdomen (due to distended gall bladder)
    - Post prandial fullness, post prandial vomiting (due to gastric outlet obstruction)
    - Patient from North India.

- **Peri-ampullary Cancer**
    - Generally painless
    - Intermittent jaundice/waxing and waning of jaundice
    - Melena/silver paint stools
    - Lump in abdomen (due to distended gall bladder)
    - Gastric outlet obstruction is unlikely, except in case of obstructing duodenal growth

- **Hilar Cholangiocarcinoma**
    - Generally painless
    - Progressive jaundice
    - Lump in abdomen is unlikely as the gall bladder is usually not distended as the block is proximal to cystic duct insertion
    - Gastric outlet obstruction is unlikely

- **Choledocholithiasis**
    - Painful intermittent jaundice
    - Cholangitis (pain, fever, jaundice: Charcot's triad; pain, fever, jaundice, altered mentation, shock: Reynolds pentad)

Format for Examination

- What is the appearance of the patient: young/middle-aged/elderly, lady/gentleman
- Whether the patient is clinically
  - Poorly/averagely/well built
  - Poorly/averagely/well nourished
- Mention height, weight, BMI
- Whether the patient is clinically
  - Conscious/stuporous
  - Co-operative/un-cooperative
  - Well/poorly oriented to time, place and person
  - Lying comfortably in bed/in discomfort/in pain (rolling in pain)
  - Well hydrated/dehydrated
  - Febrile/Afebrile.
- Mention Pulse, BP, RR and breath holding time
- Look for
  - Icterus:
    - Sites to look for icterus: sclera/bulbar conjunctiva, undersurface of tongue, soft palate, palms and soles.
    - Apart from hyperbilirubinemia, carotenemia may cause yellowish discoloration of sclera (so be aware).
    - Various color shades of icterus which help in differentiating the cause of jaundice:
      - Greenish yellow: obstructive jaundice
      - Orange yellow: hepatic cause of jaundice (alcoholic or viral hepatitis)
      - Pale yellow: hemolytic jaundice
  - Pallor, cyanosis, clubbing
  - Generalized or localized lymphadenopathy
  - Palpable left supraclavicular lymph node

- o Pedal or dependent edema
- o Skin lesions: look for scratch marks. It is not to be missed. Also look for generalized yellowish discoloration of skin.

- Look for Stigmata of chronic liver disease (top to bottom)
  - o Icterus
  - o Malar erythema
  - o Fetor hepaticus
  - o Parotid swelling
  - o Spider nevi/spider angiomata
  - o Gynecomastia
  - o Reduced chest hair
  - o Reduced axillary hair
  - o Dupuytren's contracture
  - o Palmar erythema
  - o Leukonychia
  - o Flapping tremors/Asterexis
  - o Abdominal distension
  - o Caput medusae
  - o Reduced pubic hair
  - o Testicular atrophy
  - o Pedal edema

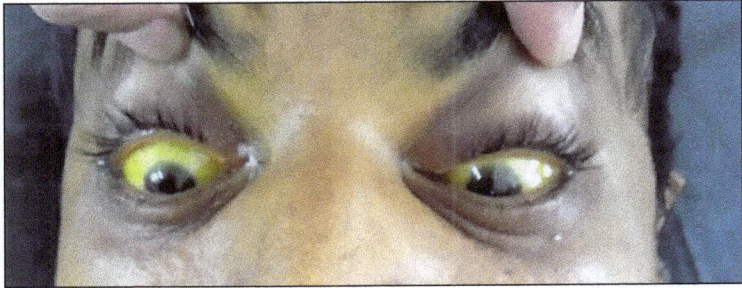

Figure 6.1: Icterus.

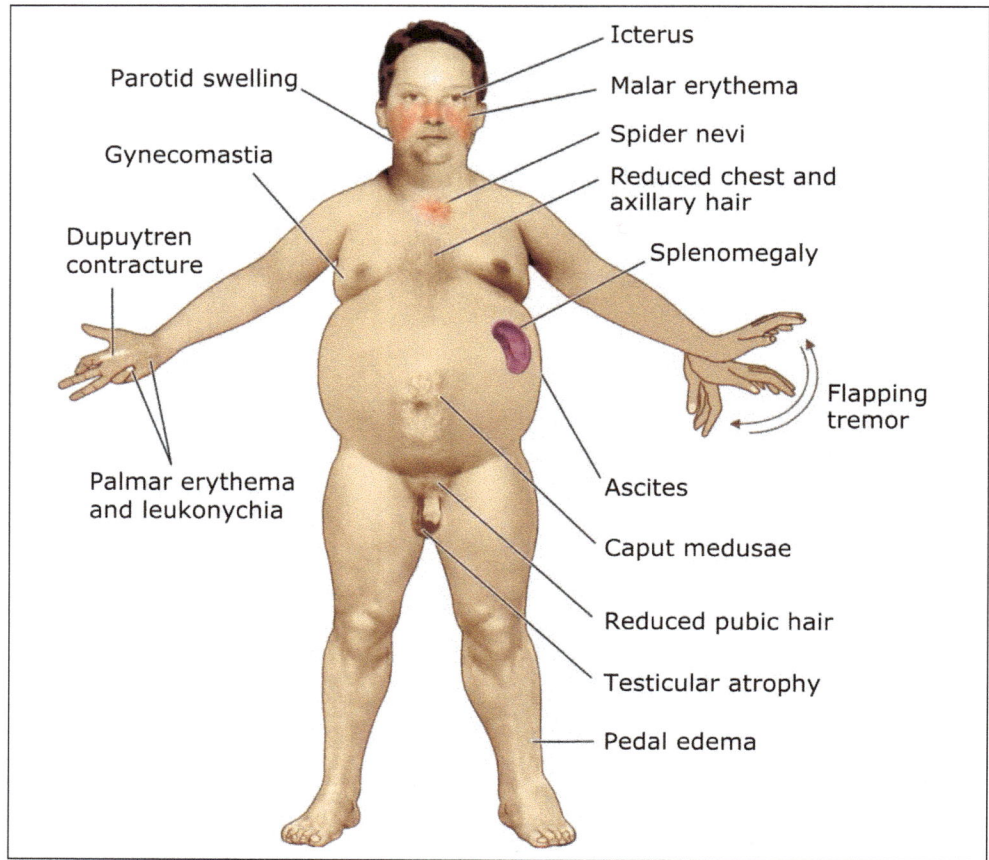

Figure 6.2: Stigmata of chronic liver disease.

- Examination of oral cavity: look for oral hygiene and any obvious mucosal lesions, apart from jaundice.
- Examination of the abdomen:
  - On Inspection: See if:
    - Abdomen is flat/distended/scaphoid
    - Umbilicus is central/displaced (upwards/downwards/sideways) inverted/everted/flat
    - All quadrants are moving equally with respiration or not
    - Look for any visible lump
      - In context of malignant obstructive jaundice distended gall bladder may be visualized in right upper abdominal quadrant on inspection as a rounded bulge just below right costal margin. Gall bladder is better seen than felt.

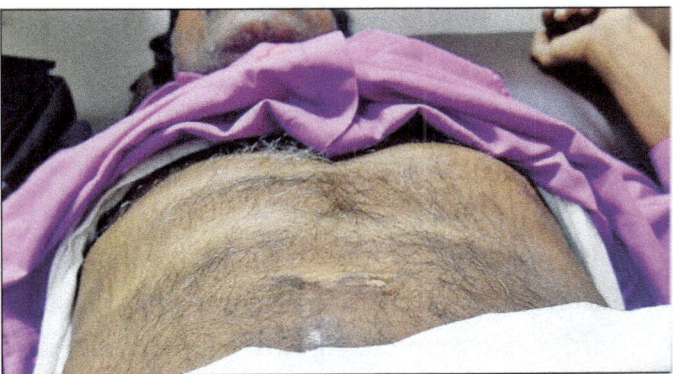

Figure 6.3: Tangential inspection of the abdomen from the leg end revealing a Right upper quadrant bulge which on palpation was confirmed to be Gall Bladder.

- Conversely, as per Courvoisiers law gall bladder will not be palpable in a patient with choledocholithiasis.
- If visible describe:
  - Size
  - Site
  - Shape
  - Surface and
  - Movement with respiration
- Occasionally in a thin built patient with bulky carcinoma head of pancreas, a lump may be visible in mid upper abdomen; in that case describe its:
  - Site
  - Size
  - Shape
  - Surface
  - Movement: pancreatic lump won't move with respiration.
- Look for visible scar (especially of previous laparoscopic cholecystectomy), sinus, engorged veins, pulsations, peristalsis or cough impulse.
- Don't forget to inspect the groin hernial sites (to look for swelling or cough impulse i.e. hernia) and genitalia.
- Inspection of renal angles to look for fullness

  o On Palpation: See if:
  - Abdomen is soft and non-tender (Alternatively abdomen could be rigid and/or tender)

- Liver: palpable or not; liver may be enlarged due to congestive hepatomegaly or metastasis.
    - If yes, measure distance of liver edge from costal margin in midclavicular line in unit of centimeter or number of fingers
    - See if:
        - It is tender/nontender
        - Surface is smooth (normal)/nodular (cirrhosis/metastasis)
        - Borders are round (congestive)/sharp (normal), regular (normal)/irregular (cirrhosis/metastasis)
        - Consistency is soft (normal)/firm (cholestatic)/hard (cirrhosis/malignancy)
- Gall bladder: palpable or not:
    - Courvoisiers law states that if gall bladder is palpable it is seldom due to gall stones.
    - In malignant obstructive jaundice there is concept of proximal block (tumor proximal to cystic duct insertion: hilar cholangiocarinoma) vs distal block (tumor distal to cystic duct insertion: carcinoma head of pancreas or periampullary tumors).
    - So gall bladder will be distended in distal blocks, whereas it tends to be collapsed in proximal blocks (although not always).
    - In case of gall bladder cancer: if it involves the neck or cystic duct then the gall bladder gets distended and on abdominal examination a cystic distended gall bladder will be palpable; whereas if the fundus or body is involved, a firm to hard lump is more likely to be palpable.
    - Describe:
        - Site: gall bladder has been characteristically described to be located at the point at which left spino-umbilical line (line from left ASIS to umbilicus) meets the costal margin. Alternatively, the point of interjunction of lateral border of rectus muscle to tip of 9th costal cartilage has also been described as a surface landmark for gall bladder.
        - Size: vertical and horizontal dimension in centimeters.
        - Shape: it is characteristically Pear shaped, globular.
        - Surface: generally smooth in distal malignant blocks. However it may be nodular in case of carcinoma of fundus/body of gall bladder.

- ♦ Margins: the lateral, medial and lower margin is generally well appreciated; the upper margin is either continuous with the enlarged liver or goes under the costal margin.
- ♦ Consistency: generally it is soft, cystic in distal malignant blocks (a tensely distended gall bladder may however have a firm consistency). It may be firm to hard in consistency in case of carcinoma of fundus/body of gall bladder.
- ♦ Tender (inflammatory) or non tender (neoplastic).
- ♦ Mobility: side to side mobility may be present but vertical mobility is unlikely.
- ♦ Movement with respiration: usually present.
- In MBBS and broad speciality exams it is better to first describe all the above points about the lump and conclude at the end that the palpable lump is probably gall bladder; whereas in superspeciality exams the candidate may directly mention that he/she could palpate the gall bladder and describe some pertinent points why it is so.
- Spleen is enlarged or not
- Any other palpable lump.
- A tumor within head of pancreas may be palpable in the form of a lump in the mid upper abdomen in a thin built patient. If palpable, describe:
  - Site
  - Size
  - Shape
  - Surface
  - Margins
  - Tenderness
  - Consistency
  - Mobility
  - Movement with respiration
  - Plane:
    - ♦ Whether the lump is intraperitoneal or not: by performing leg raising test
    - ♦ Whether the lump is retroperitoneal or not: by asking the patient to assume lateral decubitus position and palpating if the lump falls forward or not. A retroperitoneal mass won't fall ahead. Knee elbow test is no longer recommended as it would be inhuman to make a patient assume a knee-elbow position.

- Do not forget to:
  - Palpate groin hernia sites to look for cough impulse
  - Examine genitals
  - Look for tenderness in renal angles
  - Examine back and spine for tenderness/gibbus.
- On Percussion:
  - Look for upper border of liver dullness (generally in the 5th intercostal space) in midclavicular line.
  - Note the liver span (normal being 12–14 cm)
  - Percussion note over the gall bladder. Generally it is a dull note, continuous with that of liver dullness.
  - Note in the percussion note over rest of the abdomen (it is generally tympanic)
  - Tests for free fluid. Presence of free fluid i.e. ascites suggests metastatic disease in context of malignant obstructive jaundice.
- On auscultation:
  - Auscultate for bowel sounds.
  - Bruit, hum and rub
- Per rectal examination: to look for Blumer shelf (metastatic deposits in pouch of Douglas) and Clay colored stools.
- Rest systemic examination:
  - Respiratory examination in form of auscultation, assessment of breath holding time is important for clinically evaluating fitness for surgery.

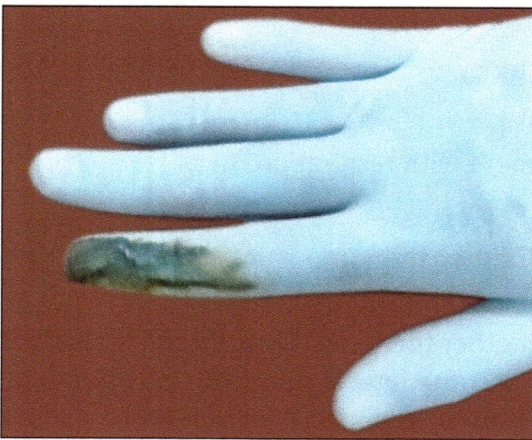

Figure 6.4: Gloved finger showing Clay Colored stools after a DRE.

EXAMPLE CASE

History

- My patient Mrs XYZ, is a 54-year-old lady hailing from Mumbai, is a homemaker.
- She presented with chief complaints of yellowish discoloration of eyes since one month.
- She was apparently alright 1 month back, when she noticed yellowish discoloration of her eyes and passage of high colored urine. It was insidious in onset, progressive in nature and was not preceded by any prodromal symptoms.
- It was associated with generalized body itching, present throughout the day, disturbing her sleep and daily routine activities.
- She gives history of passing clay colored stools since last 3 weeks.
- There is history of loss of appetite but no loss of weight.
- There is no history of
    - Pain in abdomen
    - Fever, chills
    - Nausea or vomiting
    - Hematemesis, melena or silvery paint like stools
    - Easy bruisability
    - Recent onset diabetes
    - Abdominal distension, altered sensorium
    - Respiratory discomfort, bone pain or back pain
- She seeked medical care for these symptoms for which she was evaluated with ultrasound examination
- There is no previous history of diabetes, hypertension, ischemic heart disease or TB.
- She has not undergone any major surgery in the past.
- There is no history of alcohol consumption or smoking
- She is post menopausal
- There is no history of cancer in first and second degree relatives
- She is able to perform all her daily routine activity without any difficulty and is able to easily climb 2 flight of stairs

Examination

- My patient is an elderly lady, who is averagely built, averagely nourished, with a height of 160 cm, weight of 55 kg and BMI being 21.5 kg/m^2
- She is conscious, cooperative, well oriented to time, place and person; Lying comfortably in bed; well hydrated and afebrile.
- Pulse is 72/min, BP is 110/70 mm Hg
- She is icteric and scratch marks are noted over her trunk.
- However, there is no pallor, cyanosis, clubbing, generalized or localized lymphadenopathy. There is no palpable left supraclavicular lymph node; pedal or dependent edema.
- There is no peripheral signs of chronic liver disease.
- Examination of oral cavity reveals adequate oral hygiene with no obvious mucosal lesions
- Examination of the abdomen:
  - On inspection:
    - Abdomen is flat, umbilicus is central, inverted. All quadrants are moving equally with respiration.
    - There is a visible lump in right hypochondrium. It is globular in shape, around 3 x 3 cm in size, with a smooth surface and is moving with respiration.
    - There is no visible scar, sinus, engorged veins, pulsations, peristalsis or cough impulse.
    - Inspection of groin hernial sites reveals no swelling or cough impulse and Inspection of genitalia is unremarkable. Inspection of renal angles reveals no fullness
  - On Palpation:
    - Abdomen is soft and non-tender. Liver and spleen is not palpable.
    - There is a lump palpable in the right upper quadrant just below the right costal margin, 7 cm lateral to midline, measuring 3 cm horizontally, 4 cm vertically. It is pear shaped, non tender, with a smooth surface, firm consistency, with well-defined and regular lateral, medial and inferior margins with upper part going under the costal margin. There is side to side mobility and it moves with respiration. This palpable lump is probably distended gallbladder.
    - There is no palpable cough impulse over groin hernia sites and examination

of genitals is unremarkable. There is no tenderness in renal angles. Examination of back and spine is essentially normal.

- On Percussion, upper border of liver dullness is in the 5th intercostal space in midclavicular line with liver span being 14 cm. There is dull note over the gall bladder which is continuous with the liver dullness. Rest of the abdomen is tympanic with no evidence of free fluid.
- On auscultation normal bowel sounds are heard. There is no bruit, hum or rub

- Per rectal examination is unremarkable
- Examination of the respiratory system:
  - On auscultation, air entry is bilaterally equal with normal breath sounds
  - The breath holding time is 25 seconds.
- Rest systemic examination is essentially normal

To Summarize

- My patient is a 54 year old female with no co-morbid illness with ECOG 1 performance status, presents with 1 month's history of painless progressive jaundice associated with pruritus, clay colored stools and decreased appetite
- On examination she is icteric with scratch marks present over trunk and distended gall bladder is palpable on abdominal examination.

The most probable diagnosis in my patient is malignant obstructive jaundice

The possible differential diagnosis being:

- Peri-ampullary Carcinoma
- Carcinoma head of pancreas
- Carcinoma gall bladder
- Hilar cholangiocarcinoma

How to Proceed: (Sequence and Justification)

- Review available medical records
- Routine blood investigations (Hemogram, Liver Function Test, Renal Function Test, Serum Electrolyte, INR)
  - Findings to expect:
    - Direct hyperbilirubinemia

- Raised Alkaline phosphatase (ALP)
- Mildly raised SGOT/AST and SGPT/ALP in case of cholangitis
- Deranged INR
• X-ray chest: to look for metastasis. If present, palliative treatment may be initiated and further investigation may not be warranted.

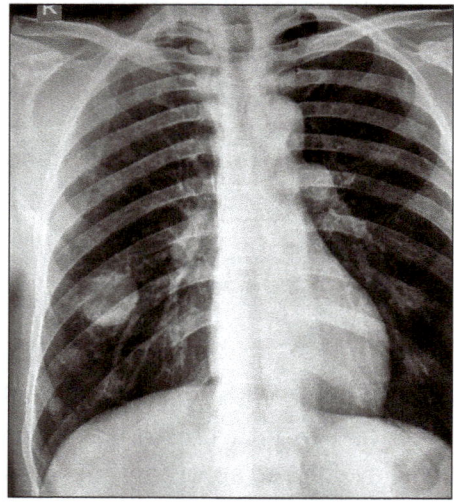

Figure 6.5: X-ray chest showing cannon ball metastasis.

• USG (A+P): It is an extension of bed side clinical evaluation, it's cheap, non invasive and easily available
    ○ To look for presence or absence of intrahepatic biliary radical dilatation (IHBRD). If present, it confirms the presence of obstructive jaundice

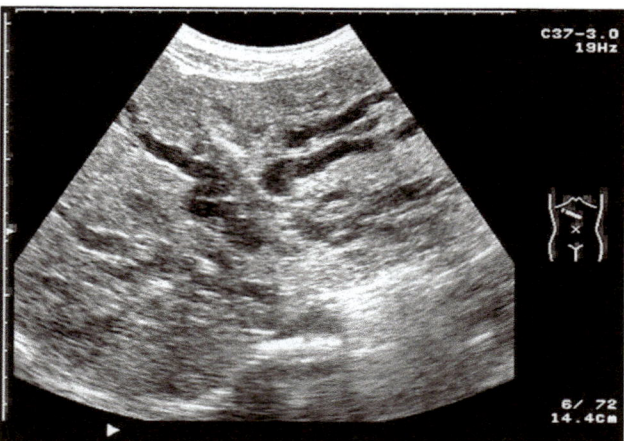

Figure 6.6: USG abdomen showing IHBRD.

- Note the Level of block: by noting the site till which the biliary system is dilated.
    - Dilated intrahepatic biliary ducts with non dilated extrahepatic biliary duct suggest block at hilar level
    - Dilated intrahepatic biliary ducts, dilated common hepatic duct with non dilated common bile duct suggests block at level of cystic duct insertion
    - Dilated intrahepatic biliary ducts, dilated common hepatic duct and dilated common bile duct suggests block at level of lower CBD
    - Dilated intrahepatic biliary ducts, dilated common hepatic duct, dilated common bile duct and dilated pancreatic duct suggests block at level of ampulla
- To look for cause of block: mass or stone.
    - If mass is present characterize it by noting its
        - Size and morphology
        - Longitudinal extent
        - Circumferential extent i.e. adjacent organ/vessel (hepatic artery, portal vein, IVC) involvement
- To examine gall bladder for stone, GB wall thickening, mass
- To look for presence of lymph nodes
- Examine liver for liver metastasis, cholangitic abscesses
- To look for free fluid
- To look for metastatic deposit elsewhere in abdomen

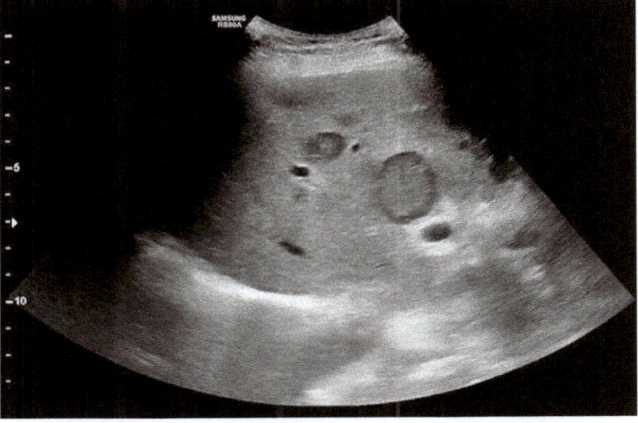

Figure 6.7: USG abdomen revealing liver metastasis.

- CECT of the chest, abdomen and pelvis: to confirm the diagnosis and stage the malignant disease
  - To note:
    - The site, size, extent and morphology of the growth
    - Involvement of adjacent organs: liver, duodenum, stomach, colon, pancreas
    - Involvement of adjacent vessels: SMA, SMV, PV, IVC, celiac artery, Hepatic artery, first jejunal artery
    - To look for lymph nodes
    - To look for liver metastasis, omental/peritoneal metastasis, ascites, lung metastasis, pleural effusion.

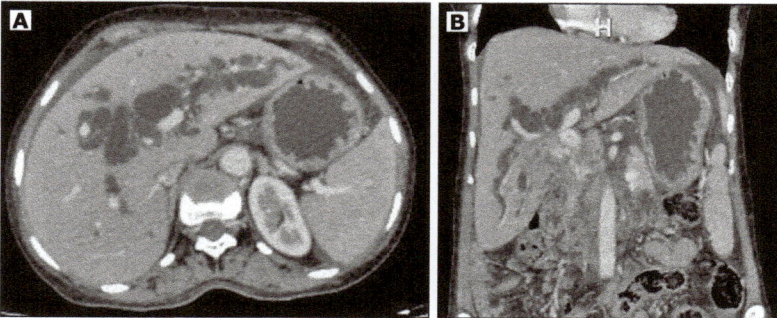

Figure 6.8: CECT showing IHBRD.

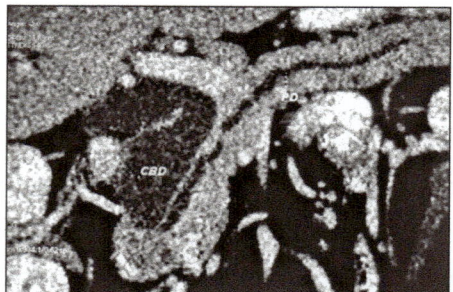

Figure 6.9: CT showing 'Double duct sign' (dilated CBD and PD) with tumor visualized in the region of the ampulla.

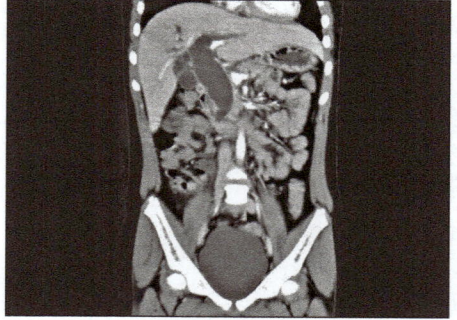

Figure 6.10: Dilated extra-hepatic bile duct without any obvious cause should suggest the diagnosis of choledochal cyst.

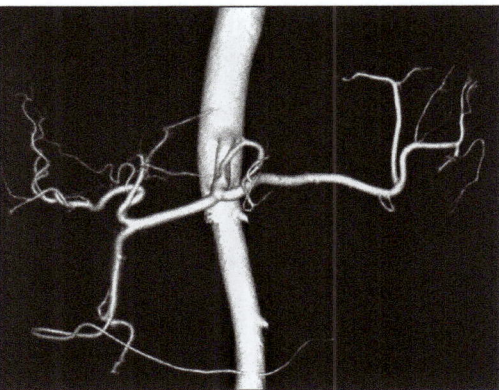

Figure 6.11: It is important to note the arterial anatomy to look for aberrant anatomy, especially replaced or accessory right hepatic artery which will have surgical implications.

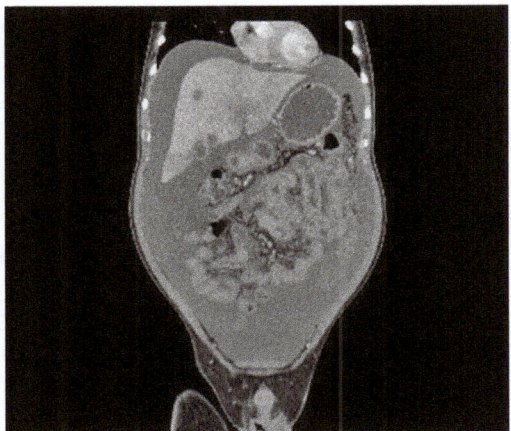

Figure 6.12: CT revealing liver metastasis and malignant ascites.

- In case of carcinoma head of pancreas (HOP) and peri-ampullary cancers a Pancreatic protocol CECT is performed.
    - 100–120 ml of iodinated contrast is injected at a rate of 3–5 ml/second.
    - Water or negative oral contrast is used to distend the stomach and duodenum.
    - It consists of non-contrast phase (optional), pancreatic parenchymal phase at 35–40 seconds and portal venous phase at 70 seconds.
    - Slice thickness is 1 mm.
    - Pancreatic cancers are hypodense in pancreatic parenchymal phase. In this phase we also assess the relation of the tumor to the arterial vessels.
    - Similarly, the relation of the tumor to the SMV-PV is evaluated in the portal venous phase.

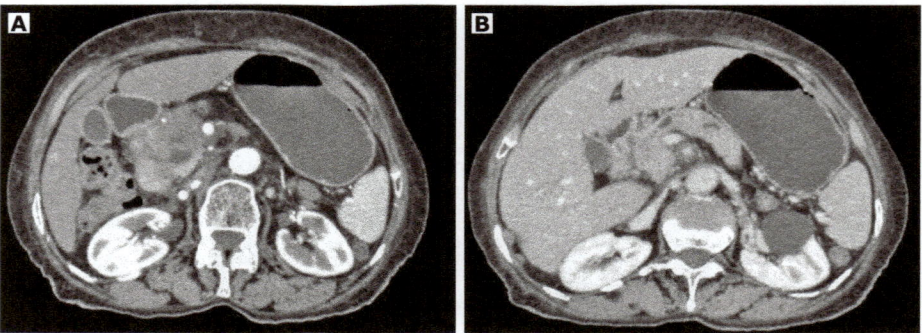

Figure 6.13: pancreatic protocol CECT. CT on left reveals hypodense lesion in head of pancreas on the pancreatic parenchymal phase; fat planes with SMA appears maintained. On venous phase (right) the tumor is now isodense; fat planes with SMV also appears maintained.

- Vessel involvement is determined, based upon the degree of contact of the tumor with the artery or vein and/or contour irregularity.

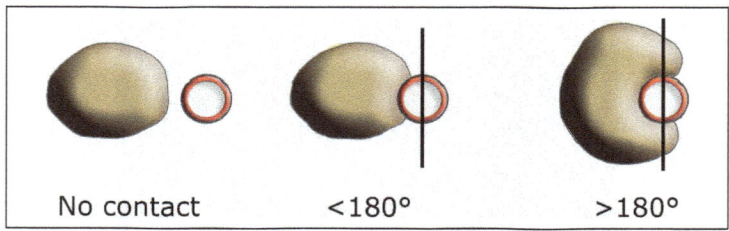

Figure 6.14: Degree of tumor contact with SMA.

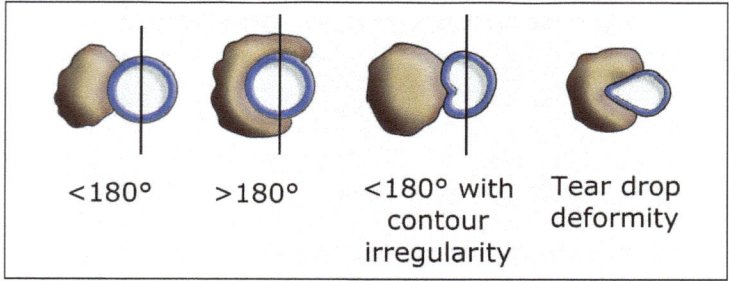

Figure 6.15: Degree of tumor contact with SMV and contour irregularity.

- Based on this, NCCN classifies the tumor as resectable, borderline resectable and unresectable.
  - Resectable:
    - Fat planes with SMA is maintained.
    - Fat planes with SMV-PV is either maintained or the degree of contact with it is </= 180 degree. And there is no contour irregularity.

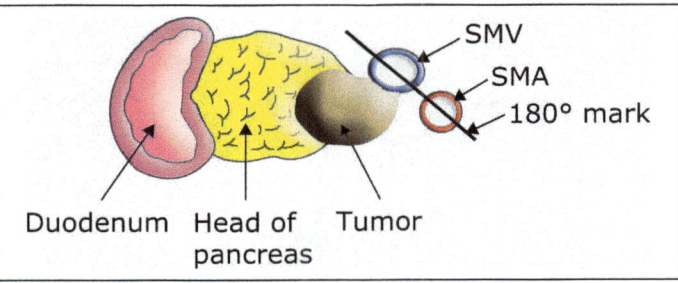

Figure 6.16: Resectable pancreatic cancer.

- Borderline resectable:
    ◆ Degree of contact with SMA </= 180 degree.
    ◆ Degree of contact with SMV-PV is > 180 degree or </= 180 degree with contour irregularity. However, vascular reconstruction is feasible.

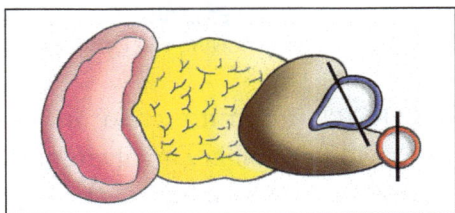

Figure 6.17: Borderline resectable pancreatic cancer.

- Unresectable:
    ◆ Distant metastasis present.
    ◆ Degree of contact with SMA > 180 degree.
    ◆ Un-reconstructible involvement/occlusion of SMV-PV.

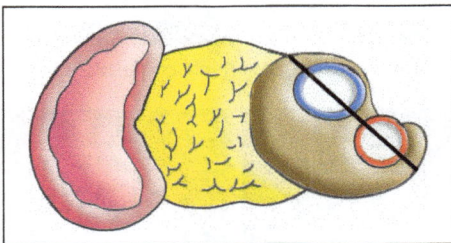

Figure 6.18: Unresectable.

○ In case of proximal growths (carcinoma gall bladder and hilar cholangiocarcinoma) conventional triple phase CECT suffices (arterial phase, portal venous phase and equilibrium phase)

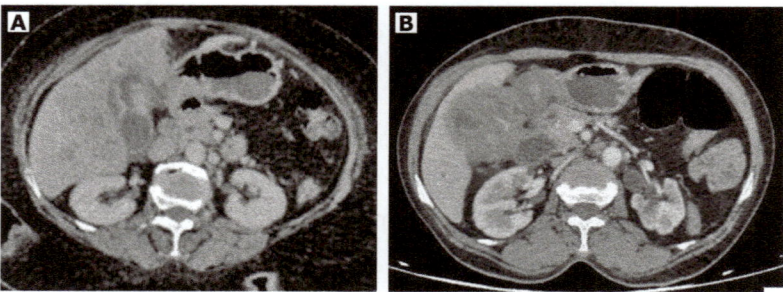

Figure 6.19: CECT images showing carcinoma gall bladder.

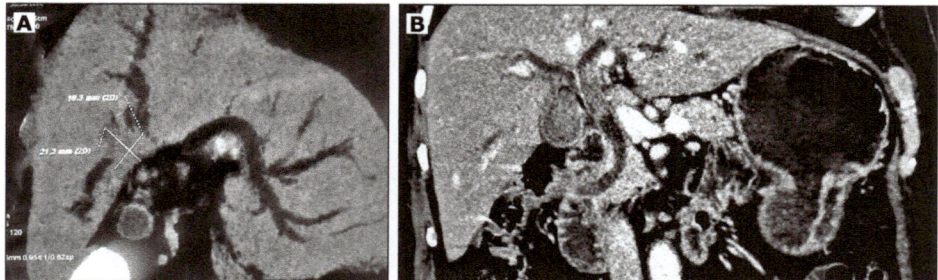

Figure 6.20: CECT images showing Hilar cholangiocarcinoma.

- MRI abdomen with MRCP: recommended in case of proximal blocks (cholangiocarcinoma or Ca GB with biliary involvement). It provides data which is complementary to CT. It provides information regarding the proximal extent of the tumor which has an implication on operative planning.

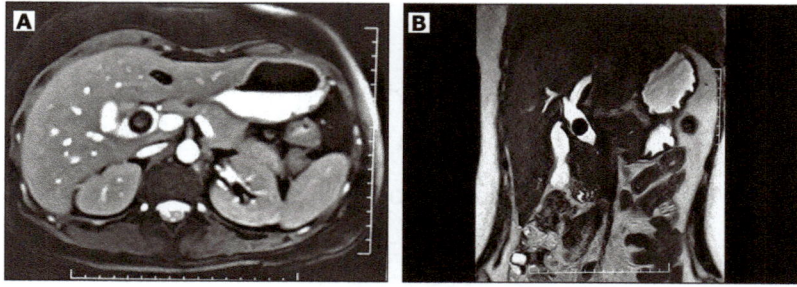

Figure 6.21: MRI revealing choledocholithiasis.

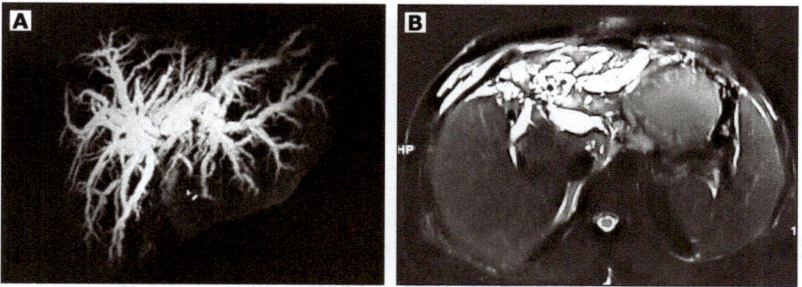

Figure 6.22: MRCP showing bilateral IHBRD with separation of right and left duct in a case of Klatskin tumor (A). MRI showing crowding of ducts in left lobe suggestive of left lobar atrophy (B).

- Blood CA 19-9 level
    - It is sialated Lewis A blood group antigen (hence levels won't rise in patients who are Lewis antigen negative)
    - Levels rise in patients with Pancreatico-biliary malignancies
    - It is however not cancer specific and CA 19-9 levels may rise in many benign HPB diseases (most importantly: Cholangitis)
    - Hence levels are best performed after achieving biliary decompression
    - Normal: < 37 U/ml
    - Role:
        - Diagnosis of Pancreatico-biliary malignancies
        - Assessing resectability
        - Assess need for staging laparoscopy (indicated if levels are > 100 U/ml as per NCCN)
        - Prognostification
        - Response assessment: post neoadjuvant therapy, post surgery, post adjuvant
        - Surveillance
- EUS:
    - Similar to CT, it can be used to characterize the growth and check for vessel involvement.
    - Additionally the most important advantage of EUS is the ability to obtain FNA or core biopsy to preoperatively establish the diagnosis of cancer
    - Has role in evaluation of patients with chronic pancreatitis with head mass and pancreatic cystic neoplasms due to its ability to perform FNA
    - Indications for biopsy:
        - Metastatic disease
        - Prior to initiating neo-adjuvant therapy
        - Case of diagnostic dilemma: chronic pancreatitis, autoimmune pancreatitis
    - Has role in evaluating periampullary tumors
- FDG-PET-CT: To rule out distant metastasis.
- Staging laparoscopy:
    - The main aim is to avoid a non-therapeutic laparotomy by looking for peritoneal metastasis/occult liver metastasis

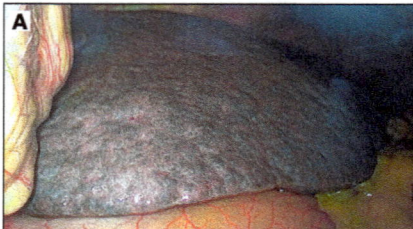 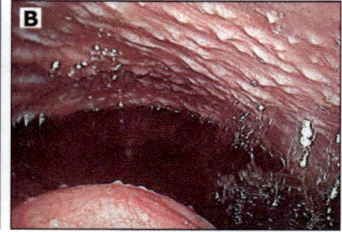 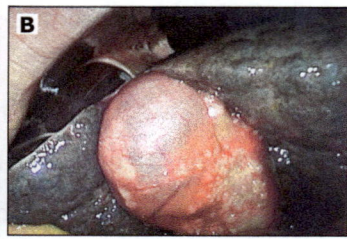

Figure 6.23: Staging laparoscopy revealing cholestatic liver (A), peritoneal metastasis with malignant ascites in a case of carcinoma pancreas (B) and carcinoma GB with serosal deposits (C).

- o It is performed as a routine in case of carcinoma gall bladder and selectively in the remaining
- o Indication in case of pancreatic cancer:
  - Borderline resectable tumor, Large tumor
  - Large regional lymph nodes
  - Tumor of the body or tail of pancreas
  - Highly symptomatic patient: severe pain, weight loss
  - Markedly elevated CA 19-9 levels (> 100U/ml as per NCCN)
- Additional investigation:
  - o Side viewing endoscopy: to visualize a peri-ampullary tumor and take biopsy from it.
  - o Cholangioscopy and Biopsy: It helps by providing direct visualization of the biliary system and facilitates targeted biopsy. It is performed with a Spy-Glass cholangioscopy system (baby scope) introduced through the ampulla into the bile duct via the the instrument channel of an ERCP scope (mother scope). Hence it is also called as the Mother-Baby technique. Biopsy is taken with help of Spy-Bite technology.
  - o Liver volumetry:
    - Surgical management of proximal blocks (Hilar CholangioCa, Ca GB with hilar involvement) usually entails a major hepatectomy, including extended right or left hepatectomy. In such cases it is important to calculate the FLR (future liver remnant) using CT or MR volumetry
    - FLR = remnant liver volume/total functional liver volume x 100
    - Target FLR:
      - o In normal liver: 20%
      - o In cholestatic/fatty liver: 30%
      - o In cirrhotic liver: 40%

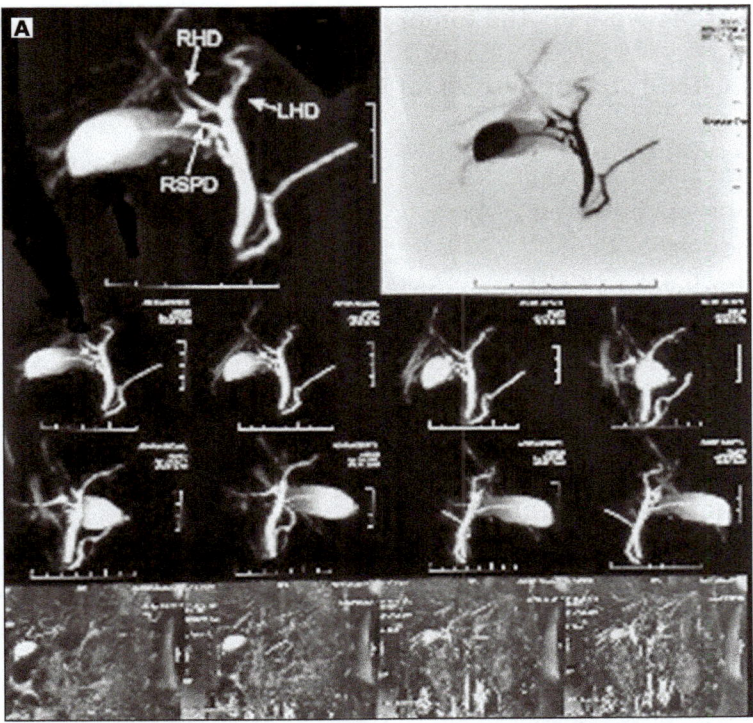
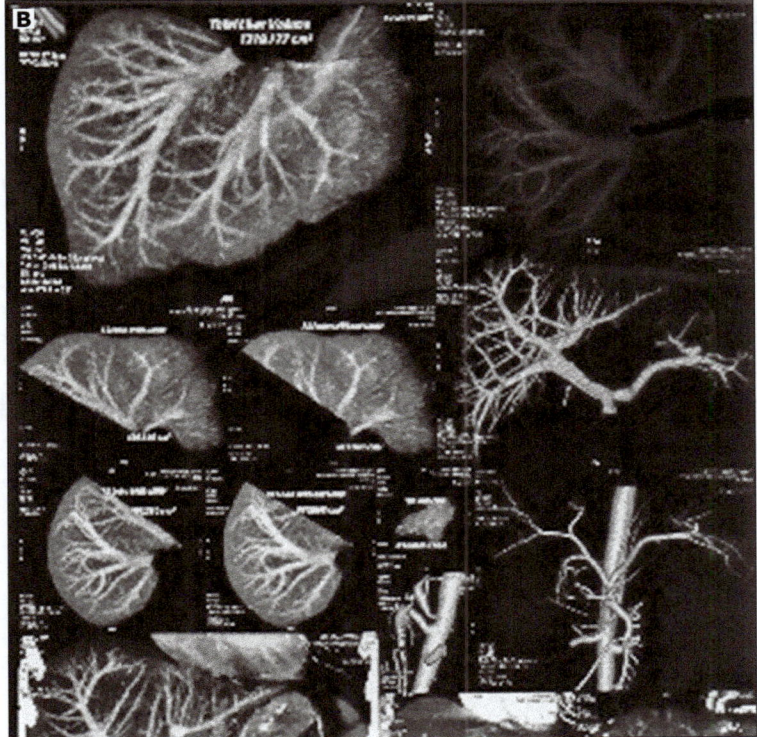

Figure 6.24: Generally before any major hepatectomy important information in the form of volumetry, cholangiogram, hepatic arteriogram and portovenogram are compiled as seen in the figure.

- At the end of the work up, the tumor is staged as per AJCC-TNM staging system

Table 6.1: AJCC-TNM staging system for Carcinoma Head of Pancreas

- T stage:
  - T1: Tumor size < 2 cm
  - T2: Tumor size between 2–4 cm
  - T3: Tumor size > 4 cm
  - T4: Tumor involves Celiac axis, SMA, CHA regardless of size
- N stage:
  - N1: Metastasis to 1–3 lymph nodes (LN)
  - N2: Metastasis to 4 or more LN
- M stage:
  - M0: No distant metastasis
  - M1: Distant metastasis present
- Staging:
  - Stage I: T1/T2
  - Stage II: T3/N1
  - Stage III: T4/N2
  - Stage IV: M1

Table 6.2: AJCC-TNM staging system for Carcinoma Gall Bladder

- T stage:
  - T1a: Tumor invades lamina propria
  - T1b: Tumor invades muscular layer (there is no sub-mucosa)
  - T2: Tumor invades perimuscular connective tissue without infiltrating serosa or liver
    - T2a: invasion on peritoneal side
    - T2b: invasion on hepatic side
  - T3: Tumor perforates the serosa and/or invades liver and/or one extra hepatic adjacent organ
  - T4: tumor invades main PV or HA or two or more extra hepatic adjacent organ
- N stage:
  - N1: Metastasis to 1–3 lymph nodes (LN)
  - N2: Metastasis to 4 or more LN
- M stage:
  - M0: No distant metastasis
  - M1: Distant metastasis present
- Staging:
  - Stage I: T1
  - Stage II: T2
  - Stage III: T3/N1
  - Stage IV: T4/N2/M1

Table 6.3: AJCC-TNM staging system for Ampullary Carcinoma

- T stage:
  - T1: Tumor limited to sphincter of Oddi or tumor invades duodenal submucosa
  - T2: Tumor invades duodenal muscularis propria
  - T3: Tumor invades pancreas
  - T4: Tumor involves Celiac axis or SMA
- N stage:
  - N1: Metastasis to 1–3 lymph nodes (LN)
  - N2: Metastasis to 4 or more LN
- M stage:
  - M0: No distant metastasis
  - M1: Distant metastasis present

Table 6.4: AJCC-TNM staging system for Hilar Cholangiocarcinoma

- T stage:
  - T1: Tumor confined to the bile duct wall
  - T2a: Tumor invades beyond bile duct wall to surrounding adipose tissue
  - T2b: Tumor invades adjacent hepatic parenchyma
  - T3: Tumor invades unilateral branches of PV or HA
  - T4: tumor invades
    - Main PV or its branches bilaterally
    - Main HA
    - Unilateral second order biliary radical with involvement of contralateral PV or HA
- N stage:
  - N1: Metastasis to 1–3 lymph nodes (LN)
  - N2: Metastasis to 4 or more LN
- M stage:
  - M0: No distant metastasis
  - M1: Distant metastasis present

- Management Principles:
  - In distal block (Ca HOP, Periampullary Ca):
    - It usually consists of upfront surgery followed by adjuvant therapy
    - Biliary drainage is done in selective patients, if indicated

- Neo-adjuvant therapy is administered selectively in borderline resectable cases
- In carcinoma gall bladder (GB) without hilar involvement:
  - It usually consists of upfront surgery followed by adjuvant therapy
  - Neo-adjuvant therapy is administered selectively in locally advanced cases (TMH criteria: T3, T4, N+)
- In proximal blocks (Hilar CholangioCa, Ca GB with hilar involvement):
  - Treatment planning is best done in the setting of a multi-disciplinary team (MDT) meeting
  - It usually consists of biliary drainage followed by liver volume augmentation followed by surgery followed by adjuvant therapy. Surgery is performed once the bilirubin level is < 2-3 mg/dl and FLR is adequate
  - Neo-adjuvant therapy may be administered in the interval period prior to surgery if deemed necessary by the MDT
- Biliary drainage:
  - Options:
    - ERCP and EBD (endoscopic biliary drainage) with stent
    - ERCP and ENBD (endoscopic naso-biliary drainage)
    - PTBD (percutaneous transhepatic biliary drainage)
  - In distal block (Ca HOP, Periampullary Ca).
    - Routine biliary drainage is not recommended for distal blocks. It is better done selectively
    - Indications:
      - Cholangitis
      - Severe pruritus
      - Coagulopathy
      - Renal insufficiency
      - Poor nutritional status
      - Surgery delayed due to any other reason
      - When neoadjuvant therapy is being planned in resectable or borderline resectable disease
      - When palliation is to be achieved in unresectable disease
    - EBD and ENBD are preferred over PTBD for distal blocks
    - Additionally, during an ERCP, bile may be procured for cytological examination and biliary brushings may be achieved for histological examination

- In proximal blocks (Hilar CholangioCa, Ca GB):
    - As treatment usually entails a hepatectomy, biliary drainage is generally performed
    - PTBD and ENBD are preferred over EBD
    - Again, bile may be procured for cytological examination and biliary brushings may be achieved for histological examination
- Liver volume augmentation
  - As discussed previously the target FLR is:
    - In normal liver: 20%
    - In cholestatic/fatty liver: 30%
    - In cirrhotic liver: 40%
  - In case the FLR is low then liver volume augmentation in form of Portal vein embolization (PVE) is generally required prior to proceeding with liver resection. ALPPS (associating liver partition with portal vein ligation for staged hepatectomy) is another option in case of low FLR

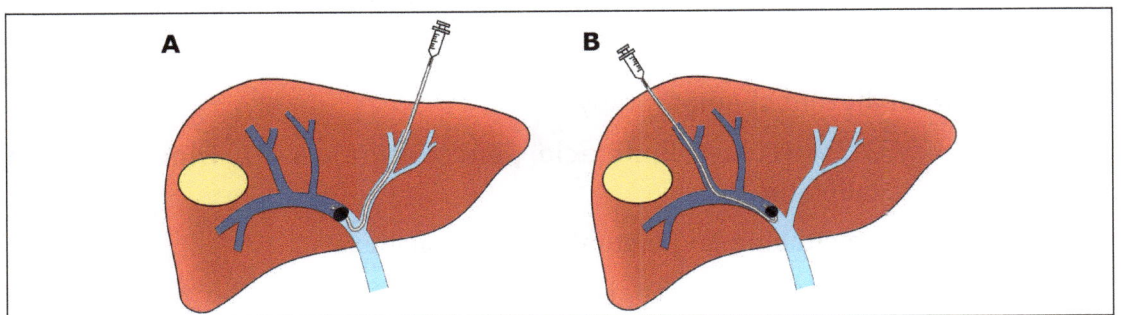

Figure 6.25: Portal Vein Embolisation (PVE); (a) Contralateral PVE, (b) Ipsilateral PVE.

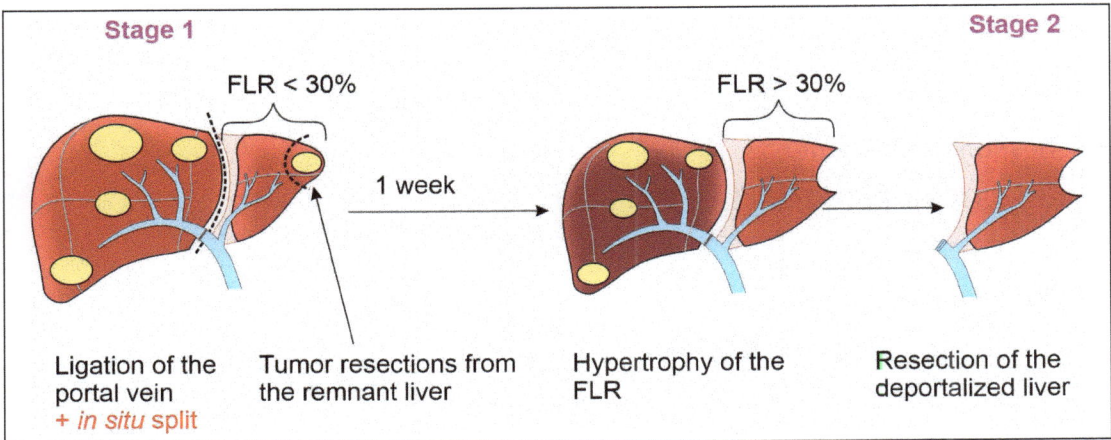

Figure 6.26: Associating Liver Partition and Portal vein Ligation for Staged Hepatectomy (ALPPS).

- Neoadjuvant therapy
  - It has a definite role in borderline resectable pancreatic cancer and locally advanced carcinoma gall bladder
  - Advantage:
    - To downstage/downsize the tumor
    - To evaluate tumor biology i.e. if the cancer progresses on therapy then it suggests aggressive tumor biology and such patients would not benefit from aggressive surgery. On the contrary good response to therapy suggests good tumor biology and hence better prognosis.
    - Therapy is given to tissues with intact vascularity and which are well oxygenated
    - Radiated tissues will be removed at surgery
    - Systemic micro-metastasis is dealt with by the systemic chemotherapy
    - Higher proportion of patients will receive chemotherapy and/or radiation
  - Disadvantage:
    - Loss of window of opportunity in case the disease progresses
  - Options
    - Neoadjuvant chemotherapy
      - FOLFIRINOX: follinic acid (leucovorine), 5-FU, irinotecan and oxaliplatin
      - Gemcitabine and albumin bound paclitaxel
      - Gemcitabine and capecitabibe
      - Gemcitabine and oxaliplatin
      - Gemcitabine and cisplatin
    - Neoadjuvant chemo-radiation
      - Gemcitabine or fluoropyrimidine based chemo-radiation
- Response assessment:
  - CT/FDG-PET-CT
  - CA 19-9 levels
- Surgery:
  - In distal block (Ca HOP, Periampullary Ca).
    - Whipples pancreatico-duodenectomy
    - Traverso-Longmire pylorus Preserving pancreatico-duodenectomy

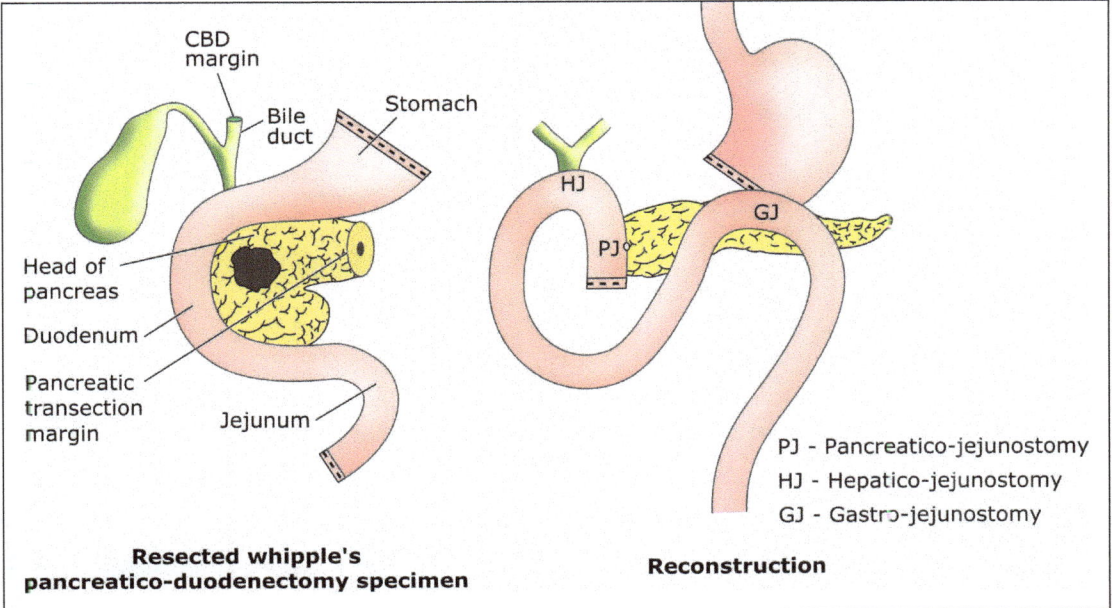

Figure 6.27: Whipple's pancreatico-duodenectomy.

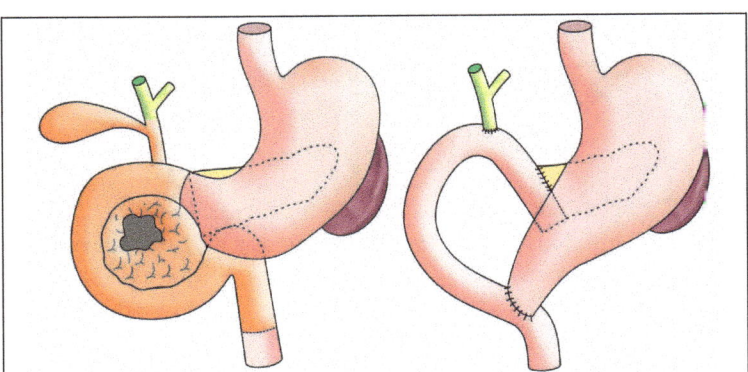

Figure 6.28: Traverso-Longmire pylorus Preserving pancreatico-duodenectomy.

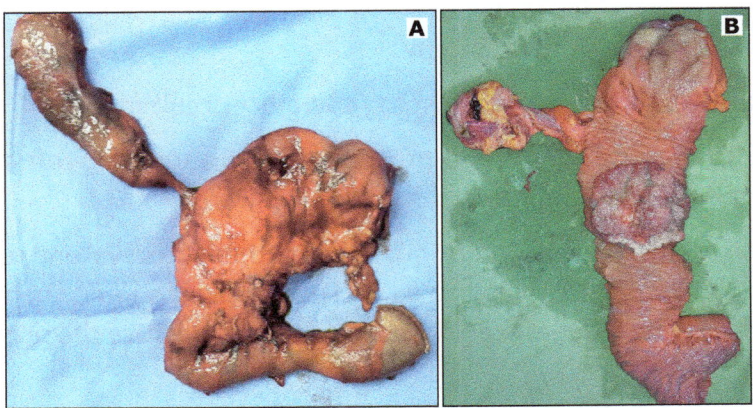

Figure 6.29: Resected Whipples PD specimen.

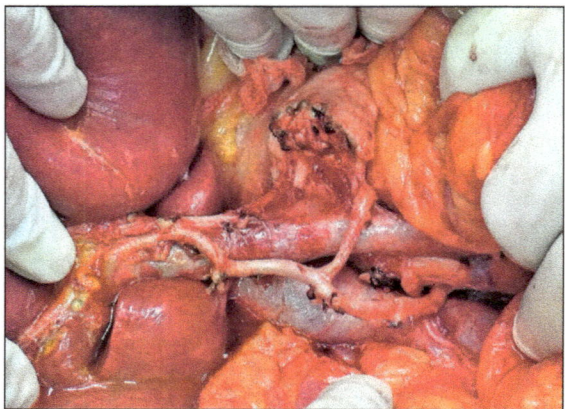

Figure 6.30: Intra-operative photo showing the surgical bed after removal of the Whipples PD specimen.

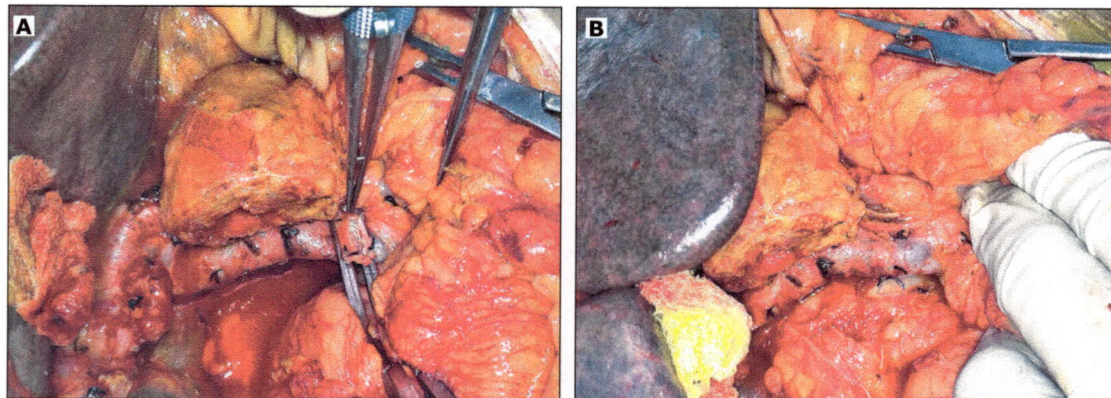

Figure 6.31: At times portal venous resection and anastomosis may be required during Whipples PD.

- In Ca GB without hilar involvement:
  - Options:
    - Extended cholecystectomy
    - Radical cholecystectomy
  - Start with a staging laparoscopy to detect occult metastasis.
  - If no metastasis is found proceed with the surgery with either open or laparoscopic technique.
  - Perform a Kocher maneuver to evaluate the aortocaval and retro pancreatic lymph nodes. Any suspicious nodes if present should then be evaluated with an intra-operative frozen section and if positive the procedure should be aborted.
  - If negative proceed with planned surgery

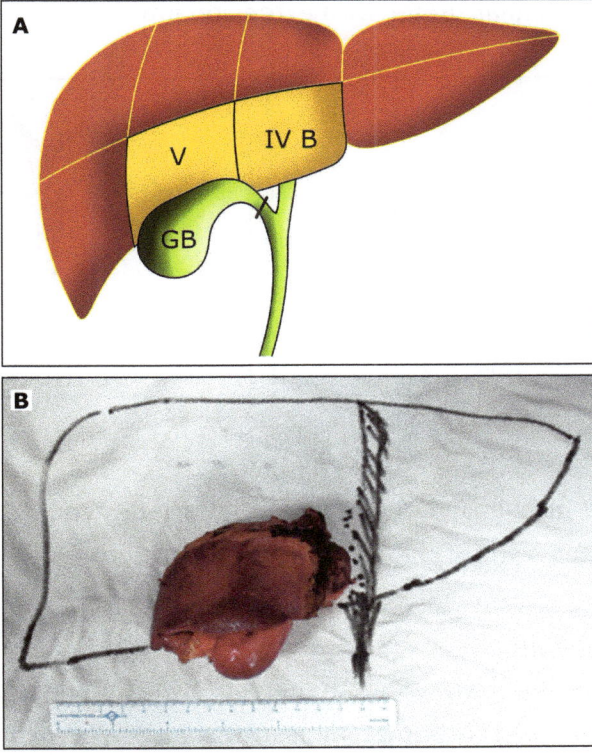

Figure 6.32: Radical cholecystectomy (A); specimen (B).

- In proximal blocks (Hilar Cholangiocarcinoma, Ca GB with hilar involvement):
    - Surgical management is very complex and would generally include some form of hepatectomy
    - Apart from extensive hepatic resection one may even have to perform portal vein resection with reconstruction.
    - There will also be some component of atrophy-hypertrophy complex which increases the level of difficulty of porta dissection.
    - Surgical management depends on the proximal extent of the biliary involvement which determines its Bismuth Corlette type:
        - Type 1: tumor limited to common hepatic duct below the level of confluence
        - Type 2: tumor involves the confluence of right hepatic duct (RHD) and left hepatic duct (LHD)
        - Type 3a: tumor involves the confluence with extension into RHD
        - Type 3b: tumor involves the confluence with extension into LHD

– Type 4: hilar tumor with extension into both RHD and LHD

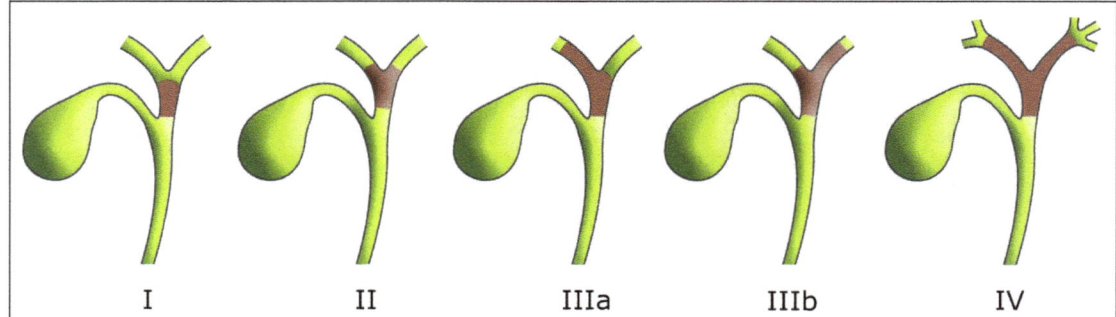

Figure 6.33: Bismuth corlette classification.

- Management based on the Bismuth Corlette type:
  – Type 1: radical choledochectomy
  – Type 2 and 3a: extended right hepatectomy including caudate lobectomy
  – Type 3b: extended left hepatectomy including caudate lobectomy
  – Type 4: usually unresectable. One may however consider liver transplant as per Mayo protocol
- Other surgical options:
  – Central or Meso hepatectomy
  – Taj-Mahal resection

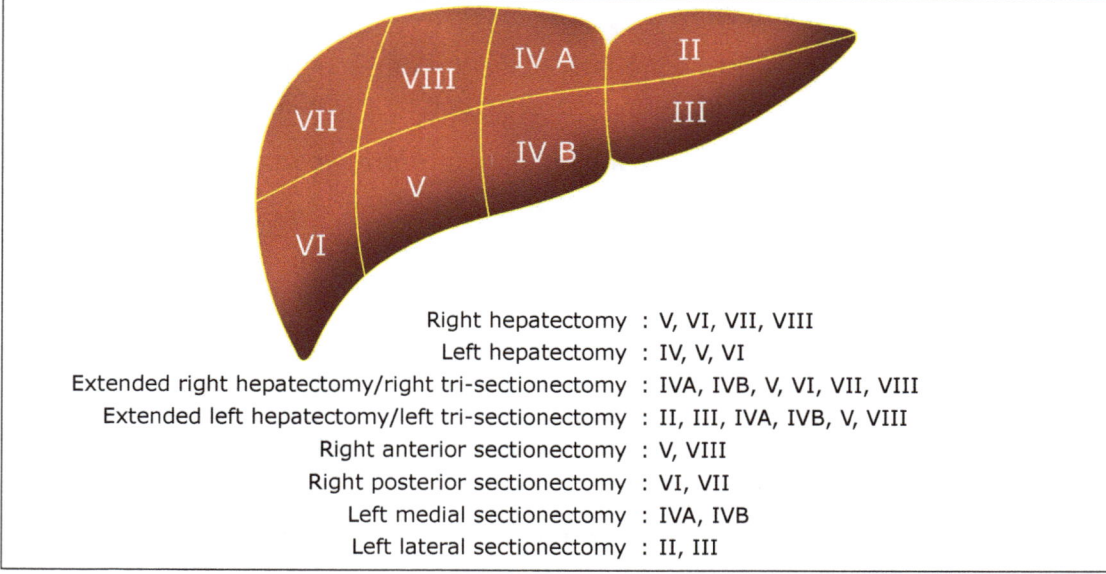

Figure 6.34: Types of hepatic resection: IHPBA/Brisbane terminology.

- Adjuvant therapy
  - Options
    - Adjuvant chemotherapy
      - Gemcitabine
      - 5-FU
      - FOLFIRINOX: follinic acid (leucovorine), 5-FU, irinotecan and oxaliplatin
      - Gemcitabine and albumin bound paclitaxel
      - Gemcitabine and capecitabibe
      - Gemcitabine and oxaliplatin
      - Gemcitabine and cisplatin
    - Adjuvant chemo-radiation
      - Gemcitabine or fluoropyrimidine based chemo-radiation
- Surveillance: modalities used:
  - History and physical examination
  - CBC, LFT and CA 19-9 levels
  - USG abdomen
  - CT chest, abdomen and pelvis
- **Go through chapter 13 for literature on the subject.**

Management of Pancreatic Head Neuroendocrine tumor in brief:

- DOTA-PET is required to stage the disease and rule out distant metastasis

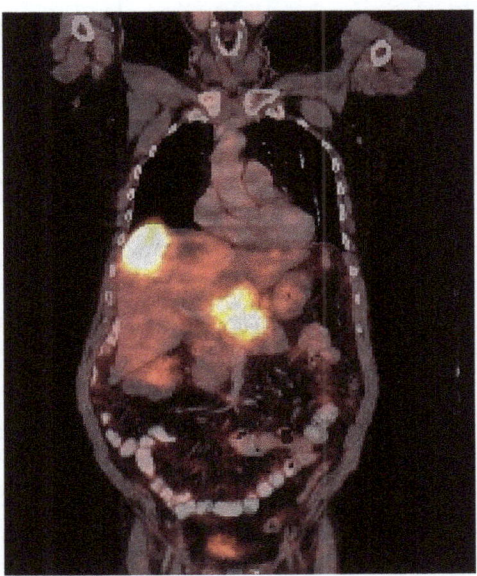

Figure 6.35: DOTA-PET CT revealing a pancreatic head NET with liver metastasis.

- NET is graded as per WHO grading system

Table 6.5: WHO Grading system for Neuro Endocrine Tumor			
Grade	Mitotic index	Ki-67 index	Differentiation
G1 NET	< 2/10 high power field	< 3%	Well
G2 NET	2–20/10 HPF	3–20%	Well
G3 NET	> 20/10 HPF	> 20%	Well
G3 NEC (NE carcinoma)	> 20/10 HPF	> 20%	Poor

- Therapeutic options for the primary:
    o Whipple's Pancreatico-duodenectomy
    o Traverso-Longmire pylorus preserving pancreatico-duodenectomy
    o Enucleation
- Therapeutic options for the Metastases:
    o Surgical Resection: Complete resection of all metastasis is preferred. In case resection of all metastasis is not surgically feasible, upto 90% debulking may provide symptomatic relief in symptomatically functional NET

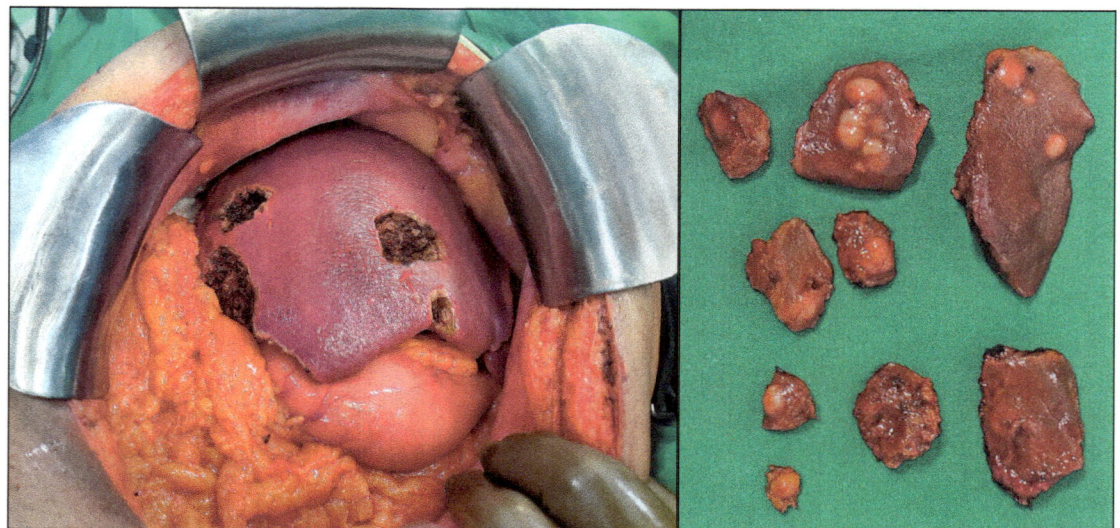

Figure 6.36: Metastatectomy in a case of metastatic NET.

- o Interventional Radiology:
    - RFA: Radio-frequency ablation
    - MWA: Microwave ablation
    - TACE: Transarterial chemo-embolisation
- TARE: Transarterial radio-embolisation
  - o Systemic Chemotherapy:
    - Cap-Tem: Capecitabine + Temozolamide
      - Alternatively: Streptozocin + 5-Fluorouracil
  - o Biological therapy: Sunitinib, Everolimus
  - o Somatostatin analogues: Octreotide
  - o PRRT: Peptide receptor radionuclide therapy
- Go through chapter 13 for literature on the subject.

Management of Choledocholithiasis in brief

- Preferred option: pre-op ERCP with biliary stone clearance and stenting followed by laparoscopic cholecystectomy followed by biliary stent removal
- Other options:
  - o Laparoscopic CBD exploration and cholecystectomy: it may be either transcystic or via a choledochotomy
  - o Open CBD exploration and cholecystectomy
  - o PTBD and biliary clearance (least preferred)

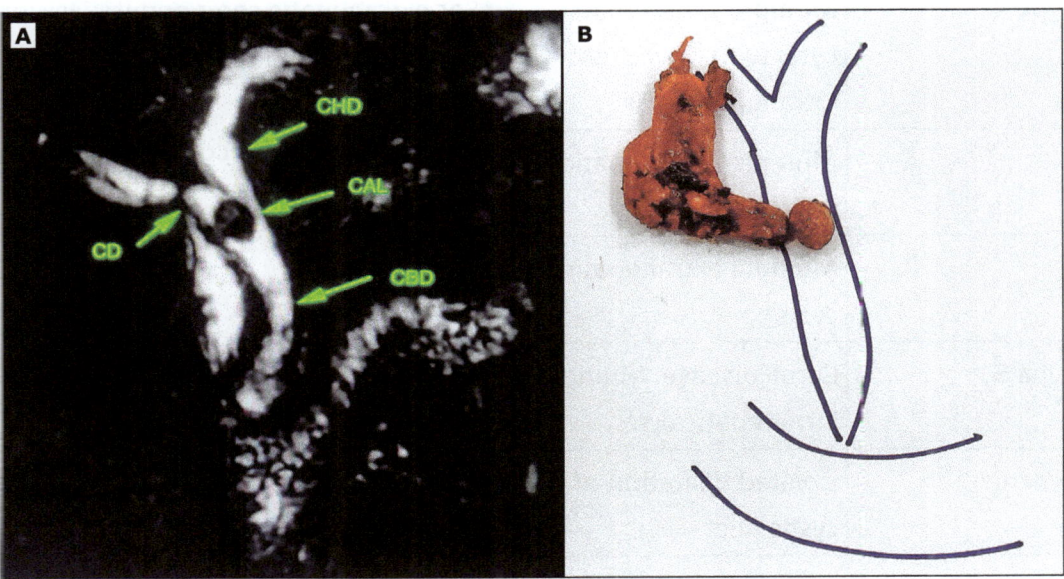

Figure 6.37: (A) MRCP Revealing Mirizzi's Syndrome, (B) Surgical specimen of Laparoscopic Cholecystectomy & CBD Exploration for Mirizzi's Syndrome.

Management of Choledochal Cyst in Brief

Table 6.6: Todani modification of Alonso Lej classification and its Management

Type	Subtype	Description	Treatment
Type 1		Solitary extrahepatic cyst	Excision with roux-en-y Hepatico-jejunostomy Or Excision and Hepatico-duodenostomy
	A	Cystic	
	B	Saccular	
	C	Fusiform	
	D	Cystic duct dilatation along with CBD dilatation	
Type 2		Extrahepatic supraduodenal diverticula	Excision
Type 3		Choledochocele: intraduodenal diverticula	Endoscopic sphincterotomy Or Surgical transduodenal excision Or Surgical transduodenal sphincteroplasty
Type 4		Multiple extrahepatic cysts with or without intrahepatic cyst	For extrahepatic component: Excision with roux-en-y Hepatico-jejunostomy Or Excision and Hepatico-duodenostomy For intrahepatic component: Hepatic resection
	A	Multiple extrahepatic and intrahepatic cysts	
	B	Multiple extrahepatic cysts	
Type 5		Caroli disease: Multiple intrahepatic cysts	Hepatic resection Liver transplant
Type 6		Isolated dilatation of cystic duct	Excision

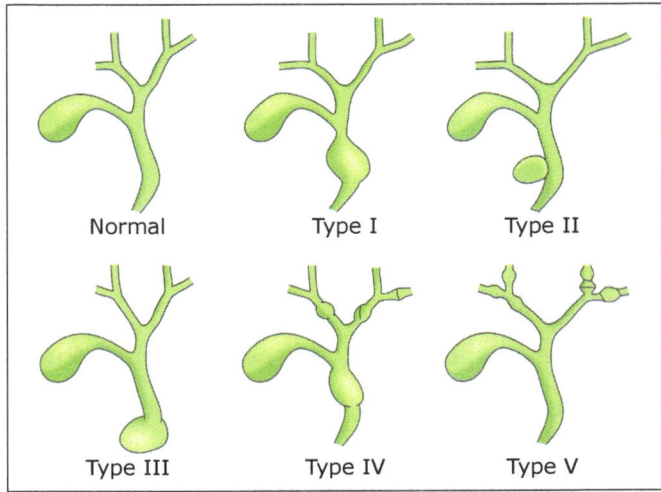

Figure 6.38

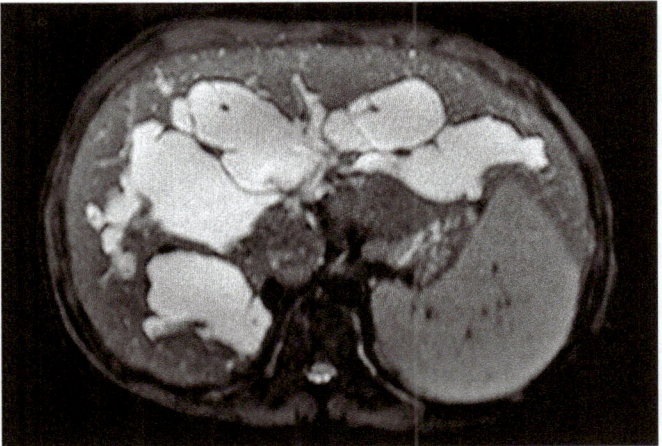

Figure 6.39: Caroli's Disease.

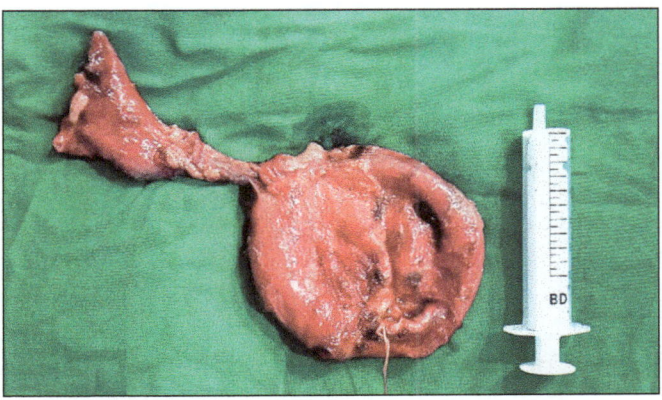

Figure 6.40: Specimen of Choledochal Cyst.

7 Case of Chronic Pancreatitis

Format for History Taking

- History of pain in abdomen:
    - Onset: insidious/sudden
    - Frequency: frequency of pain episodes per week/month/year
    - Duration: total duration, duration of each episode of pain, interval between recurring episodes of pain
    - Site
    - Nature: dull aching/colicky
    - Intensity: mild/moderate/severe
    - Radiating to back or not
    - Related to food intake or not
    - Relation with posture: relief with bending forward or not
    - Progress: intensity same as it was before or is the pain gradually intensifying
    - What does the patient require for pain relief: none/oral medication/injectable medication
    - Does the pain interfere with academics or job.
- History of vomiting:
    - Onset
    - Duration
    - Frequency
    - Quantity: small or large volume, alternatively one could describe quantity in form of cup
    - Bilious or not
    - Projectile or not
    - Related to meals or not i.e. post prandial or not
    - Is there sensation of postprandial fullness or not; is there a sense of relief after vomiting or not.

- History of fever:
    - Duration
    - Onset: insidious or sudden
    - Grade: low or high
    - Nature: intermittent or fluctuating or continuous
    - Associated chills or not.
- History of Abdominal fullness, lump or distension
- History of Jaundice, high colored urine, clay colored stools, pruritus.
- History of GI bleed: hematemesis and/or Melena. If yes: history of postural dizziness, syncope, fatigue, shortness of breath, need for blood transfusion
- History of steatorrhea: passage of frothy, oily, greasy, bulky, foul smelling stools
- History suggestive of fat soluble vitamin deficiency:
    - Vitamin A deficiency: history of decreased night vision, dryness of eyes
    - Vitamin D deficiency: bone pain, frequent fractures, muscle weakness
    - Vitamin K deficiency: history of coagulopathy such as ecchymosis; petechiae; easy bruisability
- History of diabetes mellitus:
    - Duration
    - Controlled or not
    - Medication: none/oral hypoglycemic/insulin
- History of weight loss or Loss of appetite
- History to identify etiology:
    - History of prior alcohol intake, Gall stone disease, blunt trauma abdomen, drug intake
    - History to suggest
        - Hyperparathyroidism: renal stones, painful bones, abdominal groans, psychiatric moans
        - Autoimmune pancreatitis: Age > 40, dry eyes, dry mouth
- Treatment History:
    - History of need for admissions for pain management

- History of admission to ICU
- History of evaluation with USG, CT, MRI, endoscopy
- History of PERT (pancreatic enzyme replacement therapy)
- History of endoscopic or percutaneous intervention or surgery
- Past history: Co-morbidities, previous surgeries (especially laparoscopic cholecystectomy)
- Personal history: detailed smoking and alcohol history (See chapter 2).
- Family history of pancreatitis or pancreatic cancer
- Performance history
- **Additional history in a patient with Pseudocyst**
  - History of persistence of pain or recurrence of pain weeks after initial attack of pancreatitis,
  - History of upper abdominal fullness or lump
  - History of early satiety

Justification for Each Component in History

- History of pain in abdomen: pain in pancreatitis is episodic type of pain, typically located in epigastric region, dull aching in nature, radiating to back, is precipitated by fatty meal, relieving on bending forwards
- Progress of pain: it is important to note the natural history of the disease. In the setting of chronic pancreatitis, if the pain intensity is gradually increasing, it would suggest consideration for surgery. Similarly, if the pain was previously getting relieved on oral medications but currently patient requires IV medication or opioids; this again may be considered as an indication for surgery. Interference with academics or job also suggests need for intervention.
- History of vomiting: patients with pancreatitis usually have vomiting along with pain, which usually settles with medications. history of postprandial fullness and/or postprandial voluminous vomiting is suggestive of gastric outlet obstruction which may be seen in patients with chronic pancreatitis and head mass (due to cicatrical/inflammatory narrowing of duodenum). Alternatively pancreatic cancer may arise in a patient with chronic pancreatitis which may give rise to GOO.
- History of fever: fever may be present as a part of the SIRS (systemic inflammatory response syndrome), alternatively it may be present in case of infected pseudocyst or cholangitis.

- History of upper abdominal fullness or lump: it should hint towards presence of pseudocyst.
- History of Jaundice, high colored urine, clay colored stools, pruritus: These symptoms are suggestive of obstructive jaundice. It may be seen in patients with chronic pancreatitis with head mass with cicatrical/inflammatory narrowing of intra pancreatic CBD. Alternatively pancreatic cancer may arise in a patient with chronic pancreatitis which may give rise to obstructive jaundice.
- GI bleed: it may occur due to either hemosuccus pancreaticus or sinistral portal hypertension. Hemosuccus pancreaticus results due to release of pancreatic digestive enzymes (elastase) which act on the surrounding vessels resulting in pseudoaneurysm formation, which ultimately bleed into GI tract (via the pancreatic duct: Hemosuccus pancreaticus) or into the abdominal cavity (peritoneal cavity or retroperitoneum). Alternatively, splenic vein thrombosis may occur as a sequelae of pancreatitis resulting in left sided portal hypertension or sinistral portal hypertension with subsequent variceal GI bleed.
- History of steatorrhea: chronic pancreatitis by definition includes both endocrine and exocrine deficiency. Exocrine insufficiency manifests in the form of steatorrhea i.e. malabsorption of fats resulting in excessive loss of fats in stools (> 7 grams/day). This can be corrected to some or full extent by PERT (pancreatic enzyme replacement therapy).
- History suggestive of fat-soluble vitamin deficiency: long term fat malabsorption may lead to fat soluble vitamin deficiency. Vitamin K deficiency is earliest to occur. To be mentioned, only if present.
- History of diabetes mellitus: chronic pancreatitis by definition includes both endocrine and exocrine deficiency. Endocrine insufficiency manifests in the form of diabetes mellitus.
- Loss of weight and Loss of appetite are pointers of malignancy. However, loss of weight may be seen in patients with steatorrhea. Similarly, postprandial pain may lead food fear, which may be mistaken for loss of appetite.
- History to identify etiology: history should be sought for to identify the etiology; for example: prior alcohol intake, gall stone disease, blunt trauma to upper abdomen. Also, history should be sought for to rule out hyperparathyroidism (renal stones, painful bones, abdominal groans [due to pancreatitis and ulcer disease apart from renal stones], psychiatric moans), Autoimmune pancreatitis (age > 40, dry eyes, dry mouth)

> **Table 7.1: HISORT criteria is used to diagnose Autoimmune pancreatitis**
> - H: Histology (lympho-plasmacytic sclerosing pancreatitis)
> - I: Imaging (sausage shaped pancreas with rim enhancement and narrow duct on CT)
> - S: Serology (raised IgG4 levels)
> - O: Other organ involvement (OOI). OOI includes Sjogrens syndrome manifesting as dry mouth and eyes.
> - RT: Response to steroid therapy

- History of need for admissions for pain management: it's a significant history suggesting severe disease. Multiple episodes of such admission suggests poor pain control with medical management and may be an indication for surgery.

- History of admission to ICU: It again is a significant history suggesting severe deterioration in health status. ICU admission could be due to severe disease or complications of pancreatitis: acute necrotizing pancreatitis, infected pancreatic necrosis, hemodynamic instability, sepsis, GI bleed.

- History of endoscopic or percutaneous intervention: It is usually done for pseudocyst, infected pancreatic necrosis and biliary obstruction. Procedures include percutaneous image guided drainage tube insertion, endoscopic cysto-gastrostomy, endoscopic necrosectomy, ERCP with biliary stenting.

- History of surgery: Surgery in emergency setting is done for infected pancreatic necrosis or pancreatic hemorrhage with hemodynamic instability. Surgery in semi-emergency setting includes: VARD (video assisted retroperitoneal debridement) and MIRN (minimally invasive retroperitoneal necrosectomy). Both are done as a part of step up approach (PANTER trial) in the treatment of infected pancreatic necrosis. In step-up approach, initial treatment or first step is image guided percutaneous drainage tube insertion, second step is VARD or MIRN and third step is open surgery. Conversely step down approach is open surgery (laparotomy) first.

- Past history of laparoscopic cholecystectomy: suggests that etiology of pancreatitis could be gallstone disease.

- Personal history of alcohol consumption: alcohol is an important and most common etiology for chronic pancreatitis. Similarly smoking too is an etiological factor.

- Family history of pancreatitis suggests hereditary pancreatitis. It is related to PRSS1 gene mutation. SPINK-1 gene mutation may also lead to chronic pancreatitis.

- Performance history: is important to assess fitness for surgery.

- History of persistence of pain or recurrence of pain weeks after initial attack of pancreatitis: suggests pseudocyst formation.
- History of abdominal fullness or lump: could be due to pseudocyst itself
- History of early satiety: due to gastric compression by the pseudocyst
- Patients with pseudocyst could additionally have fever due to secondary infection of pseudocyst, gastric outlet obstruction due to antral/duodenal compression, jaundice due to CBD obstruction.

Format for Examination

- At the outset, Remember:
    - Do not overlook naso-jejunal tube or drainage tube in left or right flank.
    - Patients with chronic pancreatitis are usually poorly nourished.
    - These patients generally do not have any positive findings on abdominal examination unless when they have a pseudocyst or have undergone some kind of intervention.
- What is the appearance of the patient: young/middle-aged/elderly, lady/gentleman
- Whether the patient is clinically
    - Poorly/averagely/well built
    - Poorly/averagely/well nourished
- Measure height, weight, BMI
- Whether the patient is clinically
    - Conscious/stuporous
    - Co-operative/un-cooperative
    - Well/poorly oriented to time, place and person
    - Lying comfortably in bed/in discomfort/in pain(rolling in pain). Also note patient's posture. Patient may assume a bending forward posture.
    - Well hydrated/dehydrated
    - Febrile/Afebrile.
- Mention Pulse, BP, RR
- Look for
    - Pallor, jaundice, cyanosis, clubbing

- Generalized or localized lymphadenopathy
- Palpable left supraclavicular lymph node
- Pedal or dependent edema
- Skin lesion
- Examination of oral cavity: look for oral hygiene and any obvious mucosal lesions
- Examination of the abdomen:
    - On Inspection: See if:
        - Abdomen is flat/distended/scaphoid;
        - Umbilicus is central/displaced (upwards/downwards/sideways) inverted/everted/flat.
        - All quadrants are moving equally with respiration or not
        - Look for any visible lump
            - In context of chronic pancreatitis, a pseudocyst may be visualized in the upper abdomen as a lump.
            - If visible describe: size, site, shape, surface and movement with respiration (it won't be moving with respiration).
        - Look for abdominal drain tube. If present look at the nature of fluid coming out: serous/serosanguinous/sanguinous/purulent/seropurulent. Pancreatic juice is usually cola colored.
        - Look for scars of previous surgery or drain tube insertion.
        - Look for visible sinus, engorged veins, pulsations, peristalsis or cough impulse.
        - Don't forget to inspect the groin hernial sites (to look for swelling or cough impulse i.e. hernia) and genitalia.
        - Inspection of renal angles to look for fullness
    - On Palpation: See if:
        - Abdomen is soft and non-tender (Alternatively abdomen could be rigid and/or tender; beware of well toned abdominal wall muscle in a lean patient)
        - Liver and/or spleen is palpable or not

- Any other palpable lump (especially a pseudocyst). If present describe:
  - Site
  - Size
  - Shape
  - Surface
  - Margins
  - Tenderness
  - Consistency
  - Mobility
  - Movement with respiration
  - Plane:
    - Whether the lump is intraperitoneal or not: by performing leg raising test
    - Whether the lump is retroperitoneal or not: by asking the patient to assume lateral decubitus position and palpating if the lump falls forward or not. A retroperitoneal mass wont fall ahead. Knee elbow test is no longer recommended as it would be inhuman to make a patient assume a knee-elbow position
- Do not forget to:
  - Palpate groin hernia sites to look for cough impulse
  - Examine genitals
  - Look for tenderness in renal angles
  - Examine back and spine for tenderness/gibbus.

o On Percussion:
- Look for upper border of liver dullness (generally in the 5th intercostal space) in midclavicular line.
- Note the liver span (normal being 12–14 cm)
- Percussion note over lump (pseudocyst) if any
- Note the percussion note over rest of the abdomen (it is generally tympanic)
- Tests for free fluid. Presence of free fluid i.e. ascites suggests pancreatic ascites.

- On auscultation:
    - Auscultate for bowel sounds.
    - Bruit, hum and rub
- Per rectal examination: Look for oily stools suggestive of steatorrhea
- Rest systemic examination:
    - Respiratory examination in form of auscultation, assessment of breath holding time
    - Assessment of breath holding time is important for clinically evaluating fitness for surgery

EXAMPLE CASE

History

- My patient Mr ABC, is a 34-year-old gentleman hailing from Mumbai, is an electrician by occupation.
- He presented with chief complaints of pain in mid upper abdomen since last one week.
- His history dates to 2 years back when he developed sudden onset pain in mid upper abdomen, mild to moderate in severity, dull aching in nature, radiating to back, precipitated by meals, relieving on bending forward. Initially the pain episodes were recurring at an interval of 2–3 months. Now since last one year he develops pain episodes every month, last episode occurring a week back. Previously pain used to get relieved with oral medications, however now he needs admission with injectable analgesics for pain relief.
- It is associated with nausea and small quantity bilious, non projectile vomiting
- He gives history of having lost 5–6 kg over last two years with decreased appetite during pain episodes.
- There is no history of
    - Fever, chills
    - Post prandial fullness, lump or distension
    - Jaundice, high colored urine, clay colored stools, pruritus.
    - Hematemesis, Melena.

- o Passage of frothy, oily, greesy, bulky, foul smelling stools
- o Diabetes mellitus
- He used to consume upto 100 ml of whiskey every alternate day for last 10 years. He is however abstinent since last 1.5 years
- He smokes around 8–10 bidis every day since last 10 years, he is however abstinent since last 1.5 years.
- He was evaluated for these symptoms one year back with USG and CT. He was started on capsules which were to be taken with meals, most probably PERT since last 8 months. There is no history of endoscopic or percutaneous intervention or surgery
- He has no history of any other co morbid illnesses
- Family history is not contributory
- He is able to perform all his daily routine activities.
- Remember:
  - o There are two ways of presenting history in such patients with long standing disease course
    - First, like how it has been presented here, i.e. starting HOPI (history of present illness) from the index event and then going antegrade or forward in time to the recent most event.
    - Or second, you describe the recent most episode first and then go retrograde describing the previous events.

Examination

- My patient is a young gentleman, who is averagely built, averagely nourished, with a height of 160 cm, weight of 55 kg and BMI being 21.5 kg/m^2
- He is conscious, cooperative, well oriented to time, place and person; Lying comfortably in bed; well hydrated and afebrile.
- Pulse is 72/min, BP is 110/70 mm Hg
- There is no pallor, icterus, cyanosis, clubbing, generalized or localized lymphadenopathy. There is no palpable left supraclavicular lymph node; pedal or dependent edema.
- Examination of oral cavity reveals adequate oral hygiene with no obvious mucosal lesions

- Examination of the abdomen:
    - On inspection: Abdomen is flat, umbilicus is central, inverted. All quadrants are moving equally with respiration. There is no visible lump, scar, sinus, engorged veins, pulsations, peristalsis or cough impulse.
    - Inspection of groin hernial sites reveals no swelling or cough impulse and Inspection of genitalia is unremarkable. Inspection of renal angles reveals no fullness
    - On Palpation: Abdomen is soft and non-tender. Liver and spleen are not palpable. There isn't any other palpable lump.
    - There is no palpable cough impulse over groin hernia sites and examination of genitals is unremarkable. There is no tenderness in renal angles. Examination of back and spine is essentially normal.
    - On Percussion, upper border of liver dullness is in the 5th intercostal space in midclavicular line with liver span being 14 cm. Rest of the abdomen is tympanitic with no evidence of free fluid.
    - On auscultation normal bowel sounds are heard. There is no bruit, hum or rub
- Per rectal examination is unremarkable.
- Examination of the respiratory system:
    - On auscultation, air entry is bilaterally equal with normal breath sounds
    - The breath holding time is 25 seconds.
- Rest systemic examination is essentially normal

To Summarize

- My patient is a 34 year old male with no co-morbid illness with WHO 0 performance status, was a smoker and used to consume alcohol regularly, presents with 2 years history of recurrent episodes of dull aching type of pain in the epigastric region, precipitated by meals, radiating to back, relieved on bending forwards and it is interfering with his work, it is associated with vomiting and loss of weight. He has been on PERT for the same.
- Examination is largely unremarkable

The most possible diagnosis in my patient is chronic pancreatitis with alcohol being the probable etiology

How to Proceed: (Sequence and justification)

- Review available medical records
- Routine blood investigations (Hemogram, Liver Function Test, Renal Function Test, Serum Electrolyte, INR)
- Specific blood tests: serum amylase, lipase, blood sugar level, HBa1c levels, CRP levels
- X-ray chest
- USG (A+P):
  - It is an extension of bed side clinical evaluation, it's cheap, non invasive and easily available
  - It is done:
    - To examine the pancreas; to note
      - Pancreatic size, to note if it is bulky or atrophic
      - Pancreatic echotexture
      - Pancreatic duct size and morphology
      - Presence of pancreatic stone and/or parenchymal calcification
      - Presence of pancreatic mass, lesion, cyst
    - To look for pseudocyst
    - To examine biliary system to look for cholelithiasis, choledocholithiasis, biliary dilatation, stone, mass
    - To look for Free fluid
- CECT of the abdomen and pelvis: to confirm the diagnosis and better characterize the disease
  - To note:
    - Pancreatic parenchymal morphology; whether is atrophic or bulky. To look for and characterize pancreatic head mass
    - Pancreatic duct morphology: whether it is dilated or not; duct stricture present or not; prominent/dilated side branches present or not; whether there is any ductal disruption
    - Presence of PD stone or pancreatic parenchymal calcification

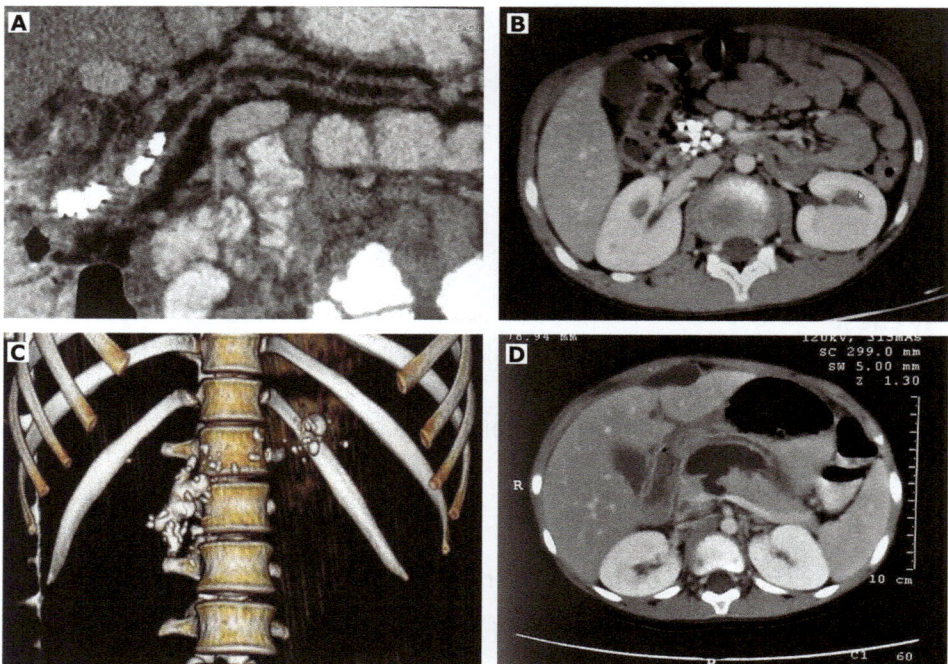

Figure 7.1: CT images showing dilated pancreatic duct with PD stones and pancreatic parenchymal atrophy (A); Inflammatory pancreatic head mass with calcification predominantly in head region (B); CT 3D reconstruction showing PD stones and pancreatic parenchymal calcification oriented along the longitudinal axis of pancreas (C); pancreatic transection due to blunt trauma abdomen causing traumatic pancreatitis (D).

- Presence of local complication:
    - Acute fluid collection
    - Pseudocyst
    - Pancreatic necrosis
    - Walled of pancreatic necrosis
    - Presence of vascular complication: Splenic vessel thrombosis, mesenteric vein thrombosis; arterial aneurysm/pseudoaneurysm.
- Presence of Feature of Sinistral portal hypertension
- Presence of pancreatic ascites, pancreatico-enteric fistula, pancreatico-pulmonary fistula
- Presence of concomitant liver cirrhosis (related to alcohol intake)

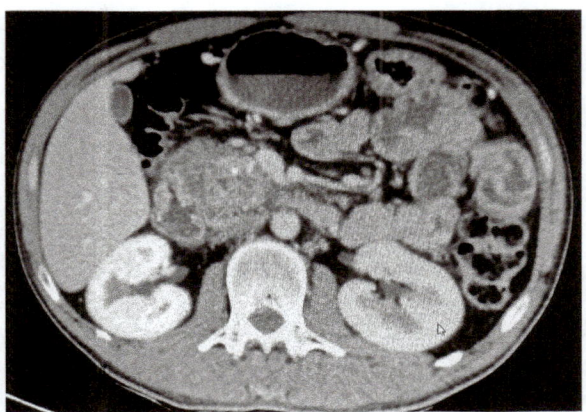

Figure 7.2: Pancreatic head mass in a patient with CCP.

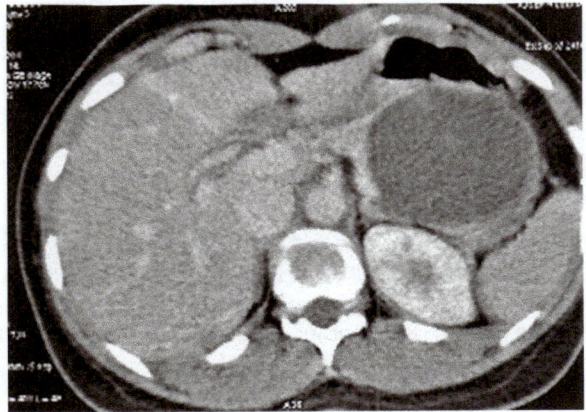

Figure 7.3: CT image showing pseudocyst.

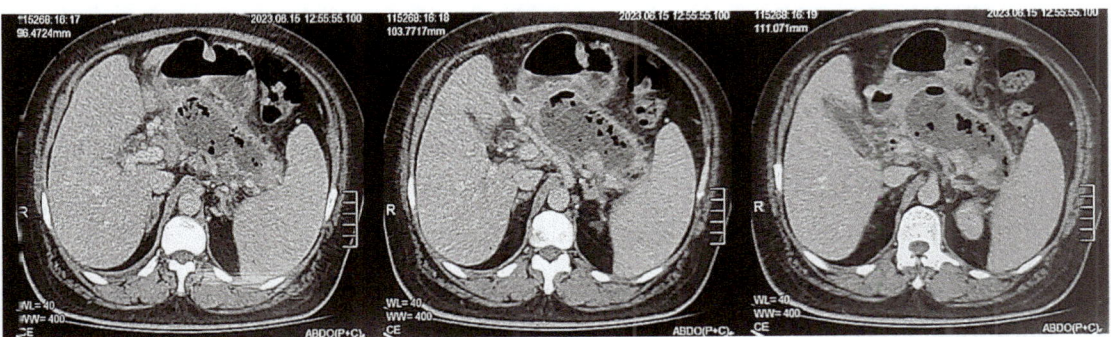

Figure 7.4: CT revealing an Infected Walled of Pancreatic Necrosis (WOPN), note the air foci within the collection.

- MRI abdomen with MRCP: It provides imformation similar to CECT. It's however better with regards to evaluation of pancreatic duct morphology

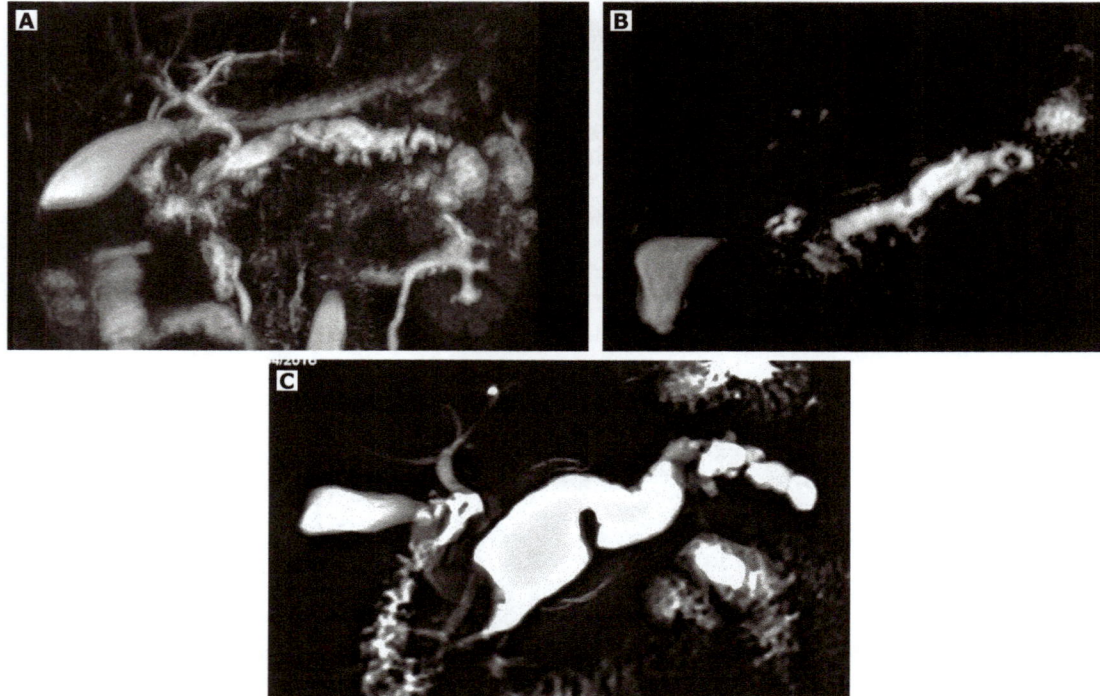

Figure 7.5: MRCP images showing dilated main pancreatic duct and side branches (A). Look for filling defects which is suggestive of stones (B). Another differential diagnosis for dilated PD is IPMN which has to be ruled out (C).

- EUS:
    - It has definite role in evaluation and diagnosis of early chronic pancreatitis which may not be detected on any other imaging modality. Rosemont criteria is used for EUS diagnosis of chronic pancreatitis.
    - It is used in evaluation of chronic pancreatitis with head mass. The most important advantage of EUS is the ability to obtain targeted FNA or core biopsy to preoperatively establish the diagnosis of cancer
    - It can be used to look for microlithiasis/sludge
    - EUS is used to perform endoscopic cysto-gastrostomy
- Additional investigation:
    - ERCP: Although ERCP is diagnostic, it is no longer routinely recommended for diagnostic purposes, but it definitely has a therapeutic role. Cambridge criteria was used for ERCP diagnosis of chronic pancreatitis.
    - Serum calcium, parathyroid hormone level: hypercalcemia and hyperparathyroidism are etiological factors for pancreatitis.

- Lipid profile: hyperlipidemia is an etiological factor for pancreatitis.
- Fecal fat estimation, fecal elastase 1 levels: to check for pancreatic exocrine function
- Blood sugar level, HBa1c: to check for pancreatic endocrine function
- FDG-PET-CT: may be used to evaluate pancreatic head mass in chronic pancreatitis
- CA19-9 level: In case malignancy is suspected

- Advise abstinence from alcohol and tobacco smoking
- PERT: pancreatic enzyme replacement therapy
  - It consists of administration of pancreatic enzymes (namely lipase, protease and amylase) in specially prepared formulations along with each meal
  - Types:
    - Non enteric coated
    - Enteric coated
    - Enteric coated microspere and minimicrospere
  - Role:
    - It is prescribed in patients with pancreatic exocrine insufficiency, to facilitate digestion
    - In pain management
- Interventional radiology:
  - Percutaneous catheter drainage (PCD) tube insertion for pseudocyst, WOPN, infected pancreatic necrosis
  - Angioembolization for pseudoaneurysm
- Endotherapy
  - ERCP and:
    - Pancreatic duct stone clearance with or without:
      - ESWL (shock wave lithotripsy)
      - Laser lithotripsy
    - Pancreatic duct stenting: indications:
      - Post PD stone clearance

- PD stricture
- Ductal disruption or disconnected duct syndrome
    - EBD (endoscopic biliary drainage) with stent: in case there is biliary obstruction and/or cholangitis
  o Endoscopic cysto-gastrostomy, Endoscopic cysto-duodenostomy: for pancreatic pseudocyst
  o Endoscopic trans mural necrosectomy: for pancreatic necrosis
  o Sinus tract endoscopy: for pancreatic necrosis
  o Endotherapy for esophago-gastric varices in case of sinistral portal hypertension
- Surgery:
  o Surgery for chronic pancreatitis:
    - Decompressive procedures:
      - Duval procedure: distal pancreatectomy with end to end pancreatico-jejunostomy: obsolete now
      - Peustows procedure: distal pancreatectomy plus longitudinal pancreatico-jejunostomy: obsolete now
      - Partington-Rochelle modification of Peustows procedure: longitudinal pancreatico-jejunostomy without distal pancreatectomy
    - Resective procedure:
      - Whipple's pancreatico-duodenectomy
      - Traverso-Longmire pylorus Preserving pancreatico duodenectomy
      - Distal pancreatectomy
      - Total pancreatectomy with islet cell transplantation
    - Hybrid procedures:
      - Beger procedure: DPPHR: duodenum preserving pancreatic head resection: pancreas is transected in the neck region followed by deep head coring leaving a sliver of pancreatic tissue along the duodenal C loop with creation of two pancreatico-jejunal anastomosis (one end to end and one side to side)
      - Berne procedure: head coring with pancreatico jejunostomy
      - Freys procedure: head coring plus longitudinal pancreatico-jejunostomy

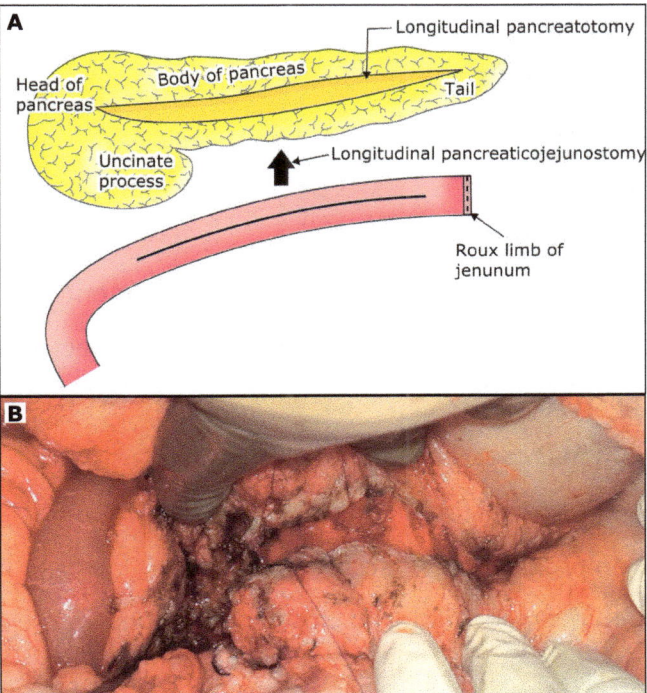

Figure 7.6: Partington Rochelle procedure.

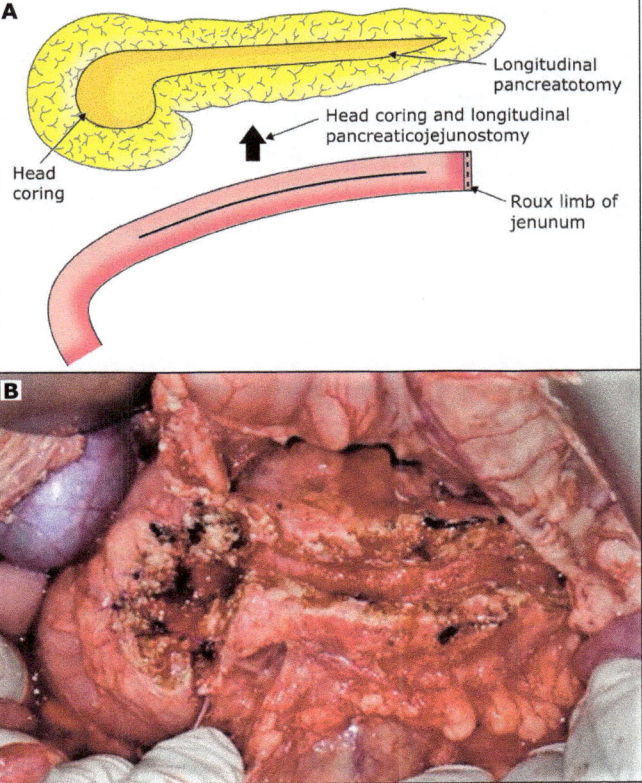

Figure 7.7: Freys procedure.

- For pseudocyst:
  - Cysto-gastrostomy
  - Cysto-duodenostomy
  - Cysto-jejunostomy
- For pancreatic necrosis:
  - VARD: video assisted retroperitoneal debridement
  - MIRN: minimally invasive retroperitoneal necrosectomy
  - Open necrosectomy
    - Open necrosectomy and open packing
    - Open necrosectomy and closed packing
    - Open programmed necrosectomy
    - Open necrosectomy and closed continuous lavage

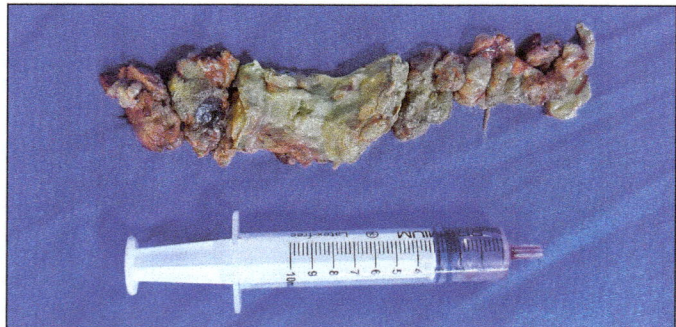
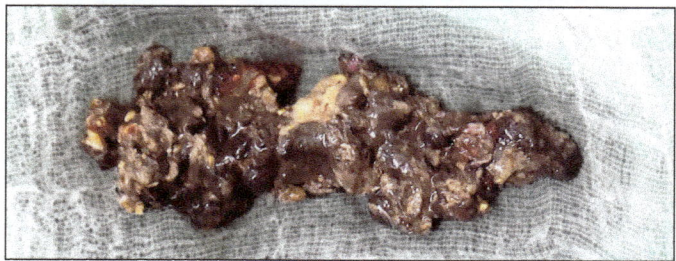

Figure 7.8: Pancreatic necrotic tissue removed during VARD.

- **Go through chapter 13 for literature on the subject.**

8 Case of Non-Cirrhotic Portal Hypertension

Introduction

- Differential diagnosis that will be discussed in this chapter:
  - EHPVO: Extra hepatic portal venous obstruction
  - NCPF: Non Cirrhotic portal fibrosis
  - Cirrhosis will be briefly discussed

Format for History Taking

- History of hematemesis:
  - Spontaneous or not
  - Number of episodes
  - Amount of bleed
  - Whether fresh blood or coffee ground
  - Blood clot present or absent
  - Whether there is history of associated melena, hematochezia
- History of fatigue, shortness of breath, postural dizziness or syncope, need for blood transfusion
- History of associated abdominal distension, jaundice, altered sensorium, decreased urine output
- History of requirement for hospitalization, blood transfusion, endoscopy and endoscopic therapy
- History of associated pain in abdomen, fever with chills
- History of lump in abdomen, left upper abdominal quadrant dragging pain or heaviness
- History to suggest hypersplenism:
  - Anemia: History of shortness of breath, fatigue
  - Leukopenia: History of repeated fever or infection
  - Thrombocytopenia: History of gum bleed, epistaxis, easy bruisability, hematuria, menorrhagia

- Brief perinatal history: History of home or hospital delivery, history of abdominal sepsis, umbilical sepsis, umbilical vein catheterization, delayed separation of cord, chronic diarrhea during infancy.
- History of delayed achievement of developmental milestones, growth retardation and poor scholastic performance
- In adult females: History of OC pill consumption, menstrual history, obstetric history (history of spontaneous abortion)
- Treatment history: History of hospital admission, ICU stay, endoscopy, cross-sectional imaging, endotherapy, surgery
- Personal history:
  - History of alcohol consumption:
    - Type of liquor
    - Frequency of consumption: per week/per month
    - Quantity
    - Total duration
    - Attempt at abstinence
  - History of smoking
- Past history: Prior history of blood transfusion, recurring jaundice, high risk behavior (promiscuity, IV drug abuse); viral hepatitis; history of DM, HTN, TB
- Family history, performance history

Justification for Each Component in History

- History of hematemesis:
  - Spontaneous or not: spontaneous bleed would suggest portal hypertensive bleed or peptic ulcer bleed, whereas hematemesis following retching would suggest bleed due to Mallory Weiss tear
  - Amount of bleed, number of episodes, blood clot present or absent: this information helps to quantify the bleed; presence of blood clots suggests significant bleed
  - Wheather fresh blood or coffee ground: vomiting fresh blood would suggest active bleed, whereas coffee ground vomitus suggest old collected blood

- o Associated melena, hematochezia: melena may be seen in any patient with upper GI bleed, however hematochezia in a patient with hematemesis would either suggest a second source of GI bleed in distal GI tract or massive upper GI bleed.
- History of fatigue, shortness of breath, postural dizziness or syncope, requirement of blood transfusion: this history helps to grade the severity of bleed and anemia.
- History of associated abdominal distension, jaundice, altered sensorium, decreased urine output:
  - o Abdominal distension suggests ascites
  - o Altered sensorium suggests hepatic encephalopathy
  - o Jaundice could suggest cirrhosis.
  - o Decreased urine output suggests hepato-renal syndrome
  - o Ascites, hepatic encephalopathy and jaundice all three individually or together points towards hepatic decompensation.
  - o Non-cirrhotic portal hypertension especially EHPVO is also associated with portal biliopathy (or more recently renamed as portal cavernoma cholangiopathy). It may lead to jaundice, cholangitis (jaundice + right upper quadrant abdominal pain + fever)
- History of associated pain in abdomen: upper GI bleed needs to be characterized, whether it's painful or painless. Variceal bleed is usually painless and peptic ulcer bleed is usually painful.
- History of lump in abdomen, left upper quadrant dragging pain or heaviness: such history would suggest splenomegaly.
- History of sudden onset left upper quadrant pain: would suggest peri-splenitis or splenic infarction
- History to suggest hypersplenism: portal hypertension, especially of the noncirrhotic type may be associated with hypersplenism, hence the need to inquire regarding related history
  - o Original definition of hypersplenism as described by Dameshek
    - Cytopenia of one or more cell lines
    - Compensatory hyperplasia of bone marrow
    - Splenomegaly
    - Correction of cytopenia after splenectomy

- So:
  - Fever could suggest either
    - Leucopenia due to hypersplenism
    - Cholangitis
  - Jaundice could suggest either:
    - Hepatic decompensation
    - Portal biliopathy
- Perinatal history: history of abdominal sepsis, umbilical sepsis, umbilical vein catheterization, delayed separation of cord and chronic diarrhea: such history is suggestive of abdominal infection during neonatal period or infancy which may lead to NCPH (EHPVO > NCPF). Hence if any such history is present it points towards the possibility of a clinical diagnosis of NCPH
- History of delayed achievement of milestones, growth retardation and poor scholastic performance: EHPVO may be associated with these
- History of OC pill consumption: OC pill consumption may lead to prothrombotic tendency
- History of spontaneous abortion: could suggest the possibility of Antiphospholipid antibody syndrome
- History of alcohol abuse: could suggest the possibility of alcoholic liver disease
- Prior history of blood transfusion, recurring jaundice or high risk behavior: could suggest viral hepatitis

Format for Examination

- What is the appearance of the patient: young/middle-aged/elderly lady/gentleman
- Whether the patient is clinically
  - Poorly/averagely/well built
  - Poorly/averagely/well nourished
  - Height, weight, BMI
- Whether the patient is clinically
  - Conscious/stuporous

- - Cooperative/un-cooperative
  - Well/poorly oriented to time, place and person
  - Lying comfortably in bed/in discomfort/in pain(rolling in pain)
  - Well hydrated/dehydrated
  - Febrile/Afebrile.
- Pulse, BP
- Look for
  - Pallor, jaundice, cyanosis, clubbing
  - Generalized or localized lymphadenopathy
  - Pedal or dependent edema
  - Skin lesions
- Stigmata of chronic liver disease (top to bottom)
  - Icterus
  - Malar erythema
  - fetor hepaticus
  - Parotid swelling
  - Spider nevi/spider angiomata
  - Gynecomastia
  - Reduced chest hair
  - Reduced axillary hair
  - Dupuytren contracture
  - Palmar erythema
  - leukonychia
  - flapping tremors/Asterexis
  - Abdominal distension
  - Caput medusae
  - Reduced pubic hair
  - Testicular atrophy
  - Pedal edema

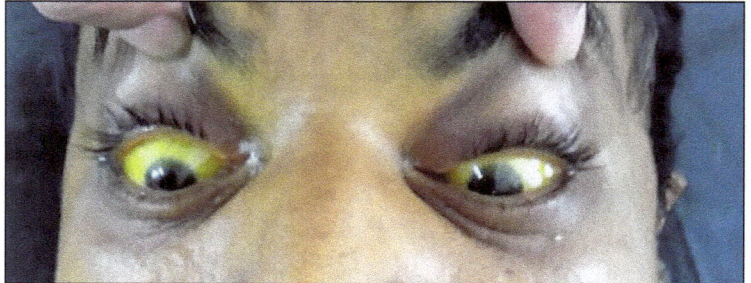

Figure 8.1: Icterus.

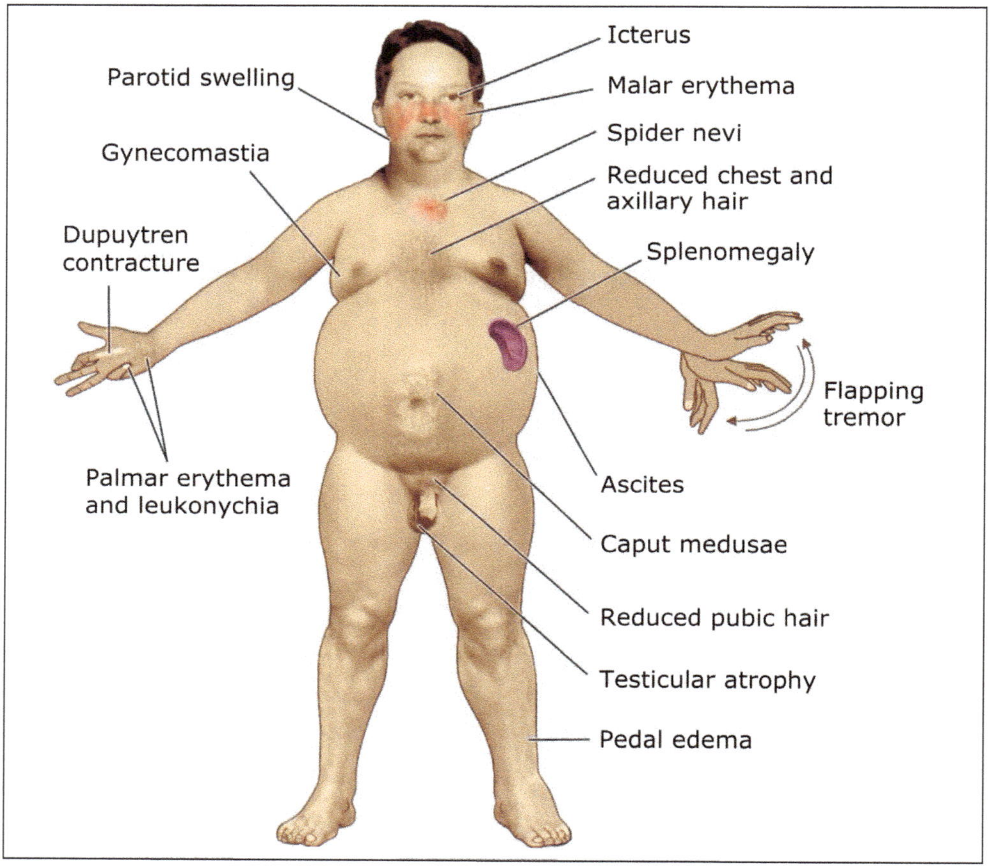

Figure 8.2: Stigmata of chronic liver disease.

- Examination of oral cavity: look for oral hygiene, any obvious mucosal lesions.
- Examination of the abdomen:
    ○ On Inspection: See if:
        ▪ Abdomen is flat/distended/scaphoid. Ascites is common in cirrhotic PH, whereas it is uncommon in NCPH. The abdomen will be distended in case ascites is present.

- Umbilicus is central/displaced (upwards/downwards/sideways) inverted/everted/flat.
- All quadrants are moving equally with respiration or not
- See if there is any visible lump. In context of portal hypertension the enlarged spleen is usually visualized as a lump in left upper quadrant
- If visible describe:
  - Size
  - Site
  - Shape
  - Surface
  - Movement with respiration

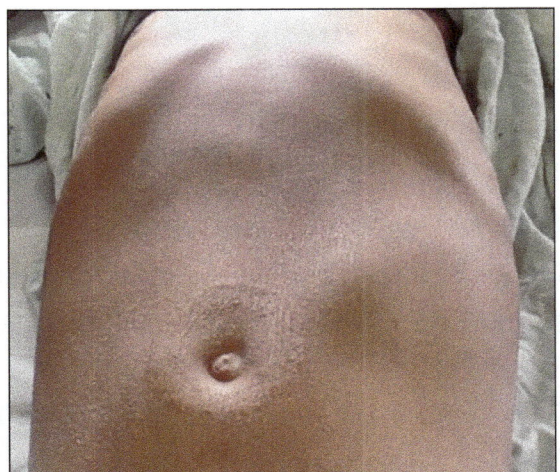

Figure 8.3: Splenomegaly seen on abdominal inspection.

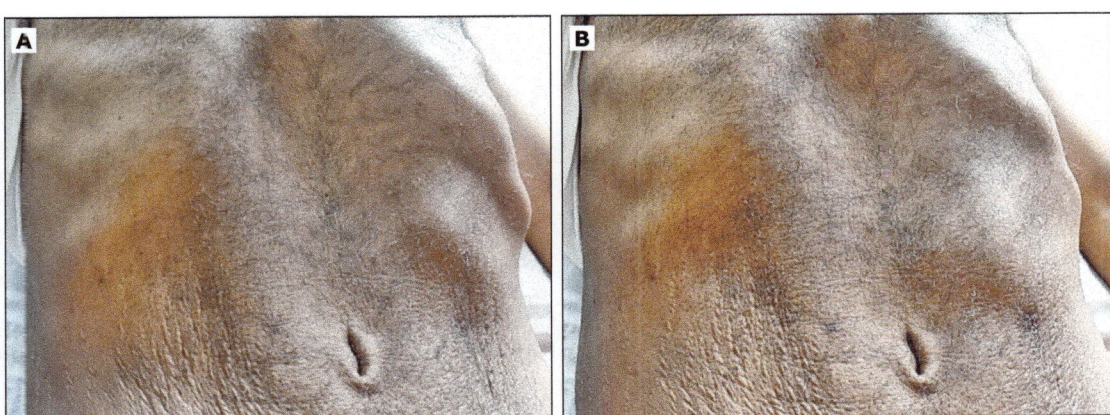

Figure 8.4: Splenomegaly seen on abdominal inspection; note the medial and caudal movement of the spleen with inspiration.

- Look for dilated or engorged veins over the abdomen or flank:
  - Dilated peri-umbilical veins radiating away from the umbilicus is suggestive of portal hypertension.
  - Dilated veins in cranio-caudal orientation in the flanks is suggestive caval obstruction
- Look for visible scar, sinus, pulsations, peristalsis or cough impulse.
- Don't forget to inspect the groin hernial sites (to look for swelling or cough impulse i.e. hernia) and genitalia.
- Inspection of renal angles to look for fullness
○ On Palpation: See if:
- Abdomen is soft and non-tender (Alternatively abdomen could be rigid and/or tender)
- Liver is palpable or not
  - If yes, measure size from costal margin in midclavicular line in unit of cm or number of fingers,
  - See if:
    ♦ It is tender/nontender
    ♦ Surface is smooth (normal)/nodular (cirrhosis)
    ♦ Borders are round (fatty liver/steatotic liver)/sharp (normal), regular (normal)/irregular (cirrhosis)
    ♦ Consistency is soft (normal)/firm (steatotic liver)/hard (cirrhotic/fibrotic liver)

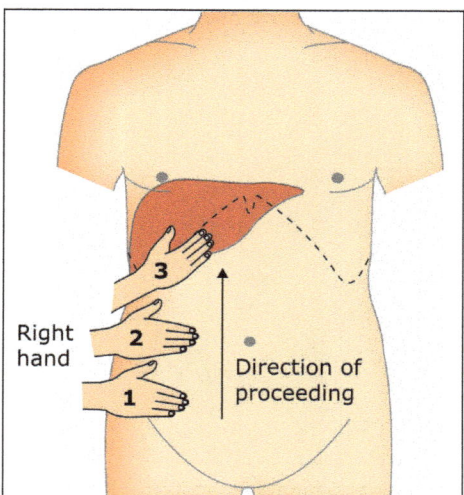

Figure 8.5: Technique of palpation of liver.

- Spleen is enlarged or not
    - If yes, measure size from costal margin along its long axis
    - Note its:
        - Extent: upto mid-clavicular line/umbilicus/beyond umbilicus
        - Surface
        - Margins; notch present or not
        - Consistency
        - Movement with respiration
        - See if it is tender/nontender

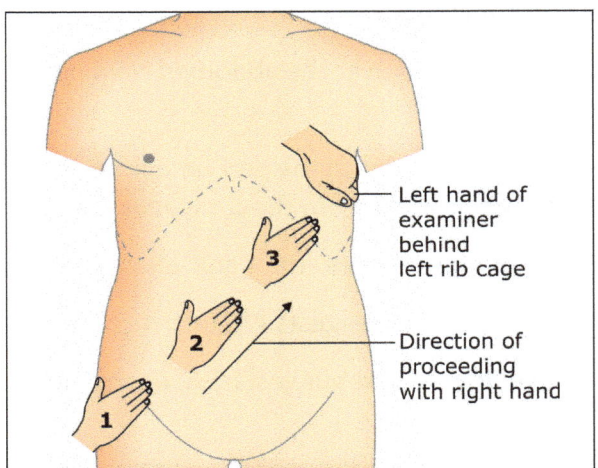

Figure 8.6: Technique of palpation of spleen.

- Grading of splenomegaly:
    - Mild: < 3 cm from costal margin
    - Moderate: 3–5 cm from costal margin
    - Massive: > 7 cm from costal margin
- Alternative method for grading:
    - Mild: < 5 cm from costal margin
    - Moderate: 5–10 cm from costal margin
    - Massive: > 10 cm from costal margin

- Alternative method for grading:
  - Hacketts method:
    - 0: unpalpable
    - 1: palpable only on deep palpation
    - 2: palpable uptil the midway point between costal margin and umbilicus
    - 3: palpable beyond the midway point between costal margin and umbilicus
    - 4: palpable beyond the umbilicus
    - 5: reaching upto the pubic symphysis
- Any other palpable lump.
- If dilated veins are seen over the abdomen then note the direction of blood flow in it:
  - Direction of blood flow in the peri-umbilical veins in patients with portal hypertension is away from the umbilicus.
  - Direction of blood flow in the flank veins:
    - Below upwards suggests IVC obstruction
    - Above downwards suggests SVC obstruction

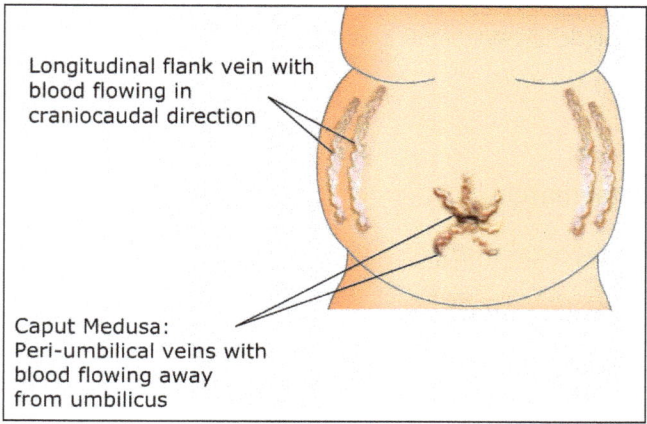

Figure 8.7: Abdominal veins.

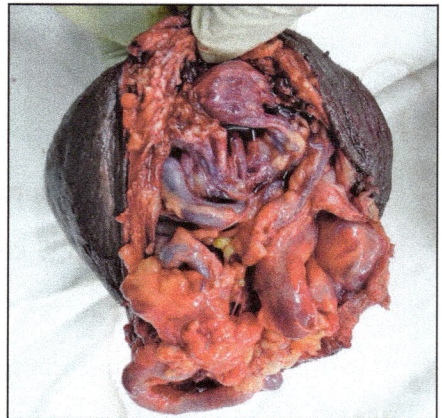

Figure 8.8: Surgical specimen showing tuft of venous collaterals in an umbilical hernial sac.

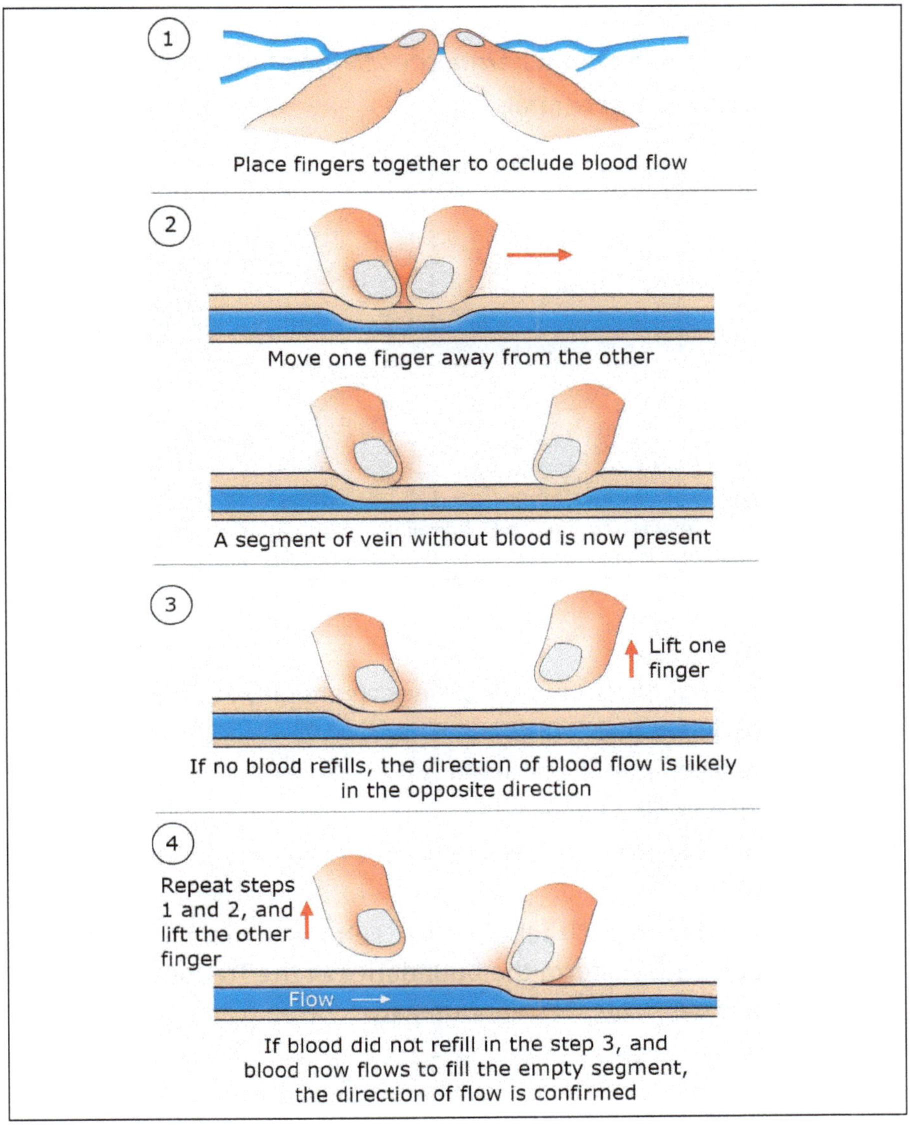

CHAPTER 8: CASE OF NON CIRRHOTIC PORTAL HYPERTENSION

Technique to identify direction of Blood Flow in a vein

1 Place fingers together to occlude blood flow

2 Move one finger away from the other

A segment of vein without blood is now present

3 Lift one finger

If no blood refills, the direction of blood flow is likely in the opposite direction

4 Repeat steps 1 and 2, and lift the other finger

Flow →

If blood did not refill in the step 3, and blood now flows to fill the empty segment, the direction of flow is confirmed

Figure 8.9: Technique to identify direction of Blood Flow in a vein.

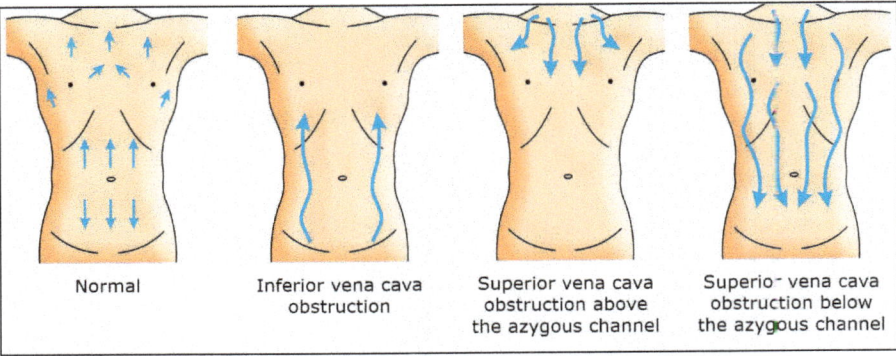

Normal | Inferior vena cava obstruction | Superior vena cava obstruction above the azygous channel | Superior vena cava obstruction below the azygous channel

Figure 8.10: Direction of blood flow in Abdomino-Thoracic veins and its significance.

- Do not forget:
  - To palpate the groin hernia sites to look for cough impulse
  - Examination of genitals
  - To look for tenderness in renal angles
  - Examination of back and spine for tenderness/gibbus.

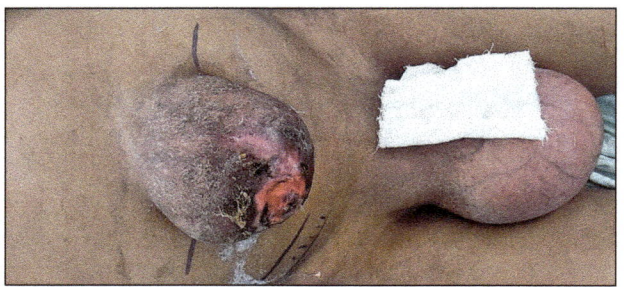

Figure 8.11: Do not forget examination of the genitalia as you may miss out on findings like hernia, hydrocele or scrotal wall edema in a patient with Portal hypertension; also note the ruptured umbilical hernia in this cirrhotic patient.

o On Percussion:
  - Look for upper border of liver dullness (generally in the 5th intercostal space) in midclavicular line.
  - Note the liver span (normal being 12–14 cm)
  - Length of splenic dullness
  - In case the spleen is not palpable but there is a strong clinical suspicion then perform:
    - Percussion in the Traube's space: Left costal margin, left anterior axillary line and 6th rib form the boundaries of the Traube's space. Dull note in this space suggests splenomegaly.

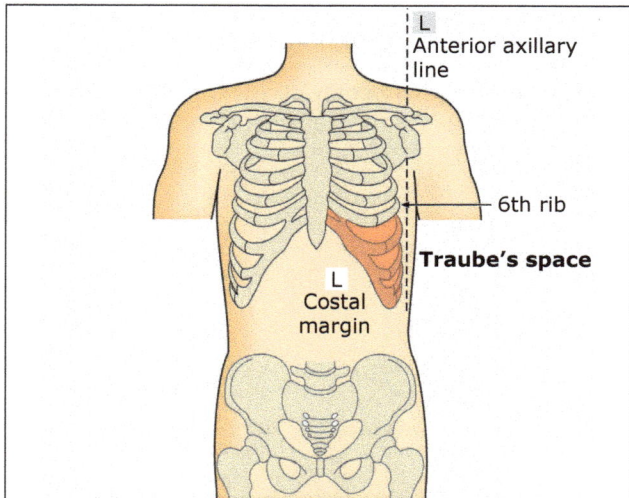

Figure 8.12: Traube's space.

- Castell sign: It involves percussion in the lowest intercostal space (8th or 9th) in the left anterior axillary line in inspiratory and expiratory phases. If a resonant note is heard in the expiratory phase and a dull note is heard in the inspiratory phase then it suggests splenomegaly. If resonant note is found in both phases then it suggests the contrary.
          - Nixon's sign: with the patient in right lateral decubitus, start percussion from the midpoint of left costal margin and proceed in a direction perpendicular to the left costal margin. Splenomegaly is said to be present if dullnes is present within 8 cm from the costal margin.
    - Note in the rest of the abdomen
    - Tests for free fluid
  - On auscultation:
    - Look for bowel sounds, bruit, hum and rub
    - Look for:
          - Cruveilher Baumgarten sign: venous hum in the umbilical region due to flow in recanalised umbilical vein
          - Kenawy sign: venous hum in the epigastric region due to flow in splenic vein
- Do not forget per rectal examination: mainly to look for melena or fresh blood
- Proctoscopic evaluation: to look for rectal varices
- Rest systemic examination

How to Reach a Clinical Diagnosis

- EHPVO: young patients in 1st or 2nd decade presenting with well tolerated upper GI bleed with massive splenomegaly and/or hypersplenism, portal biliopathy and no ascites. Minimal hepatic encephalopathy (MHE) may be present. History of abdominal sepsis, umbilical sepsis, umbilical vein catheterization, delayed separation of cord and chronic diarrhea may be present
- NCPF: patient in 3rd or 4th decade presenting with well tolerated upper GI bleed with massive splenomegaly and/or hypersplenism and no ascites. Portal biliopathy is less common
- Cirrhosis: patient who is middle-aged or elderly presents with poorly tolerated upper GI bleed associated with features of hepatic decompensation i.e. ascites, jaundice, hepatic encephalopathy. Splenomegaly is generally mild to moderate.

Portal biliopathy is rare. Etiological history may be present e.g. alcohol, high risk behavior, recurrent jaundice etc.

Format for presenting the Diagnosis

- Case of portal hypertension; cirrhotic/non cirrhotic; bleeder/non bleeder; underwent endotherapy or not and whether it was successful or not; symptomatic/asypmtomatic splenomegaly present or not; hypersplenism present or not; portal biliopathy present or not; growth retardation present or not (to be mentioned in pediatric cases of EHPVO)
- Differential diagnosis include:
  - NCPF
  - EHPVO
  - Cirrhosis

EXAMPLE CASE

History

- My patient Mr XYZ, an 18-year-old gentleman, hailing from Mumbai, is a 2nd year engineering student.
- He presented with chief complaints of having vomited blood twice in last 2 days.
- He was apparently alright until 2 days back, when he vomited small quantity of bright red blood on two occasions.
- It was spontaneous, not preceded by nausea or retching, not associated with Melena
- It was not associated with postural dizziness, syncope, fatigue or shortness of breath
- On further enquiry, he gives history of having noticed a lump in his left upper abdomen since 1 month. The lump has not changed in size since first noticed. There is also a sensation of heaviness in left upper abdomen.
- There is no history of
  - Abdominal pain
  - Abdominal distension, altered sensorium
  - Jaundice, fever with chills,
- There is no history to suggest Hypersplenism
- On enquiring with mother regarding perinatal history, she says that he was delivered at hospital. There is no history to suggest abdominal sepsis, umbilical

sepsis, umbilical vein catheterization, delayed separation of cord, and chronic diarrhea during infancy.
- There is no history to suggest growth retardation or poor scholastic performance
- For these symptoms he seeked medical care, following which he was admitted, transfused one bag of blood and then was evaluated with endoscopy and underwent an endoscopic procedure, most probably endoscopic variceal banding. There is no history of hematemesis since then.
- There is no past history of alcohol consumption, recurring jaundice, blood transfusion or high risk behavior.
- There is no history of any co-morbid illness or previous surgeries
- There is no history of smoking
- Family history is not significant
- He is able to perform all his daily routine activity without any difficulty

Examination

- My patient is a young gentleman, who is averagely built, averagely nourished, with a height of 172 cm, weight of 60 kg and BMI being 20.3 kg/m^2
- He is conscious, co-operative, well oriented to time, place and person; Lying comfortably in bed; well hydrated and afebrile.
- Pulse is 72/min, BP is 110/70 mm Hg
- There is no pallor, jaundice, cyanosis, clubbing, generalized or localized lymphadenopathy. There is no palpable left supraclavicular lymph node; pedal or dependent edema, skin lesions or **stigmata of chronic liver disease.**
- Examination of oral cavity reveals adequate oral hygiene with no obvious mucosal lesions
- Examination of the abdomen:
  - On inspection: Abdomen is flat, umbilicus is central, inverted. All quadrants are moving equally with respiration. There is no visible lump, scar, sinus, engorged veins, pulsations, peristalsis or cough impulse.
  - Inspection of groin hernial sites reveal no swelling or cough impulse and Inspection of genitalia is unremarkable. Inspection of renal angles reveals no fullness
  - On Palpation: Abdomen is soft and non-tender. Liver is palpable upto 2 cm below costal margin in midclavicular line, is non-tender, with smooth surface, firm consistency with sharp, regular border moving with respiration. Spleen is enlarged, palpable 10 cm below the costal margin, extending up to umbilicus,

- is nontender, having smooth surface, firm consistency with rounded regular margins, moving with respiration. There isn't any other palpable lump.
  - There is no palpable cough impulse over groin hernia sites and examination of genitals is unremarkable. There is no tenderness in Renal angles. Examination of back and spine is essentially normal.
  - On Percussion, upper border of liver dullness is in the 5th intercostal space in midclavicular line with liver span being 14 cm. Length of splenic dullness is 20 cm. Rest of the abdomen is tympanitic with no evidence of free fluid.
  - On auscultation normal bowel sounds are heard. There is no bruit, hum or rub
  - Per rectal examination is unremarkable
- Rest systemic examination is essentially normal

To Summarize

- My patient is 18 year old engineering student, with no comorbid illnesses, WHO 0 performance status, presents with history of 2 episodes of spontaneous painless hematemesis since 2 days associated with a sensation of lump in left upper quadrant. He gives no history of abdominal distension or altered sensorium or history to suggest hypersplenism. He neither smokes nor consumes alcohol. For these symptoms he was admitted, received a blood transfusion and underwent endoscopic variceal banding.
- On examination there are no signs of CLD. There is hepatomegaly and massive splenomegaly

The most probable diagnosis in my patient is non cirrhotic portal hypertension due to EHPVO, with an episode of well tolerated bleed, with asymptomatic splenomegaly with no features of hypersplenism or portal biliopathy and has undergone successful endotherapy

How to Proceed: (Sequence and justification)

- Review available medical records
- Hemogram, LFT, INR and other routine blood investigations (Renal Function Test, Serum Electrolyte).
  - Hemogram to look for anemia, leucopenia and thrombocytopenia
  - LFT to look for bilirubin levels, albumin levels and liver enzyme levels (SGOT/AST,SGPT/ALT, ALP). Hyperbilirubinemia could suggest hepatic

decompensation due to cirrhosis (Indirect hyperbilirubinemia) or bile duct block due to portal biliopathy (Direct hyperbilirubinemia). Raised ALP suggests cholestasis which again could be due to portal biliopathy
- INR to look for coagulopathy
- RFT to look for raised creatinine which would suggest hepato-renal syndrome
- SE to look for hyponatremia
- Bilirubin level, albumin level and INR is required for calculation of Child Pugh score. Creatinine, bilirubin and INR is required for calculation of MELD score. Creatinine, bilirubin, INR and sodium level is required for calculation of MELD-Na score. All three of these are used for grading the severity of the cirrhotic liver disease.

Table 8.1: Child Turcot Pugh score

- Parameters:
  - Bilirubin:
    - 1 point: < 2 mg/dl
    - 2 point: 2–3 mg/dl
    - 3 point: > 3 mg/dl
  - Albumin:
    - 1 point: > 3.5 g/dl
    - 2 point: 2.8–3.5 g/dl
    - 3 point: < 2.8 g/dl
  - INR:
    - 1 point: < 1.7
    - 2 point: 1.7–2.3
    - 3 point: > 2.3
  - Ascites:
    - 1 point: absent
    - 2 point: controlled with medication
    - 3 point: refractory
  - Hepatic encephalopathy:
    - 1 point: none
    - 2 point: grade 1–2
    - 3 point: grade 3–4
- CTP A: score 5–6
- CTP B: score 7–9
- CTP C: score 10–15

- Additional blood tests:
  - Serum ammonia: in case patient has clinical features of hepatic encephalopathy
  - ABG (arterial blood gas) and serum lactate levels
- X-ray chest: as a routine
- Upper GI endoscopy:
  - To identify cause for upper GI bleed:
    - Portal hypertensive bleed:
      - Varix: esophageal and/or gastric varices
      - Portal hypertensive gastropathy
    - Non-Portal hypertensive bleed:
      - Peptic ulcer
      - Mallory Weiss tear
      - Angiodysplasia
      - Dieulafoy lesion
      - Malignancy
  - Presence of varices confirms the presence of portal hypertension
    - Esophageal varices if present: note its grade, extent and look for presence of stigmata of recent bleed
    - Baveno classification for grading of esophageal varices
      - I: small straight varices
      - II: enlarged tortuous varices occupying less than 1/3rd of the esophageal lumen
      - III: enlarged tortuous varices occupying more than 1/3rd of the esophageal lumen
    - Sarin classification of gastric varices
      - Gastro-esophageal varices (GOV)
        - GOV1: esophageal varices extending onto lesser curve of stomach
        - GOV2: esophageal varices extending into gastric fundus

- Isolated gastric varices (IGV):
    - IGV1: Isolated fundic varices
    - IGV2: Isolated gastric varices elsewhere in stomach

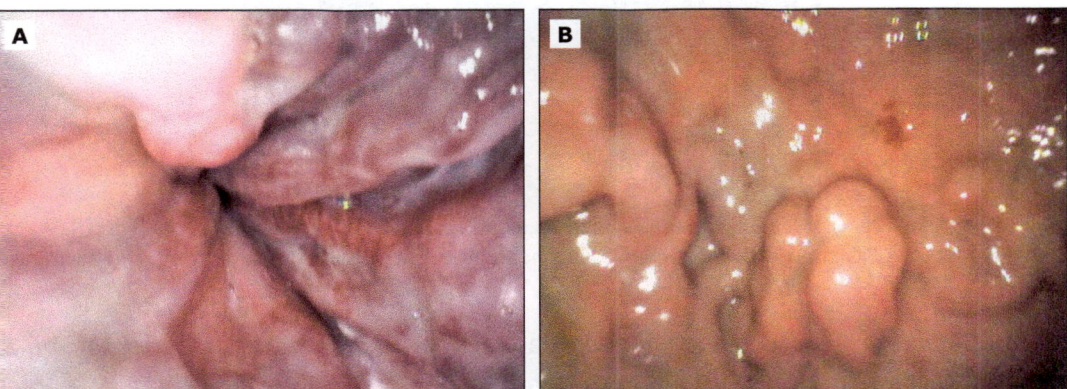

Figure 8.13: Upper GI endoscopy showing esophageal varices (A) and gastric varices (B).

- USG (A+P): it is an extension of bed side clinical evaluation, it's cheap, non invasive and easily available
    - To examine the liver to see:
        - Its size: increased (fatty liver), normal or shrunken (cirrhosis)
        - Echotexture: normal or altered (diseased)
        - Surface: normal or wavy/nodular (cirrhosis)
        - Hepatic vasculature: PV, hepatic artery, hepatic vein
            - Portal veins: its size, wall thickness, flow velocity, direction of blood flow, flow pattern, presence or absence of any thrombus
                - Findings to suggest portal hypertension: Increase in PV diameter and flow velocity, reversal of PV flow
                - Findings to suggest NCPF: Increased PV wall thickness, peripheral pruning of PV branches
                - Findings to suggest EHPVO: Presence of portal cavernoma
            - Hepatic veins: its size, flow velocity, flow pattern, presence or absence of any thrombus
                - Lack of flow or thrombus in hepatic vein or adjacent IVC could suggest Budd Chiari syndrome

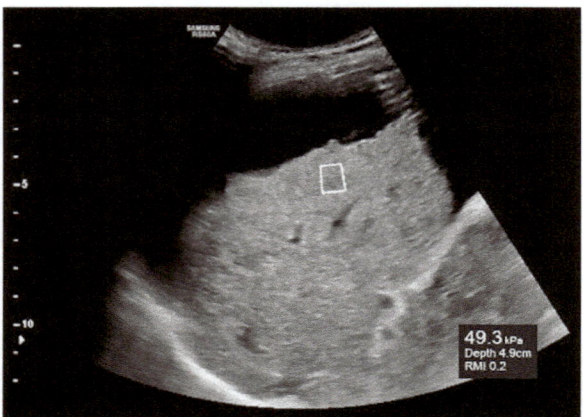

Figure 8.14: USG showing cirrhotic liver with nodular surface, altered echotexture and ascites.

- o Biliary system: to see for cholelithiasis, choledocholithiasis, intrahepatic biliary radical dilatation (IHBRD), extrahepatic bile duct (EHBD) dilatation
    - Dilated bile duct in setting of EHPVO would suggest portal cavernoma cholangiopathy (previously called as portal biliopathy)
- o SMV, splenic vein (SV): its size, flow velocity, flow pattern, presence or absence of any thrombus
    - It is important to examine SMV and SV for surgical planning
    - In case there is an SV or SMV thrombosis spleno-renal shunt and meso-caval won't be feasible.
    - SV size of 7 mm is required for PSRS (proximal spleno renal shunt) to be feasible
    - Also splenic vein thrombosis with splenic hilar collaterals with normal liver and liver vasculature would suggest Sinistral portal hypertension
- o Left Renal vein: It is important to note for surgical planning (PSRS, DSRS)
- o Spleen: its size, presence of infarct or hematoma
- o Presence of intra-abdominal collaterals elsewhere
- o Presence of free fluid
- CECT and/or MRI with IV contrast of the abdomen and pelvis:
    - o To obtain a road map to plan shunt surgery
    - o It provides anatomic information about PV-SMV-SV and renal vein and thus helps with surgical planning

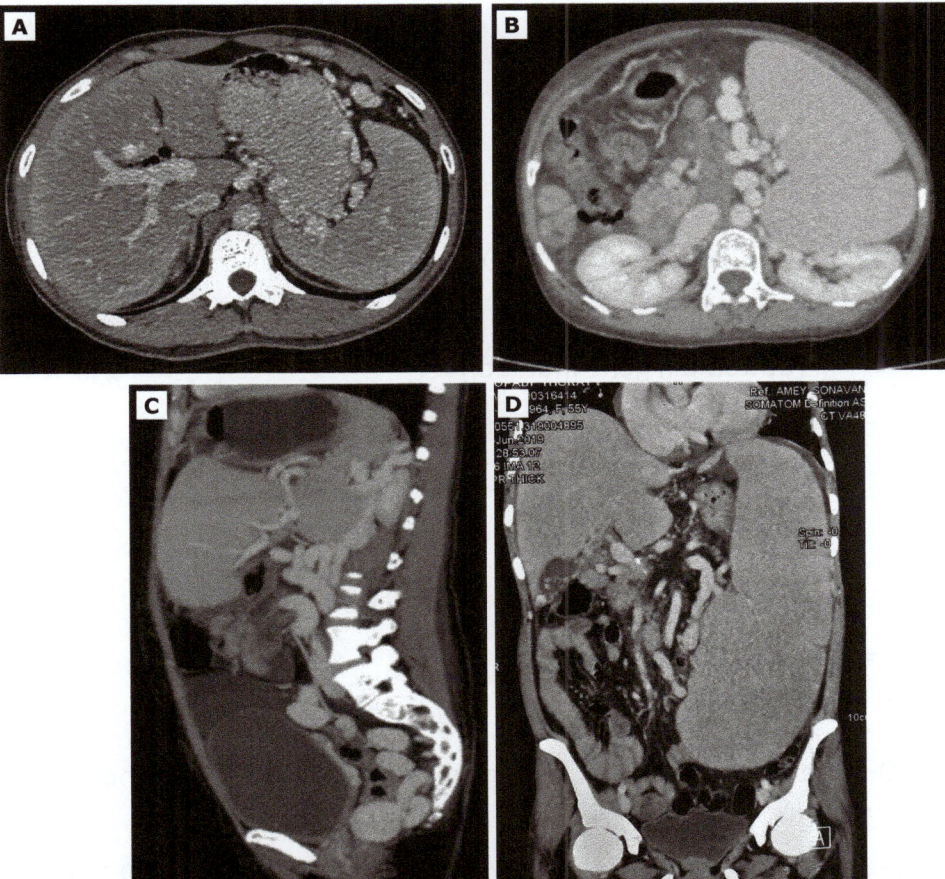

Figure 8.15: CT images showing enlarged spleen with multiple dilated, tortuous venous collaterals in hepato-duodenal ligament, peri-gastric, peri-esophageal and splenic hilar regions.

- Optional investigation
  - Interventional radiology:
    - Transjugular catheterization of the hepatic vein and:
      - Measurement of Hepatic venous pressure gradient (HVPG)
      - TJLB: Transjugular liver biopsy
  - Fibroscan, transient elastography
  - Spleno-portogram: it is invasive and rarely performed now a days. But it can provide splenic pulp pressure
  - Thrombophilia work-up for Inherited or Acquired Thrombophilias or Hypercoaguable states

- Thrombophilic work-up
  - They include:
    - Protein C deficiency
    - Protein S deficiency
    - Anti-thrombin 3 deficiency
    - Factor 5 Leiden mutation
    - Prothrombin gene mutation
    - Tests for Antiphospholipid antibodies:
      - Anti-cardiolipin
      - Lupus anticoagulant
      - Anti β2-glycoprotein I antibodies
    - Homocysteine levels
    - JAK-2 mutation
- A D-dimer assay is useful as a general test for verifying the presence of thrombosis
- The majority of patients with venous thromboembolism (VTE) need not be tested for thrombophilia as the data supporting its clinical usefulness and benefits are limited or nonexistent.
- Indications for testing:
  - Recurrent thromboembolic episodes
  - Thromboembolism at a young age (i.e. < 40 y)
  - A family history for thromboembolism
  - Thrombosis in an unusual site, e.g. cerebral, splanchnic veins (Hepatic, Mesenteric).
- Do not perform thrombophilia testing at the time of a VTE event, as it can be inaccurate (often false positive).
- Tests should be performed at least 4–6 weeks after an acute thrombotic event or discontinuation of anticoagulant/thrombolytic therapies including warfarin, heparin, direct thrombin inhibitors (DTIs), direct factor Xa inhibitors, and fibrinolytic agents

- o Do not perform thrombophilia testing while a patient is receiving anticoagulation. Instead,
  - – Wait until 2 weeks after discontinuing warfarin, or
  - – 2 days for direct oral anticoagulants and heparin.
- o The exception is DNA analysis for genetic mutations, which is not generally affected by other medical issues or anticoagulant therapy.
- o If abnormal results are found during acute illness or anticoagulant therapy, testing should be repeated in a new specimen when the patient is stable and after anticoagulant therapy is discontinued.
- o The goal of thrombophilia testing should be to aid decision making regarding future VTE prophylaxis, to guide testing of family members, and to determine the cause in severe or fatal VTE. Test results alone should not be used to decide on the duration of anticoagulation therapy.

- Pharmacotherapy
  - o Options
    - Beta blocker: propranolol, nadolol, carvedilol
    - Octreotide
    - Terlipressin
    - Somatostatin
    - Vasopressin
  - o Pharmacotherapy is usually considered as the initial treatment modality in case of acute variceal bleed before endoscopy and endotherapy can be arranged for. Its role is complementary to that of endotherapy.
  - o Additionally propranolol is used for long term primary and secondary prophylaxis

- Endotherapy
  - o Primary modality for management of variceal bleed
  - o Options:
    - Endoscopic variceal band ligation (EVL)
    - Endoscopic sclerotherapy (EST)
    - Endoscopic glue injection: cyanoacrylate

- o EVL is preferred over EST for esophageal varices
- o Glue injection is the preferred endotherapeutic modality for gastric varices

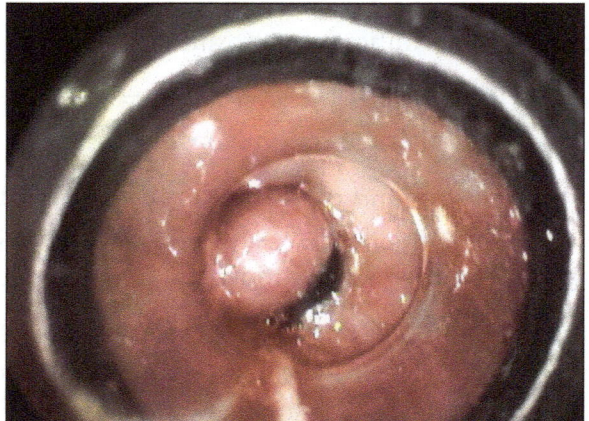

Figure 8.16: Endoscopic variceal band ligation.

- Interventional Radiology:
  - o Options:
    - TIPS: transjugular intrahepatic porto-systemic shunt
    - DIPS: Direct intrahepatic porto-systemic shunt
    - Angioembolization with coil, autologous clot or glue
    - BRTO: balloon occluded retrograde transvenous obliteration of varices
    - PARTO: plug assisted retrograde transvenous obliteration of varices

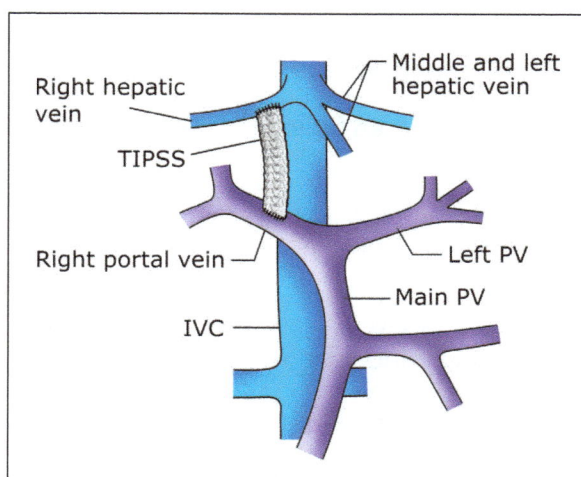

Figure 8.17: TIPSS between right portal vein and right hepatic vein.

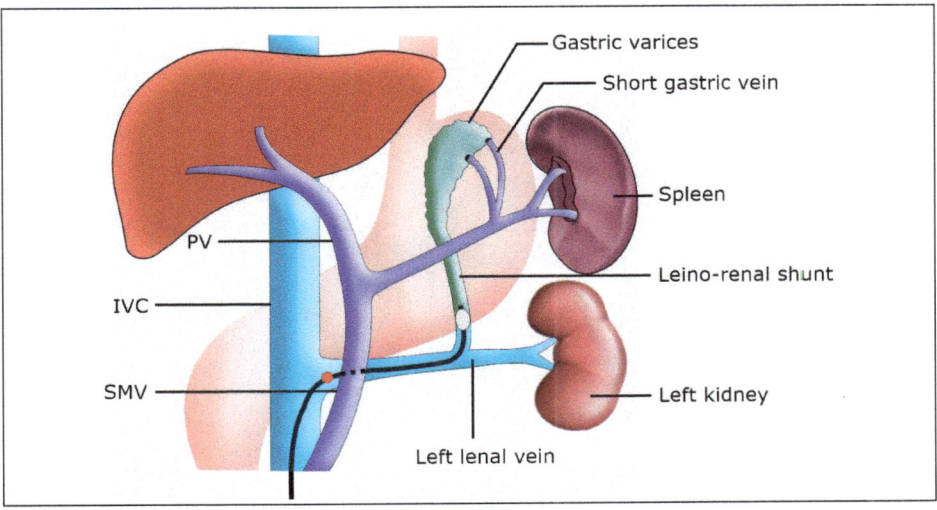

Figure 8.18: Balloon-occluded Retrograde Transvenous Obliteration of varices (BRTO).

- Surgery
  - Options:
    - Surgical shunts
      - Non selective shunt:
        - PSRS: linton shunt: proximal spleno-renal shunt
        - PCS: porto-caval shunt: end to side (Eck fistula) or side to side. Shunt diameter in this case is generally more than 10 mm
        - MCS: meso-caval shunt
        - Mitra shunt: Side to side spleno-renal shunt

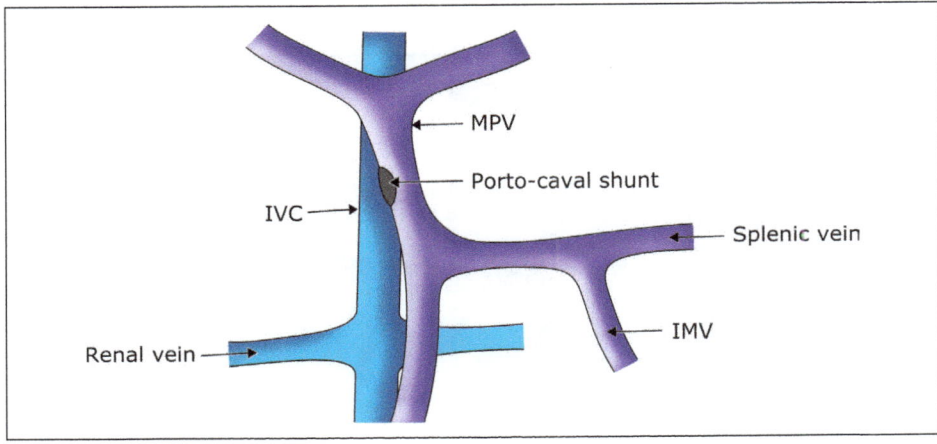

Figure 8.19: Side-to-side porto-caval shunt.

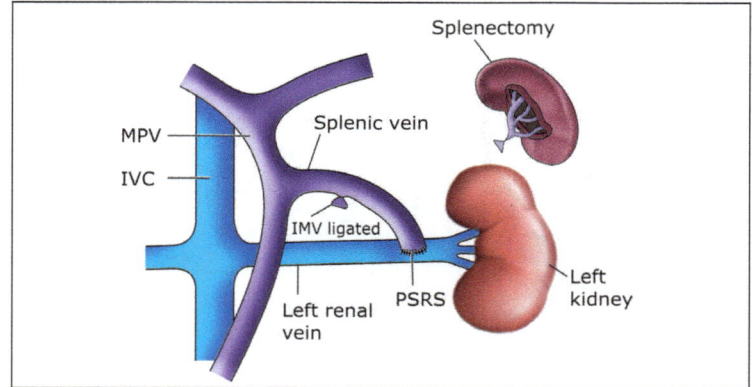

Figure 8.20: Proximal splenorenal shunt.

- Selective shunt:
    ♦ DSRS: warren shunt: distal spleno-renal shunt
    ♦ Ionokuchi shunt: coronary-caval shunt

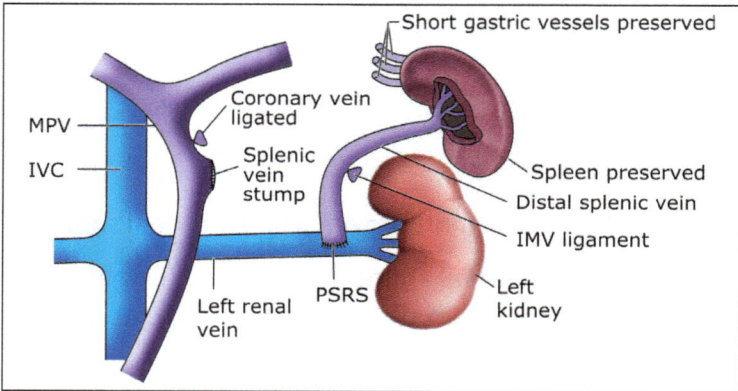

Figure 8.21: Warren/distal splenorenal shunt.

- Partial porto-caval shunt: Sharfeh shunt (shunt diameter < 8 mm)

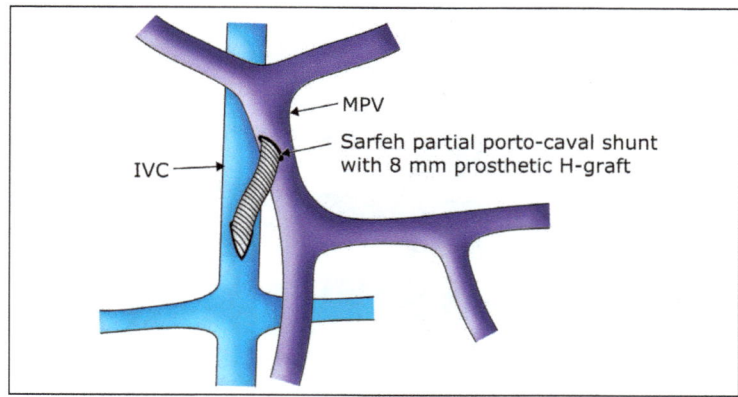

Figure 8.22: Sarfeh partial porto-caval shunt.

- Devascularization surgery:
  - Sugiura-Futugava surgery and its modification
  - Hassabs surgery

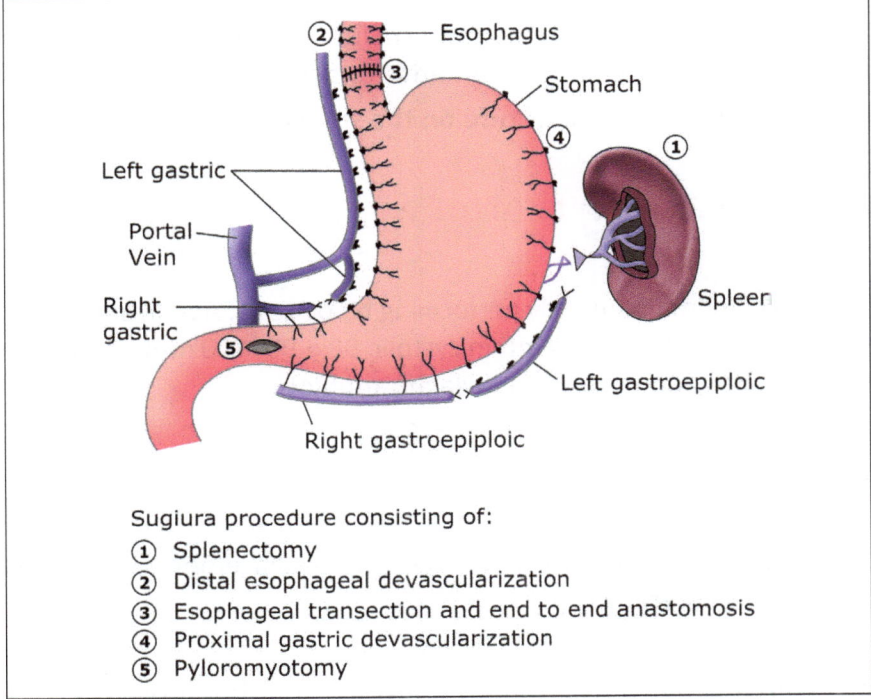

Figure 8.23: Devascularization surgery.

- Liver transplantation
○ Generally PSRS is the preferred shunt surgery in NCPH. Whereas Sharfehs shunt and warren shunt are preferred shunt in cirrhotics

Table 8.2: Indication for surgery in NCPH
- Refractory variceal bleed
- Secondary prophylaxis in NCPH
- Symptomatic slpenomegaly, hypersplenism
- Ectopic varices
- Portal biliopathy
- Growth retardation
- Patients from rural areas who lack basic medical facility
- Rare blood group type

- Surveillance/follow-up
  - Non selective beta blocker (propranolol): for long term primary or secondary prophylaxis
  - Surveillance endoscopies and SOS endoscopic variceal band ligation in case varices are identified
- Remember conservative management including Endoscopic surveillance with endotherapy and propranolol is alternative to surgery.
- **Go through chapter 13 for literature on the subject.**

PRINCIPLE OF MANAGEMENT OF ACUTE VARICEAL BLEED: (IN SHORT)

- Admit
- Resuscitate while simultaneously performing blood tests. Administer crystalloids and blood products (target is to maintain systolic BP > 90–100 mm Hg and hemoglobin levels > 8 mg/dl). Administer prophylactic antibiotic
- Perform blood tests. Plan urgent endoscopy
- Initiate pharmacotherapy
- Perform endotherapy
- Consider esophageal tamponade with Sengstaken-Blakemore tube in case of bleed refractory to endotherapy
- Consider TIPS in case of refractory bleed
- Emergent surgery: portocaval shunt or devascularization surgery is considered as the last resort in case of refractory variceal bleed

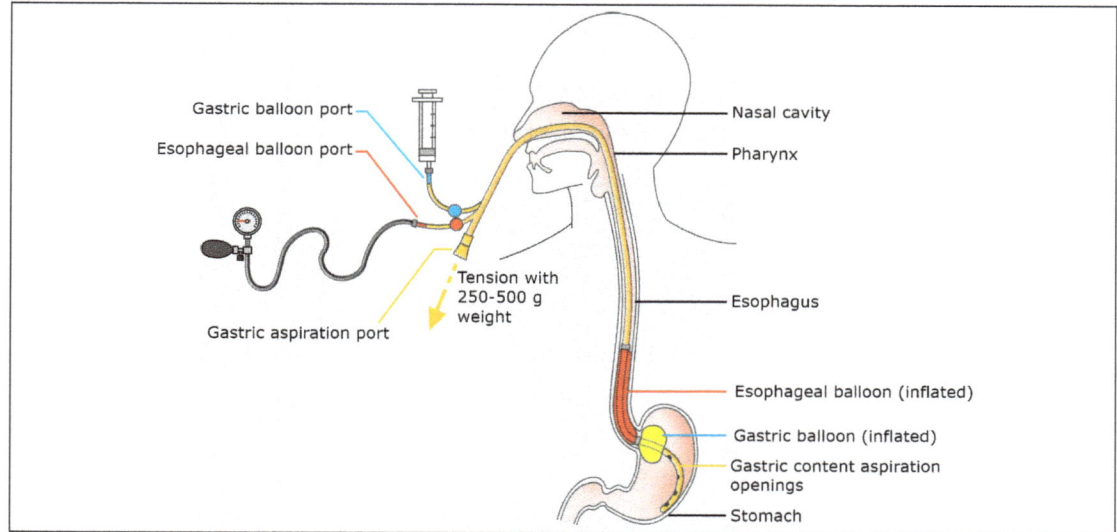

Figure 8.24: Sengstaken-Blakemore tube used in refractory Variceal Bleed.

9 Case of Bile Duct Injury

Format for History Taking

- History prior to surgery:
  - History of right upper quadrant abdominal pain
  - Fever
  - Jaundice
  - Whether the patient has undergone ERCP or not
  - Total duration of symptoms prior to surgery
- Surgical details:
  - Whether cholecystectomy procedure was done on elective or emergency basis
  - Whether it was done via laparoscopic/open technique or is there history of conversion from laparoscopy to open
  - Duration of surgery
  - History of post-operative ICU stay
  - History of intra-or post-operative blood transfusion
  - Was any event/complication mentioned/explained in post-operative briefing
  - Was the gall bladder and stones shown or not
  - Whether any abdominal drainage tube was placed or not.
- Immediate post-operative details:
  - Was patient comfortable and symptom free in the immediate post-operative period, if not what symptoms she had (pain, fever, jaundice, nausea and vomiting).
  - If a drain tube was placed, what was the color of the effluent coming out, its amount and trend
  - Was the drain tube removed within first 2-3 post-operative days or was it retained.
  - Was any cross sectional imaging (USG, CT, MRI) performed
  - Was any post-operative percutaneous/endoscopic/surgical intervention done; in case of surgical or percutaneous intervention was any tube inserted into

the abdomen, if yes what was the color/nature, amount and trend of the fluid coming out
  - When was the patient discharged, was he/she discharged with drain tube in situ.
- Later post-operative/disease course:
  - History of yellowish discoloration of sclera and high colored urine:
    - Duration
    - Onset: Insidious or sudden onset
    - Nature: Intermittent or persistent or progressive.
  - History of pruritus (itching): generalized or localized to certain body part; Present throughout the day or at certain point of the day (as in, more towards the night); disturbing lifestyle or not; disturbing sleep or not.
  - Color of stools: Cholic or acholic, i.e. note whether stool is normal brown colored or clay coloredl.
  - History of pain:
    - Site
    - Onset: insidious or sudden
    - Nature: intermittent/continuous
    - Duration
    - Character of pain: Dull aching or colicky
    - Intensity: mild/moderate/severe
    - Radiation to mid back or right infrascapular region: present or not
    - Related to meals or not
    - Related to posture or not
  - History of fever:
    - Duration
    - onset: insidious or sudden
    - Grade: low or high
    - Nature: intermittent or fluctuating or continuous
    - Associated chills or not.
  - History of vomiting:
    - Quantity
    - Bilious or not

- Projectile or not
- Related to meals or not.
  - History of hematemesis or Melena; postural dizziness, syncope, fatigue, shortness of breath, need for blood transfusion.
  - History suggestive of fat soluble vitamin deficiency:
    - Vitamin A deficiency: history of decreased night vision, dryness of eyes
    - Vitamin D deficiency: bone pain, frequent fractures, muscle weakness
    - Vitamin K deficiency: history of coagulopathy such as ecchymosis; petechiae; easy bruisability.
  - History suggestive of chronic liver disease:
    - Abdominal distension
    - GI bleed
    - Altered sensorium
    - Decreased urine output
    - History to suggest Hypersplenism
  - History of loss of weight; loss of appetite
- Past history: History of co-morbid illness, any other surgery
- History of smoking or alcohol consumption.
- Treatment history: history of any cross sectional imaging, percutaneous/endoscopic/surgical intervention done; in case of surgical or percutaneous intervention was any tube inserted into the abdomen, if yes what was the color/nature, amount and trend of the fluid coming out.
- Family history
- Performance history

Justification for Each Component in History

- **Firstly, Understanding classification of bile duct injury (BDI):**
  - Bismuth classification was described during the era of open cholecystectomy when most common type of BDI were Biliary stricture. Hence Bismuth classification is mainly about types of biliary strictures. Later on, with the advent of Laparoscopic cholecystectomy, newer variants of BDI were noticed which have been included in the more recent Strasberg Classification. Bismuth Classification of biliary strictures is incorporated into the Strasberg classification.

Table 9.1: Bismuth-Strasberg Classification

- Type A: Cystic duct stump leak
- Type B: Ligation of Right posterior sectoral duct
- Type: C: Bile leak from a divided right posterior sectoral duct
- Type D: lateral bile duct injury
- Type E: bile duct strictures resulting from bile duct transection (as classified by Bismuth)
  - E1: stricture in CHD > 2 cm away from hilum
  - E2: stricture within 2 cm from the hilum
  - E3: Stricture at the hilum; however communication between right and left duct is maintained
  - E4: Stricture at the hilum with separation of right and left ducts; i.e. communication between right and left duct is not maintained
  - E5: combined stricture of main bile duct and right sectoral duct.

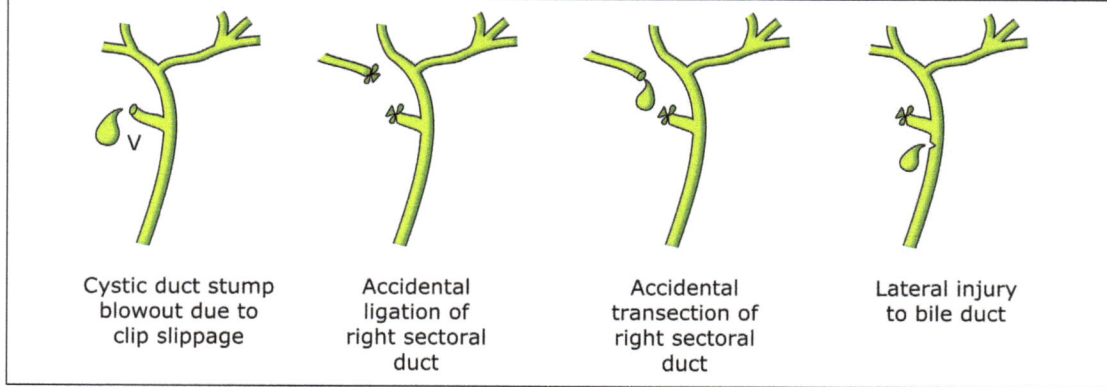

Figure 9.1: Bismuth strasberg classification of bile duct injury.

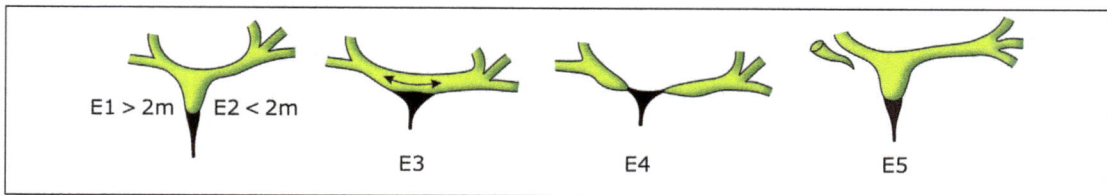

Figure 9.2: Bismuth-Strasberg classification of biliary stricture.

- Type A BDI results due to slippage of ligature or clip used to obliterate the cystic duct. There is no loss of bilio-enteric continuity.
- Type D BDI results due to lateral injury to main bile duct. It may be due to excessive traction or thermal injury (due to cautery) to the main bile duct. There is no loss of bilio-enteric continuity.
- Due to anomalous anatomy, Right posterior sectoral duct may lie very close to the area of dissection in the Calot's triangle. The same may be miss identified as cystic duct and may be ligated during surgery resulting in type B injury. If it is divided without ligation it results in bile leak due to type C BDI.
- Type E BDI results due to Classical BDI involving bile duct transection. There is loss of bilio-enteric continuity.
- Significance of bilio-enteric continuity:
  - Bilio-enteric continuity is maintained in type A and D BDI; whereas it is lost in type E injury.
  - Significance lies in the fact that ERCP and stenting is possible (and potentially curative) in patients with maintained Bilio-enteric continuity; whereas it won't be possible in those without.
- Mechanism of "Classical BDI" as described in literature: CBD is miss identified as cystic duct, dissected, clipped and cut. Then as the dissection is carried proximally in the presumed gall bladder fossa the common hepatic duct is cut with resultant leak of golden bile. Thus as a result CBD is clipped, CHD is cut open and there is loss of a segment of the main bile duct. So there is loss of bilio-enteric continuity.

Now Let's Start

- History prior to surgery:
  - This is to basically get an idea about the condition which patient had due to which he had to undergo cholecystectomy.
    - History of right upper quadrant abdominal pain precipitated by meals radiating to right infrascapular region, not related to posture, may or may not be associated with vomiting usually suggests symptomatic biliary colic without cholecystitis. When there is associated fever, it suggests cholecystitis. If there is radiation of pain to back with relief of pain with bending forward, it suggests gall stone pancreatitis. And when Charcot triad (pain, fever and jaundice) is present, then the patient usually has cholangitis.
    - Surgery is anticipated to be relatively straight forward in patients with biliary colic. Whereas in patients with cholecystitis, cholangitis, pancreatitis and those who have undergone ERCP, surgery is anticipated to be difficult.

- If the total duration of symptoms is long, consider chronic cholecystitis which again increases the complexity of the surgery.
- Surgical details:
  - Elective or Emergency basis: emergency surgery is usually performed for complicated disease such as gall bladder perforation or gangrenous or emphysematous cholecystitis, which again hints towards a difficult surgery.
  - Whether it was done via laparoscopic/open technique: in today's times most of the cholcystectomies are done laparoscopically. So, if the surgery was done via open technique, consider it to be an anticipated difficult surgery.
  - History of conversion from laparoscopy to open: suggests difficult surgery or occurrence of an intra-operative complication such as bleeding or bile duct injury.
  - Duration of surgery: on an average, laparoscopic cholecystectomy takes anywhere between 1–1.5 hours. Longer duration of surgery suggests more difficult surgery.
  - History of post-operative ICU stay: patients are generally shifted to the ward after an uneventful laparoscopic cholecystectomy. Patients are shifted to ICU if patients have severe comorbid illness or if surgery was difficult or a surgical complication has occurred or if a complication is anticipated in the post-operative course.
  - History of intra or post-operative blood transfusion: need for blood transfusion during or after cholecystectomy is highly unusual and should raise alarm about intra operative hemorrhage.
  - Was any event/complication mentioned/explained in post-operative briefing: it is very important to be truthful to the patient or relatives if any complication occurs. However, many a times facts are purposefully hidden. Mention what was explained to the patient in brief.

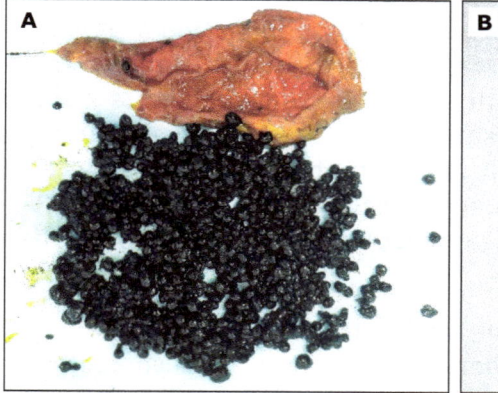
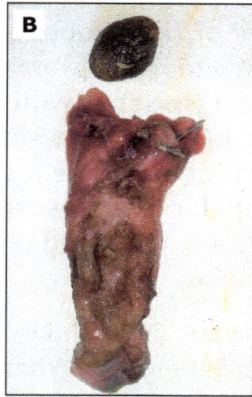

Figure 9.3: Multiple tiny gall stones (A) vs solitary large gall stone (B). The risk of residual CBD stones is higher in the first case.

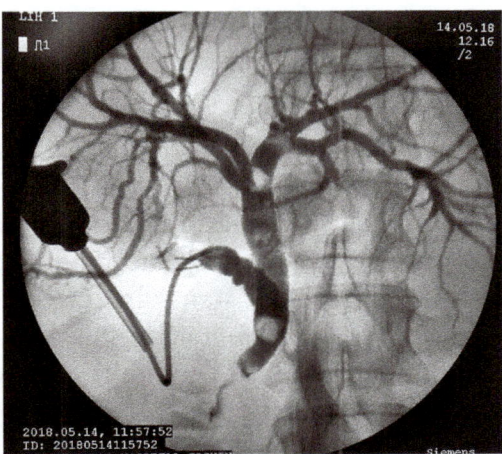

Figure 9.4: Intra-operative cholangiography revealing CBD store.

- o Whether any abdominal drainage tube was placed or not: drains are usually selectively placed in difficult surgery or in case where complication such as bile leak or bleeding is being anticipated or has occurred.
- Immediate post-operative details:
  - o Was patient comfortable and symptom free in the immediate post-operative period: it is generally said that a patient who has undergone an uneventful laparoscopic cholecystectomy should be up and around on the next day after surgery. That is, they are comfortable, pain free, out of the bed having breakfast. Any deviation from such normal course should suggest further evaluation.
  - o Patients may have mild suture site pain and anesthesia drug related post-operative nausea and vomiting. Undue pain, fever, jaundice suggests deviation from normal post-operative course and suggests further evaluation.
  - o Drain details:
    - Color of the effluent: straw colored fluid suggests serous discharge, red colored fluid suggests sanguineous (bloody) discharge. Generally the effluent is sero-sanguinous i.e. light red watery. Greenish or yellowish effluent suggests bile leak (See Fig. 2.15: Types of drain fluid effluent; Page number 14).
    - The amount of fluid coming out (especially if bilious) is to be noted. Also note the trend of the amounting draining, whether it is decreasing, stable or increasing. Stable or increasing trend suggests biliary fistula.
    - Was the drain tube removed within first 2–3 post-operative days or was it retained: normally it is removed within first 2–3 post-operative days. Retention of drain suggests otherwise.

- Performance of cross-sectional imaging (USG, CT, MRI): It is usually performed in order to evaluate a post-operative complication such as bilioma, retained stone, hemorrhage.
- Post-operative percutaneous/endoscopic/surgical intervention: percutaneous intervention in the early post-operative course is most probably a PCD (percutaneous catheter drainage) insertion to drain a bilioma. An ERCP (endoscopic retrograde cholangio pancreaticography) or rarely a PTBD may be done to extract a retained stone or stent the CBD in case of Strasburg type A or D bile duct injury (BDI). Successful biliary stenting via ERCP suggests there is no CBD cut off and the bilioenteric continuity is maintained (Strasburg type A or D). Surgery in the early post-operative course is done for two reasons. First, to perform lavage in case, sepsis source control cannot be achieved with percutaneous drain tube insertion alone. Secondly for performing immediate or early BDI repair which is performed in select centers only.
- Details of drain inserted at time of intervention: same like previously discussed (see above).
- Was the patient discharged with drain tube in situ: this is usually done if the drain effluent is bilious.

- Later post-operative/disease course:
  - History of yellowish discoloration of sclera and high colored urine: it suggests obstructive jaundice. This is usually due to formation of biliary stricture (Strasburg type E BDI) as a sequelae of major bile duct injury.
  - Onset and nature of jaundice: generally, jaundice in patient with post cholecystectomy bile duct stricture is insidious in onset and progressive in nature. Onset is more rapid if the CBD has been clipped or ligated at time of cholecystectomy. Intermittent type of jaundice may be seen in choledocholithiasis.
  - History of pruritus in a jaundiced patient suggests obstructive pathology.
  - Color of stools: Cholic or acholic:
    - Passage of clay colored stools in the setting of BDI suggests biliary stricture formation with obstruction to the flow of bile.
    - Whereas passage of cholic stools (normal brown colored) could suggest that either:
      - There is no obstruction to flow of bile.
      - Or the patient has developed an internal bilio-enteric fistula (choledocho-duodenal, choledocho-gastric fistula). Therefore, inspite of there being a biliary stricture, patient continues to pass cholic stools.

- o History of fever: suggests presence of collection, persistence of biliary fistula or cholangitis/cholangiolytic abscess.
- o History suggestive of fat soluble vitamin deficiency: may be found in patient with long standing obstructive jaundice. Vitamin K deficiency is earliest to occur.
- o History suggestive of chronic liver disease: Long standing obstructive jaundice (> 6 months) may result in secondary biliary cirrhosis. This may consequently lead to portal hypertension and hepatic decompensation:
  - GI bleed: Variceal bleed
  - Abdominal distension: ascites
  - Altered sensorium: hepatic encephalopathy
  - Decreased urine output: hepatorenal syndrome
- Treatment history in later disease course: patient with post cholecystectomy bile duct stricture is generally evaluated using MRCP, CT and PTC (percutaneous transhepatic cholangiogram). Patients may need PTBD insertion for relieving obstructive jaundice and its consequences. Or PTBC (percutaneous transhepatic biliary catheter) insertion may be done a day before planned reparative surgery to help facilitate intra op. identification of bile ducts.
- History of co-morbid illness: to see tolerance for surgery
- Smoking history: patients who smoke do not tolerate surgery well
- Family history: usually insignificant
- Performance history: to see tolerance for surgery

Format for Examination

- What is the appearance of the patient: young/middle-aged/elderly, lady/gentleman
- Whether the patient is clinically
  - o Poorly/averagely/well built
  - o Poorly/averagely/well nourished
- Measure height, weight, BMI
- Whether the patient is clinically
  - o Conscious/stuporous
  - o Co-operative/unco-operative

- Well/poorly oriented to time, place and person
- Lying comfortably in bed/in discomfort/in pain(rolling in pain)
- Well hydrated/dehydrated
- Febrile/Afebrile
- Mention Pulse, BP
- Look for
    - Icterus:
        - Sites to look for icterus: sclera/bulbar conjunctiva, undersurface of tongue, soft palate, palms and soles.
    - Pallor, cyanosis, clubbing,
    - Generalized or localized lymphadenopathy,
    - Pedal or dependent edema,
    - Peripheral signs of chronic liver disease
    - Skin lesions: look for scratch marks in a patient with pruritus
    - Stigmata of chronic liver disease

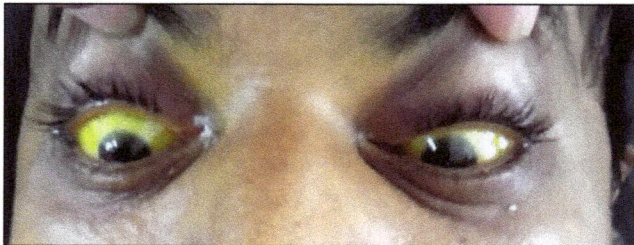

Figure 9.5: Icterus.

- Examination of oral cavity: look for oral hygiene and any obvious mucosal lesions
- Examination of the abdomen:
    - On Inspection: See if:
        - Abdomen is flat/distended/scaphoid;
        - Umbilicus is central/displaced (upwards/downwards/sideways) inverted/everted/flat.
        - All quadrants are moving equally with respiration or not
        - Look for any visible lump

- Look for visible scar: of cholecystectomy, drain tube exit site. Describe:
  - Type:
    ♦ Laparoscopic cholecystectomy (LC) port sites: typical LC port sites are umbilical, epigastric, right hypochondriac and right lumbar
      □ In case of LC, see if the port positions are alright.
      □ At times an additional port may be inserted on the left side of the midline for additional retraction or to facilitate intracorporeal suturing

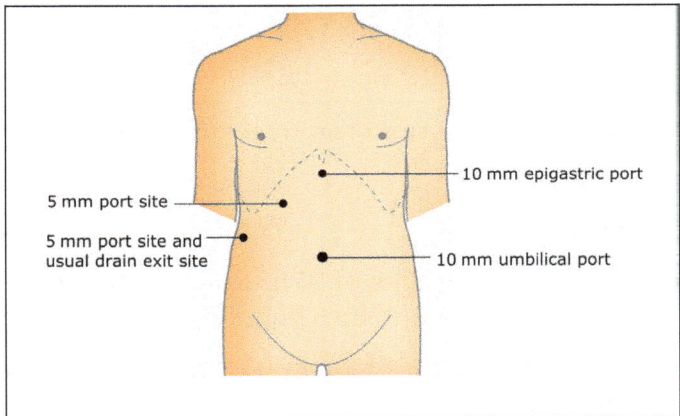

Figure 9.6: Scars to expect in laparoscopic cholecystectomy.

   ♦ Scar of open cholecystectomy which generally is a right subcostal incision; less commonly right para-median or midline.

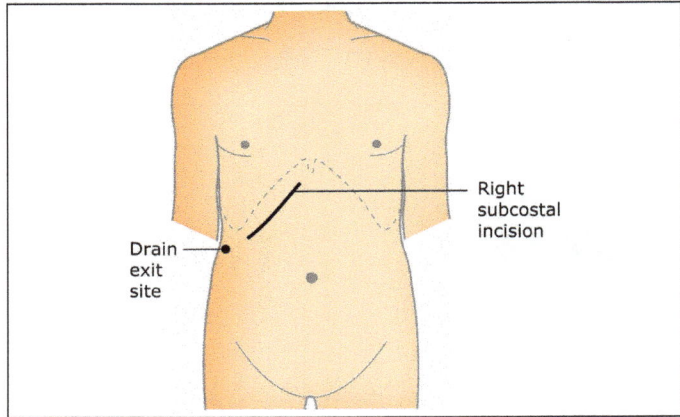

Figure 9.7: Scars to expect in open cholecystectomy.

♦ In case of laparoscopy converted to open, there will be umbilical port site scar apart from the right subcostal incision.

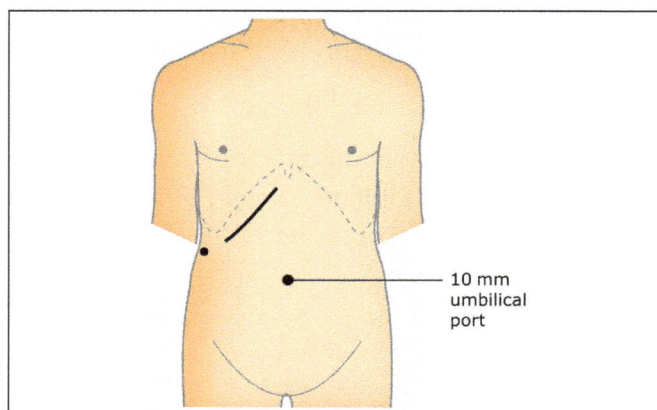

Figure 9.8: Scars to expect in laparoscopy converted to open cholecystectomy.

- Drain site:
  ♦ Drain placed at time of LC is usually exited from the right lumbar port, so there won't be 5 but only 4 scars
  ♦ Whereas in case of open cholecystectomy drain sites will be separate from the main incision
- See if the scar is well or poorly healed
- See if there is any cough impulse over the scar.
- Look for any drainage tube, if present note its:
  - Site
  - Nature of effluent: serous/serosanguinous/sanguinous/bilious/enteric/purulent.

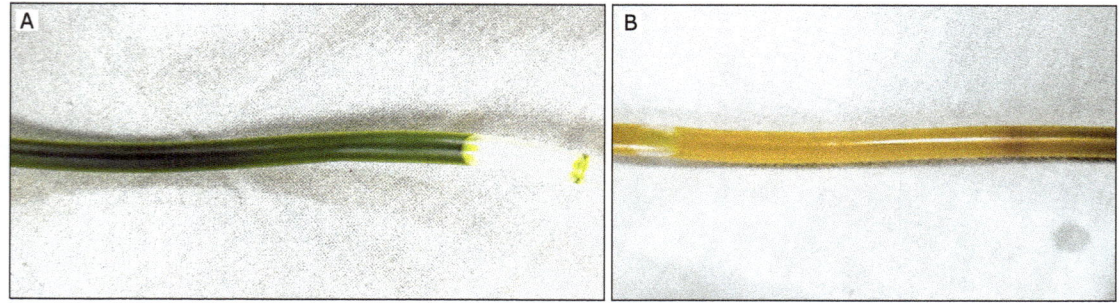

Figure 9.9: Different colors of Bilious Drain Effluent; (A) Green bile, (B) Golden bile.

- Look for sinus, engorged veins, pulsations, peristalsis or cough impulse.
- Don't forget to inspect the groin hernial sites (to look for swelling or cough impulse i.e. hernia) and genitalia.
- Inspection of renal angles to look for fullness
- On Palpation: See if:
  - Abdomen is soft and non-tender (Alternatively abdomen could be rigid and/or tender)
  - Liver is palpable or not
  - Spleen is enlarged or not
  - Any other palpable lump.
  - Examine scar for any tenderness, induration, bogginess or cough impulse.
- Do not forget to:
  - Palpate groin hernia sites to look for cough impulse
  - Examine genitals
  - Look for tenderness in renal angles
  - Examination of back and spine
- On Percussion:
  - Look for upper border of liver dullness (generally in the 5th intercostal space) in midclavicular line.
  - Note the liver span (normal being 12–14 cm)
  - Note the percussion note over rest of the abdomen (it is generally tympanic)
  - Tests for free fluid. Presence of free fluid suggests ascites
- On auscultation:
  - Auscultate for bowel sounds.
  - Bruit, hum and rub
- Per rectal examination. On DRE note the stool color to see if it is cholic or acholic
- Rest systemic examination:
  - Respiratory examination in form of auscultation
  - Assessment of breath holding time is important for clinically evaluating fitness for surgery.

EXAMPLE CASE

History

- My patient Mr ABC, is a 34-year-old male hailing from Mumbai, is an electrician by occupation.
- He presented with chief complaints of yellowish discoloration of eyes of one month duration.
- My patient's history dates back to 3 months, back when he developed right upper quadrant abdominal pain, mild to moderate in severity dull aching and intermittent in nature, precipitated with meals, non radiating, not associated with meals, relieved with oral medications; associated with occasional vomiting.
- For these symptoms he was evaluated, found to have gall stones for which he underwent laparoscopic surgery for removal of gall bladder. Surgery was done on elective basis on __/__/____, 2 months back. Surgery lasted for around 3 hours. At the end of surgery relatives were briefed that the surgery was difficult. Following surgery patient was kept in ICU and a drain tube was placed in the abdomen. However no blood transfusion was given.
- On the next day after surgery patient had pain in right upper quadrant of abdomen. The drain was draining greenish fluid. A USG was done following which another drain tube was percutaneously inserted which also drained greenish fluid. The quantity of effluent gradually decreased over time. Patient was discharged 2 weeks after the surgery with 2 drain tubes in situ. The drain output reduced to nil by the 4th week after surgery following which both of them were removed.
- Now, since last one-month patient developed yellowish discoloration of sclera and high colored urine, which was insidious in onset and progressive in nature
- It was associated with generalized pruritus since last 3 weeks which does not interfere with his sleep
- Patient is passing normal colored stools
- It is associated with intermittent mild right upper quadrant abdominal pain, dull in nature, mild in intensity, non radiating, not related with meals or posture, relieved with oral medications.
- Patient has lost around 2 kg weight over last one month and his appetite is decreased.
- There is no history of:
    - Fever, chills
    - Nausea, vomiting
    - Easy bruisability

- o Abdominal distension, hematemesis, melena or altered sensorium
- o Loss of weight; loss of appetite
- For these symptoms patient was evaluated with MRI
- There is no previous history of diabetes, hypertension or TB.
- He has not undergone any other major surgery in the past.
- He used to previously smoke around 10 cigarettes per day and occasionally consume alcohol, both for the last 10 years.
- Family history is not contributory
- He is able to perform all his daily routine activity without any difficulty

Examination

- My patient is a young gentleman, who is averagely built, averagely nourished, with a height of 160 cm, weight of 55 kg and BMI being 21.5 kg/m^2
- He is conscious, co-operative, well oriented to time, place and person; Lying comfortably in bed; well hydrated and afebrile.
- Pulse is 72/min, BP is 110/70 mm Hg
- He is icteric and scratch marks are noted over his trunk.
- However, there is no pallor, cyanosis, clubbing, generalized or localized lymphadenopathy, pedal or dependent edema.
- There is no peripheral signs of chronic liver disease.
- Examination of oral cavity reveals adequate oral hygiene with no obvious mucosal lesions
- Examination of the abdomen:
    - o On inspection: Abdomen is flat, umbilicus is central, inverted. All quadrants are moving equally with respiration.
    - o 4 port site scars of laparoscopic cholecystectomy are seen. It is well healed and there is no cough impulse over it. Additionally, the scar of the previously placed percutaneous drain tube is also noted in the right hypochondrium.
    - o There is no visible lump, sinus, engorged veins, pulsations, peristalsis or cough impulse.
    - o Inspection of groin hernial sites reveals no swelling or cough impulse and Inspection of genitalia is unremarkable. Inspection of renal angles reveals no fullness
    - o On Palpation: Abdomen is soft and non-tender. Liver and spleen are not palpable. There isn't any other palpable lump.
    - o There is no tenderness, induration, bogginess or cough impulse over the scar.

- There is no palpable cough impulse over groin hernia sites and examination of genitals is unremarkable. There is no tenderness in renal angles. Examination of back and spine is essentially normal.
- On percussion, upper border of liver dullness is in the 5th intercostal space in midclavicular line with liver span being 14 cm. Rest of the abdomen is tympanitic with no evidence of free fluid.
- On auscultation normal bowel sounds are heard. There is no bruit, hum or rub
- Per rectal examination is unremarkable and the gloved finger is stained with normal colored stool.

- Examination of the respiratory system:
  - On auscultation, air entry is bilaterally equal with normal breath sounds heard
  - The breath holding time is 25 seconds.
- Rest systemic examination is essentially normal

To Summarize

- My patient is a 34 year old male with no co-morbid illness with WHO 0 performance status. He underwent a difficult laparoscopic cholecystectomy 3 months back for symptomatic cholelithiasis following which the intraoperatively placed drain started draining bilious effluent. An additional drain tube was inserted percutaneously which again drained bilious fluid. Now since one month he has developed features of progressive obstructive jaundice which is associated with right upper quadrant abdominal pain and loss of weight
- On examination he is icteric with scratch marks present. Scars of laparoscopic cholecystectomy and additional drain is seen

The most probable diagnosis in my patient is benign biliary stricture due to bile duct injury

How to Proceed in a case of BBS: (Sequence and justification)

- Review available medical records
- Liver Function Test and other Routine blood investigations (Hemogram, Renal Function Test, Serum Electrolyte, INR).
  - LFT to look for direct hyperbilirubinemia and raised alkaline phospatase levels.
  - Mild elevation of SGOT/SGPT in the setting of obstructive jaundice would suggest cholangitis
  - Raised INR is suggestive of coagulopathy

- X-ray chest as a part of routine work up
- USG (A+P): it is an extension of bed side clinical evaluation, it's cheap, non invasive and easily available
    - To look for presence or absence of intrahepatic biliary radical dilatation (IHBRD). If present it confirms the presence of obstructive jaundice

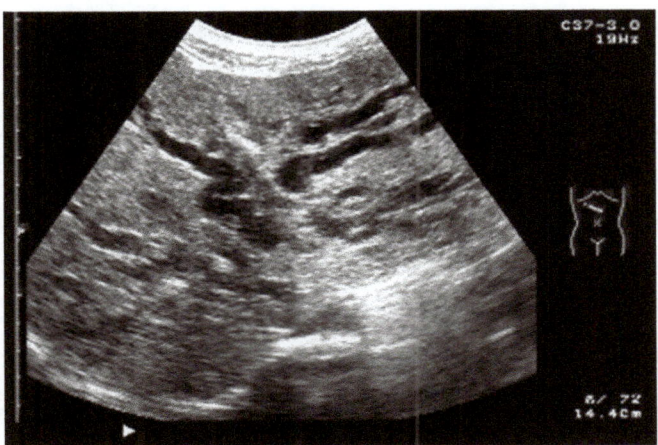

Figure 9.10: USG abdomen showing IHBRD.

    - To note the level of block: by noting the site till which the biliary system is dilated.
        - Dilated intrahepatic biliary ducts with non dilated extrahepatic biliary duct suggest block at hilar level. If present check if the right and left ductal systems are in continuity or are separated
        - Dilated intrahepatic biliary ducts, dilated common hepatic duct with non dilated common bile duct suggests block at level of cystic duct insertion
        - Dilated intrahepatic biliary ducts, dilated common hepatic duct and dilated common bile duct suggests block at level of lower CBD
        - Dilated intrahepatic biliary ducts, dilated common hepatic duct, dilated common bile duct and dilated pancreatic duct suggests block at level of ampulla.
    - To look for cause of block: in this case possibilities are stricture or residual/recurrent CBD stone
    - To look for presence of residual gall bladder with or without stone within it, cystic duct stump stone
    - To look for presence of collection/bilioma, cholangitic abscess

- To look for presence of stent/PTBD tube in situ
    - To look for presence of pneumobilia
    - To examine the vessels (hepatic artery, portal veins) for features of injury: lack of flow, altered flow velocity and pattern, thrombosis
    - Examine liver for features of cirrhosis
- CECT of the abdomen and pelvis:
    - To confirm presence of OJ by looking for IHBRD
    - To find the level of block to know of the Bismuth-Strasberg type of benign biliary stricture (BBS)
    - To examine the vessels (hepatic artery, portal vein) to rule out concomitant vascular injury. It is of medico-legal importance to rule out associated vascular injury prior to planning a reparative surgery.
    - To look for local complication: collection/bilioma, cholangitic abscess
- MRI abdomen with MRCP:
    - To obtain a cholangiogram to delineate the biliary anatomy
    - To classify the Bismuth-Strasberg type of BBS
    - It helps to better characterize the BBS, to note its proximal and distal extent. In case of hilar strictures it helps to note if there is separation of right and left ductal systems (type E4) or whether the continuity is maintained (type E3)
    - To look for associated vascular injury
    - Provides a road map for surgery

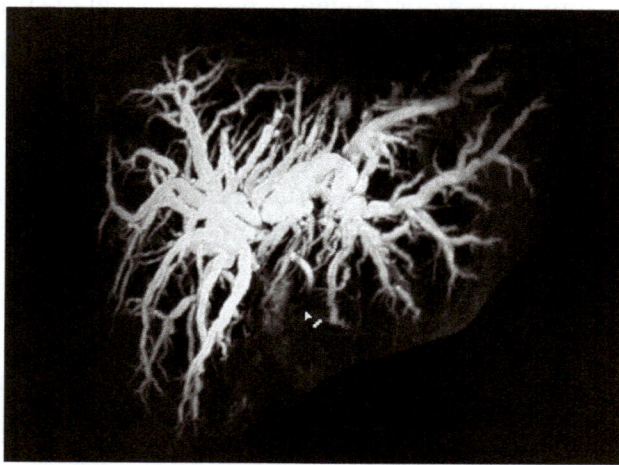

Figure 9.11: MRCP image revealing type E4 biliary stricture with separation of right and left main duct.

- Generally CECT is performed in the acute setting whereas MRI with MRCP is performed in the chronic setting
- ERCP (endoscopic retrograde cholangio-pancreaticography)
  - Provides cholangiogram
  - However, role in BBS is generally limited as bilio-enteric continuity is generally lost. In such a situation cut off will be present on cholangiogram and proximal bile duct wont get opacified
  - Hence it cannot provide roadmap for surgery
  - Additionally, it is invasive and associated with the risk of complications (e.g. cholangitis, pancreatitis)
  - However, on the contrary, if bilio-enteric continuity is maintained, therapeutic modality such as biliary stenting, stricture dilatation may be considered
- PTC (percutaneous transhepatic cholangiogram):
  - Provides cholangiogram and information about the proximal limit of the stricture thus helps in classifying the Bismuth-Strasberg type of BBS
  - However it is invasive and hence not routinely performed
  - It is only performed in case a PTBD (percutaneous transhepatic biliary drainage) is otherwise indicated (the most common indication being cholangitis)

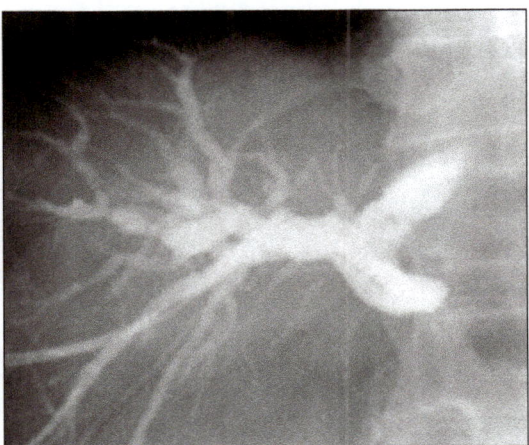

Figure 9.12: PTC showing type E1/E2 biliary stricture.

- Fistulogram:
  - May be performed in case a drain tube is present in situ. It involves injection of radio-opaque dye through it under fluoroscopy.
  - It is a cheaper alternative to MRCP and may give all the information necessary

- Biliary drainage:
  - Options:
    - PTBD: percutaneous transhepatic biliary drainage is the preferred mode of achieving biliary drainage in BBS
    - ERCP and biliary stenting may be alternatively considered if bilio-enteric continuity is maintained as previously discussed
  - Indications:
    - Cholangitis
    - Severe pruritus
    - Coagulopathy
    - Renal insufficiency
- Pre-op PTBC (percutaneous transhepatic biliary catheter) insertion may be selectively performed in difficult strictures (E4, E3) to facilitate identification of duct at surgery. It doubles as a trans-anastomotic stent post-op. It is usually inserted on or the day before planned surgery.
- Surgery:
  - Roux en y hepaticojejunostomy: Well vascularized, tension free, wide, side to side Roux en y hepaticojejunostomy performed using Kelly-Blumgart technique with fine absorbable sutures

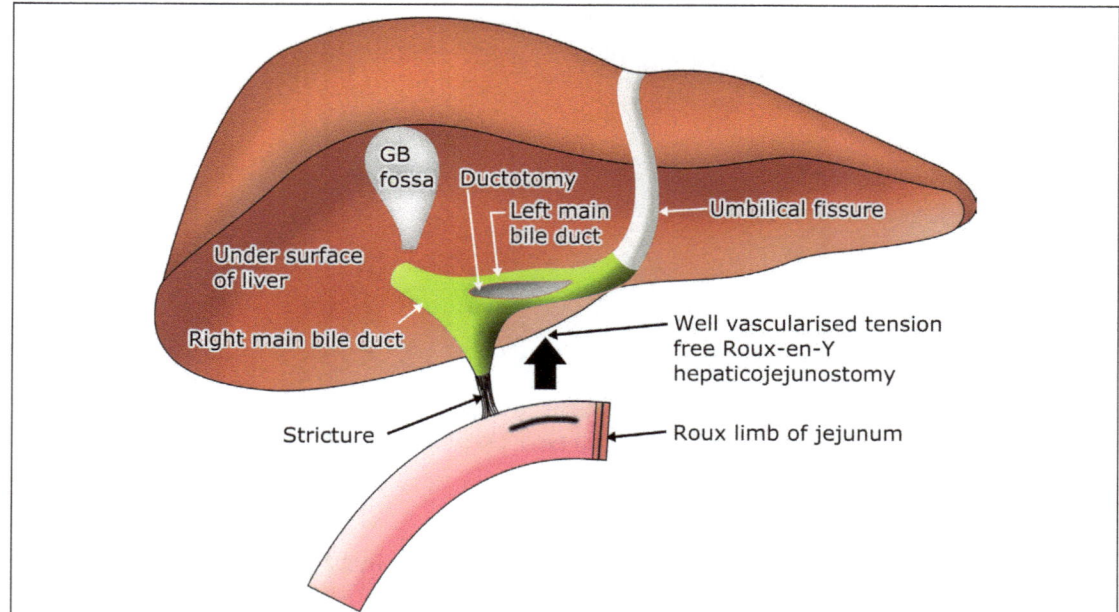

Figure 9.13: Roux-en-Y hepaticojejunostomy.

- Surveillance
- **Go through chapter 13 for literature on the subject.**

Principles of Management in the Acute Setting

- In the acute setting patients usually present with bile leak/bile in drain
- First step: blood tests including LFT followed by:
- USG A+P: to mainly look for:
    - Biloma/collection
    - IHBRD
    - Residual stone
- CECT A+P may be considered to give additional information, more than what we get on USG. It also gives information about concomitant vascular injury, if any.
- If a collection is present, one can proceed with USG guided tapping of the collection to confirm whether it is bile or not. If it's bile then USG/CT guided percutaneous catheter drainage of the collection should be considered. If there are multiple pockets of collection or bilious ascites laparoscopy/laparotomy with lavage and drain placement may have to be considered for source control.

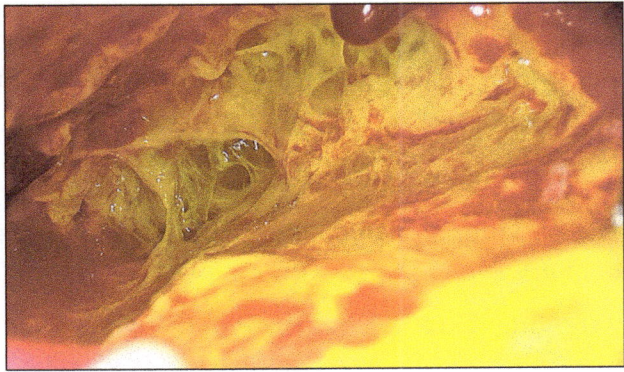

Figure 9.14: Intra-operative picture revealing an Organised Bilioma in a case of Bile Duct Injury.

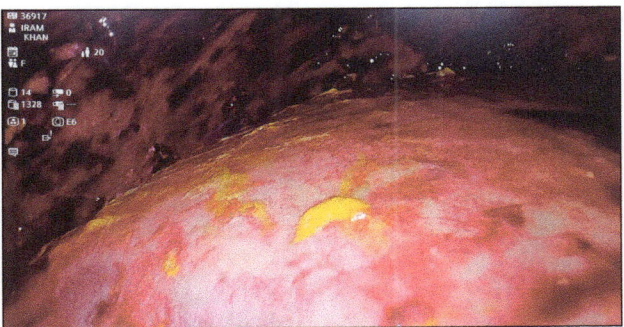

Figure 9.15: Intra-operative picture of after Laparoscopic Debridement, Lavage and Drainage.

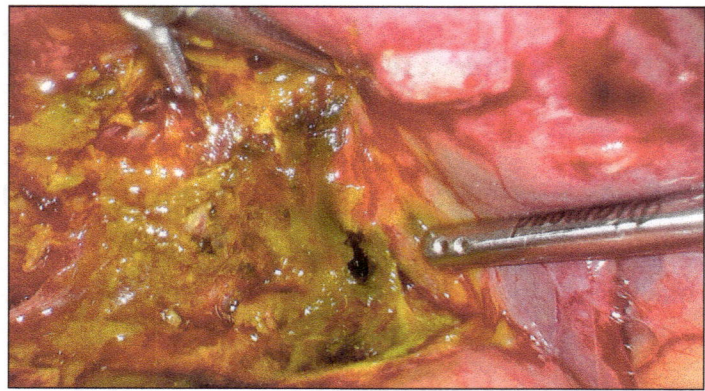

Figure 9.16: Intra-operative picture revealing the site of Bile Duct Injury.

- Next step in the management is to look at the trend of the drain;
  - Whether
    - It is high or low
    - Increasing or decreasing
    - Remaining bilious or becoming serous
  - Management changes accordingly
  - If drain output is high or increasing: investigate further with a cholangiogram (ERCP/MRCP) and proceed accordingly.
  - If it is low or decreasing: wait and watch
- MRI with MRCP: it provides cholangiogram and helps in identifying the Bismuth Strasberg type of injury and further treatment planning
- ERCP and biliary stenting: ERCP will help in identifying the Bismuth Strasberg type of injury.
  - In case where bilio-enteric continuity is maintained (i.e. type A and type D) biliary stenting may be performed which may be potentially therapeutic.
  - It is not feasible in classical injury where main bile duct is either clipped or ligated (i.e. type E) in which case a cut off will be seen on cholangiogram. In this situation MRCP may need to be considered.

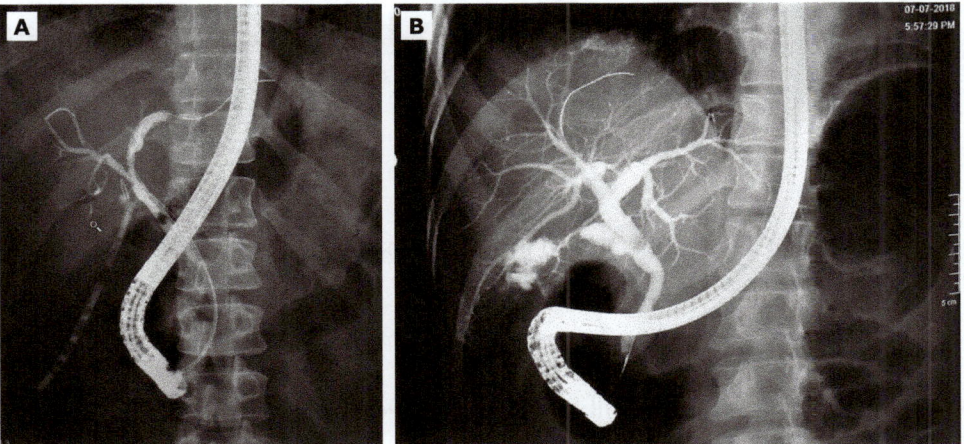

Figure 9.17: ERCP images showing type A injury (A) and type D injury (B).

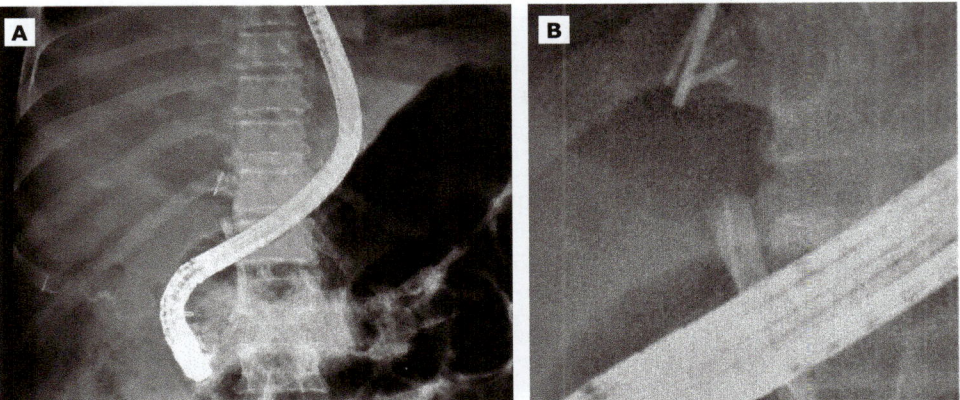

Figure 9.18: ERCP image showing complete 'Cut off' due to CBD clipping.

- If it is a case of type A or D injury: biliary stenting may suffice
- If it is a case of type B or C injury: wait and watch
- If it is a case of type E injury, the patient will in due course of time develop a BBS, management of which has been previously discussed.
- **Go through chapter 13 for literature on the subject.**

10 Case of Inflammatory Bowel Disease

Introduction

- Differentials that will be discussed in this chapter:
  - Ulcerative colitis
  - Crohn's disease
- Main focus of this chapter will be on ulcerative colitis. This is because UC is more likely to be kept in examinations.

Format for History Taking

- History of diarrhea/loose stools:
  - Volume: small or large quantity
  - Frequency of stools per day
  - Consistency of stools: watery/liquid/semi solids/solid (see Bristol Classification)
  - Foul smelling or not
  - Mixed with blood or not
  - Mixed with mucus or not
  - Total duration of disease

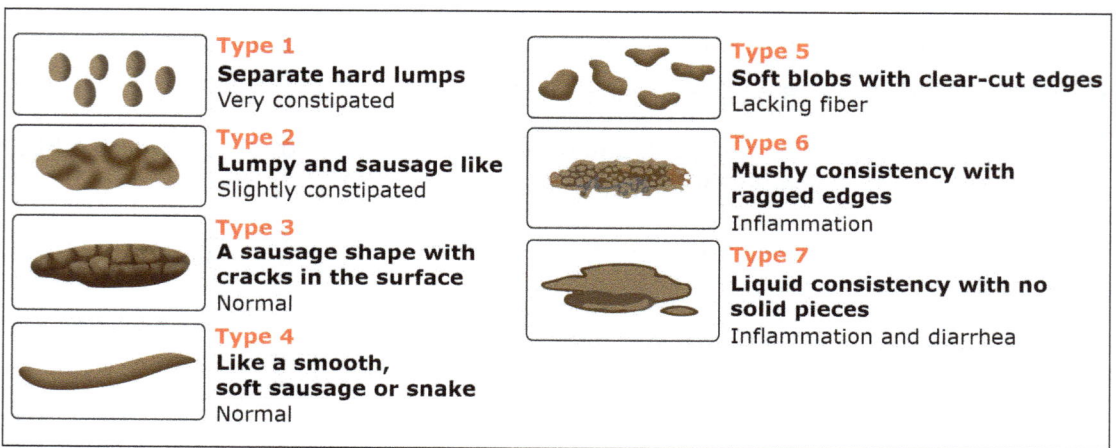

Figure 10.1: Bristol Stool Chart.

- History of sensation of incomplete evacuation, tenesmus, urgency; spurious diarrhea; nocturnal defecation.
- History of perianal pain; discharge; mass coming out per rectum; incontinence
- History of associated abdominal pain: crampy abdominal pain; left iliac fossa pain relieved by defecation
- History of Fever
- History of nausea, vomiting, abdominal distension, ball rolling sensation, borborygmi
- History of food intolerance
- History of remission and relapse of symptoms
- History of severe exacerbation in symptoms
- History suggestive of Extraintestinal manifestations:
  - Joint pain
  - Skin lesion: tender nodule or ulcers on leg or trunk
  - Red/watery eyes
- Presence of pruritus, fatigue, jaundice
- History of weight loss, Loss of appetite
- History of smoking, appendicectomy
- If presenting for first time with history of loose stools, ask for history of recent travel or outside food intake, radiation exposure, preceding antibiotic use
- Brief treatment history: evaluation with endoscopy, biopsy, cross sectional imaging. History of treatment with steroids, Azathioprine (azoran), Meslamine (mesocol) and biologicals. Additionally, history of hospital admission, ICU stay, need for blood transfusion and surgery need to be inquired.
- History suggestive of complications of Steroids: frequent infection, weight gain, facial puffiness, diminished vision because of cataract formation, fracture with trivial injury, new onset diabetes, dyspepsia (steroids induced gastric ulcers), psychiatric problems (depression)
- Past history of comorbid illness and surgery
- Personal history: alcohol history, red meat consumption, married or unmarried, family completed or not.
- Menstrual history
- Family history of IBD
- Performance history: ability to perform daily routine activities.

Justification for Each Component in History

- History of diarrhea/loose stools: patients with UC and Crohn's colitis present with symptoms of passage of loose stools multiple times per day, which is usually mixed with blood and mucus. Based on frequency, volume, consistency and smell one can differentiate between small and large bowel diarrhea.

- Large bowel diarrhea: Frequent passage of small volume, non offensive, semi solid stools mixed with blood and mucus suggests large bowel diarrhea.
- Small bowel diarrhea: Infrequent, large volume, foul smelling, watery diarrhea suggests small bowel diarrhea.
- Also frequency of bloody stools is one of the factors included in Truelove and Witts criteria used to grade severity of ulcerative colitis:

Table 10.1: True-Love and Witts criteria

- Frequency of bloody stools:
  - Mild: upto 4 stools/day with or without blood
  - Moderate: 4–6 stools/day
  - Severe: > 6 bloody stools/day
- Fever:
  - Mild: < 37.5°C
  - Moderate: 37.5–37.8°C
  - Severe: > 37.8°C
- Pulse:
  - Mild: < 90 bpm
  - Moderate: </= 90 bpm
  - Severe: > 90 bpm
- Hemoglobin:
  - Mild: > 11.5 g/dl
  - Moderate: 10.5–11.5 g/dl
  - Severe: < 10.5 g/dl
- ESR:
  - Mild: < 20 mm/h
  - Moderate: 20–30 mm/h
  - Severe: > 30 mm/h
- CRP:
  - Mild: normal
  - Moderate: </= 30 mg/L
  - Severe: > 30 mg/L

- Total duration of diarrhea: patients with IBD will have a prolonged disease course with onset in the 2nd or 3rd decade of life. Second peak is in 4th–5th decade. Natural history consists of episodes of disease relapse and remission. A small proportion of patients with UC will have acute severe colitis at index presentation necessitating emergency surgery.

- History of sensation of incomplete evacuation: It is a pointer towards rectal malignancy.

- Urgency and tenesmus are irritative rectal symptom. It could be suggestive of an inflammatory disease process in rectum (e.g. Inflammatory bowel disease) or rectal malignancy. Tenesmus has been variably defined as "the sensation of incomplete defecation" or "a repeated painful urge to defecate without excreting stool". Urgency refers to the urgent urge to pass stools.

- Nocturnal defecation is again an irritative rectal symptom suggestive of rectal inflammation seen in UC

- History of spurious diarrhea: (spurious=not real) it is a condition in which patient attempts to empty rectum several times a day, often passing flatus and a little amount of blood stained mucus or liquid mucus mixed feces. It is seen in carcinoma rectum and fecal impaction.

  Patients with long standing UC are at risk of developing malignancy, hence symptoms of sensation of incomplete evacuation, urgency, tenesmus, spurious diarrhea should all be asked for

- History of perianal pain: It suggests fissure in ano, peri anal abscess. Perineal involvement in form of fissure, fistula, abscess and skin tags is more commonly seen in Crohn's colitis compared to ulcerative colitis and its presence points towards the diagnosis of Crohn's disease.

- History of discharge: it suggests fistula in ano, ruptured peri anal abscess.

- History of mass per rectum: it could suggest either tumor, prolapsed internal hemorrhoids, external hemorrhoids, skin tag and rectal prolapse. To differentiate inquire if it is soft (benign) or firm (neoplastic), prolapsing with straining (hemorrhoids/rectal prolapse) or not, reducible (hemorrhoids/rectal prolapse) or not.

- History of incontinence: it can either be true incontinence due to sphincter damage as in perineal involvement by Crohn's disease or less commonly UC (such as fistula or abscess). Alternatively sphincter may get damaged during surgical management of fistula or abscess. Also, the sphincter may be infiltrated in patients with ano-rectal malignancy resulting in incontinence. Frequent passage of loose stools may lead to occasional seepage of liquid stools. Presence of incontinence has surgical implications. If incontinence is present, an end ileostomy may be preferable to a sphincter saving surgery such as ileal pouch anal anastomosis after a total proctocolectomy.

- History of urinary symptoms, especially fecaluria, if present, suggests recto-urinary fistula.
- History of associated abdominal pain: patients with UC may have crampy abdominal pain and left iliac fossa pain relieved by defecation.
- History of colicky abdominal pain, nausea, vomiting, abdominal distension, ball rolling sensation, borborygmi: all are suggestive of intestinal obstruction. This is especially true in patients with Crohn's disease where small bowel involvement is more common.
- History of Fever: fever may be present as a part of systemic inflammatory response syndrome. Or it may be a pointer towards presence of an intraabdominal inflammatory pathology such as abscess, phlegmon.
- History of food intolerance: could suggest allergy as cause for diarrhea, for example lactose intolerance, gluten enteropathy.
- History of severe exacerbation in symptoms: suggests an episode of acute severe colitis.
- History of joint pain suggests extraintestinal manifestation of IBD namely arthritis and ankylosing spondylitis.
- History of skin lesion: presence of tender nodule on leg or trunk suggests erythema nodosum. Presence of ulcers on leg or trunk suggests pyoderma gangrenosum. Both of which are extraintestinal manifestations of IBD.
- History of red/watery eyes suggests extraintestinal manifestation of IBD namely iritis and uveitis.
- Presence of pruritus, fatigue, jaundice: suggests presence of Primary Sclerosing Cholangitis.
- History of postural dizziness, syncope, fatigue, shortness of breath, need for blood transfusion: to quantify the blood loss.
- History of weight loss, Loss of appetite: weight loss could be due to chronic inflammation, decreased food intake or malignancy. Decreased food intake may be due to loss of appetite (due to SIRS) or food fear.
- History of smoking: smoking is considered to be an etiological factor for Crohn's disease and is known to aggravate disease severity. Whereas it is protective in case of UC.

- History of appendicectomy: appendicectomy at early age is considered to be protective against UC.
- History of recent travel or outside food intake could suggest infective etiology for diarrhea.
- History of radiation exposure: could suggest radiation enteritis as cause for diarrhea.
- History of preceding antibiotic use could suggest Clostridium deffcile as the cause for diarrhea (pseudomembranous colitis).
- Brief treatment history: patients diagnosed with IBD will be started on steroids, Azathioprine (azoran), Meslamine (mesocol) or biologicals (infliciximab or adalimumab) either individually or in combination. If patient is on long term steroids inquire about history suggestive of complications of Steroid.
- History of hospital admission, ICU stay, need for surgery all suggest severe disease. Surgery if performed, note: if it was an emergency or elective surgery. Was it done as a part of staged surgery and whether a stoma was created.
    - Surgery in UC is curative and is usually performed as a staged procedure: 3 stage, 2 stage, modified 2 stage or less commonly single staged.
    - 3 staged: usually done in emergency setting. Colectomy with ileostomy > completion proctectomy with ileal pouch anal anastomosis with diverting ileotomy > stoma reversal.
    - 2 staged: total proctocolectomy with IPAA with diverting ileostomy > stoma reversal.
    - Modified 2 stage: colectomy with ileostomy > completion proctectomy with IPAA without diverting stoma.
    - Single stage: total proctocolectomy with IPAA. Usually done in elective setting in a well preserved patient.
- Personal history: history of red meat consumption: red meat consumption is an etiological factor for IBD. Also note if patient is married or not and if family is completed or not. This has surgical implications as proctectomy may lead to infertility. Hence if the patient is unmarried or if family is not complete then surgery needs to be deferred, if possible. If surgery cannot be deferred option of sperm or ovum banking needs to be explained to the patient.
- Family history of IBD: IBD has a genetic component, for example NOD2 gene mutation.
- Performance history: to clinically assess fitness for surgery.

- Remember:
  - The clinical presentation of Crohn's disease is different than that of UC. UC presents as described above with bloody loose stools and systemic symptoms. This is because UC is limited to colon.
  - Crohn's disease on the other hand may have a more varied presentation because CD may involve any part of the GI tract (anywhere from the mouth to anus). Also, the manifestation varies with the pattern of the disease.

> **Table 10.2: Montreal classification for Crohn's disease**
>
> - Age of onset:
>   - A1: < 17 years
>   - A2: 17–40 years
>   - A3: > 40 years
> - Location:
>   - L1: Terminal ileum with or without cecum
>   - L2: Colon
>   - L3: Ileum plus colon
>   - L4: Proximal small bowel
> - Pattern:
>   - B1: Non structuring non penetrating
>   - B2: Stricturing
>   - B3: Penetrating

  - So, a patient with L1, B2 disease will have features of intestinal obstruction such as colicky abdominal pain, abdominal distension, nausea, vomiting, ball rolling sensation and borborygmi.
  - Patient with L2 disease will have features similar to UC
  - Patient with L3 disease will have features of UC and additionally will also have features of L1 disease such as colicky abdominal pain, abdominal distension, nausea, vomiting, ball rolling sensation and borborygmi.
  - As discussed previously patient with B2 pattern of disease will usually have feature of intestinal obstruction. Patients with B1 pattern of disease will present with pain, fever, GI bleed. B3 disease pattern results in either free bowel perforation, contained bowel perforation, Abscess formation, phlegmon

formation, internal fistula or external fistula. Free perforation is an emergency situation and such patient won't be kept in exams. Patient with phlegmon/abscess formation present with pain, fever and lump in abdomen with or without features of intestinal obstruction. Internal fistulas manifest variably, patient may even be asymptomatic. Entero/colo vesical fistula present with features of urinary tract infection. Cardinal feature is fecaluria. External fistula or entero/colo cutaneous are usually post surgical, and manifest with discharge of pus/stools from the skin.

Format for Examination

- What is the appearance of the patient: young/middle-aged/elderly, lady/gentleman: generally young
- Whether the patient is clinically
    - Poorly/averagely/well built
    - Poorly/averagely/well nourished
    - Generally poorly built and nourished
- Measure height, weight, BMI
- Whether the patient is clinically
    - Conscious/stuporous
    - Co-operative/unco-operative
    - Well/poorly oriented to time, place and person
    - Lying comfortably in bed/in discomfort/in pain(rolling in pain)
    - Well hydrated/dehydrated (important to mention as patient may be dehydrated due to frequent passage of loose stools)
    - Febrile/Afebrile
- Mention Pulse, BP
- Look for
    - Pallor, jaundice (primary sclerosing cholangitis), cyanosis, clubbing
    - Generalized or localized lymphadenopathy
    - Palpable left supraclavicular lymph node
    - Pedal or dependent edema
    - Skin lesions: look for skin lesions like erythema nodosum, pyoderma gangrenosum, both of which are extra-intestinal manifestation of IBD. Also look for scratch marks (suggestive of primary sclerosing cholangitis)

- o Joints: look for inflamed, erythematous, swollen joints with restricted movements suggesting arthritis
- o Signs of chronic liver disease (primary sclerosing cholangitis)
- Examination of oral cavity: look for apthous ulcers which may be seen in patients with Crohn's disease.
- Examination of the abdomen:
  - o On Inspection: See if:
    - Abdomen is flat/distended/scaphoid
    - Umbilicus is central/displaced(upwards/downwards/sideways) inverted/everted/flat.
    - All quadrants are moving equally with respiration or not (there may be localized or generalized restriction to abdominal wall movement with respiration in case of localized or generalized peritonitis)
    - See if there is any visible lump
    - Look for visible scar, sinus, engorged veins, pulsations, peristalsis or cough impulse.
    - Mention scars of previous surgeries (generally vertical midline)
    - Describe stoma if any:
      - Describe its site:
        - Right lower quadrant fossa (ileostomy)
        - Right upper quadrant (transverse colostomy)
        - Left lower quadrant (sigmoidostomy)
      - Pouting (ileostomy) or flush with skin (colostomy)
      - Whether there is single lumen (end stoma) or two lumen visible (loop or double barreled stoma)
      - Effluent: Enteric (small bowel) or fecal (colon)
      - Look for any mucosal lesion as in erythema, granularity, erosion or ulcer
      - Health of surrounding skin (whether there is any excoriation).
      - Look for complications: common ones are:
        - Prolapse
        - Sunken stoma
        - Peri-stomal hernia
      - Based on these we can guess whether it is an ileostomy or colostomy

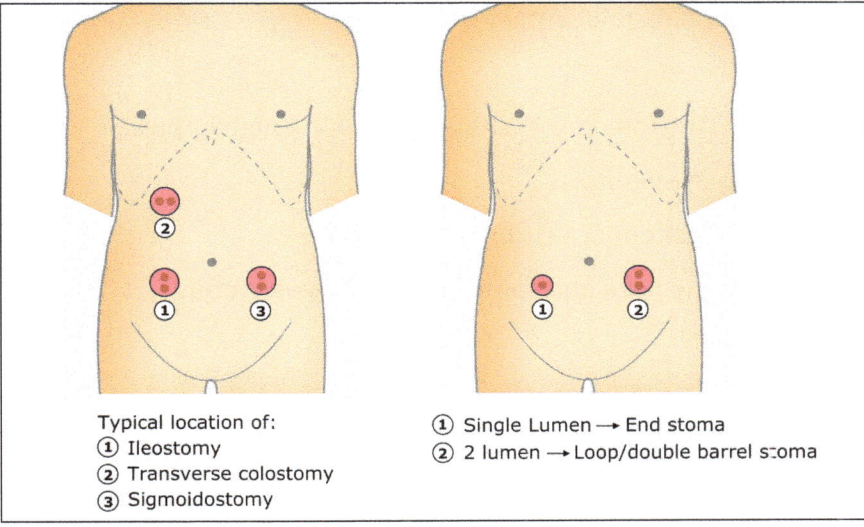

Figure 10.2: Stoma.

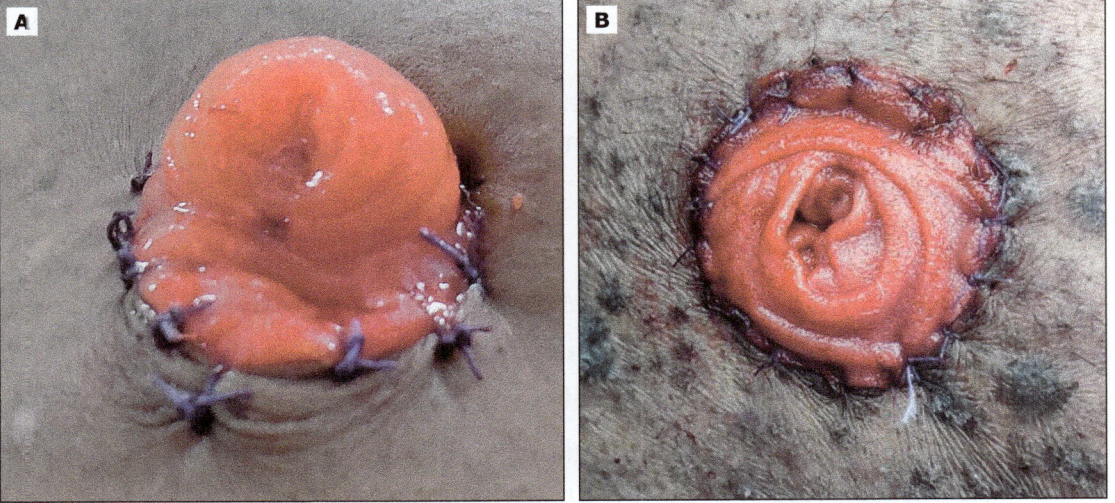

Figure 10.3: (A) Pouting Ileostomy; (B) Flush Colostomy.

- Don't forget to inspect the groin hernial sites (to look for swelling or cough impulse i.e. hernia) and genitalia.
- Inspection of renal angles to look for fullness

o On palpation: See if:
  - Abdomen is soft and non-tender (Alternatively abdomen could be rigid and/or tender)
  - Liver is palpable or not
  - Spleen is enlarged or not

- Any other palpable lump.
- Do not forget to:
  - Palpate groin hernia sites to look for cough impulse
  - Examine genitals
  - Look for tenderness in renal angles
  - Examine back and spine for tenderness/gibbus.
- On Percussion:
  - Look for upper border of liver dullness (generally in the 5th intercostal space) in midclavicular line.
  - Note the liver span (normal being 12–14 cm)
  - Note in the rest of the abdomen (generally tympanitic)
  - Tests for free fluid
- On auscultation:
  - Auscultate for bowel sounds. Hear for hyperperistaltic bowel sounds, if there is clinical suspicion of intestinal obstruction
  - Bruit, hum and rub

- Per rectal examination: The format is as follows:
  - Examination of perianal area: Look for fissure, skin tag, external hemorrhoids, external opening of fistula in ano, perianal abscess, sinus, growth or prolapse
  - Note if patient is using any kind of diaper or pad
  - Do not forget to look for excoriation of perianal skin due to feces in a patient with incontinence or in a patient using diaper.
  - Digital rectal examination: with a gloved finger: to note tone, to palpate for any mucosal lesion
  - If present, note:
    - The distance of the growth from anal verge.
    - The longitudinal extent in cm
    - Circumferential extent to be mentioned as extending from …..'O' clock to …..'O' clock
    - Proximal extent of the growth
    - Consistency: soft/firm/hard

- Form: Ulcerative/proliferative/ulcero-proliferative/polypoidal
- Fixity: Fixed or not
- Do not forget to note tone and squeeze pressure and mention it as first point in DRE. This is of importance in operative planning. If the sphincter function is poor sphincter salvage may not be possible.
- Also note what is seen on the gloved finger: normal stool/blood/mucus/pus.
  - Perform proctoscopy if available. In case of IBD you can expect to look for erythematous, inflamed, granular, friable mucosa with ulcers or erosion

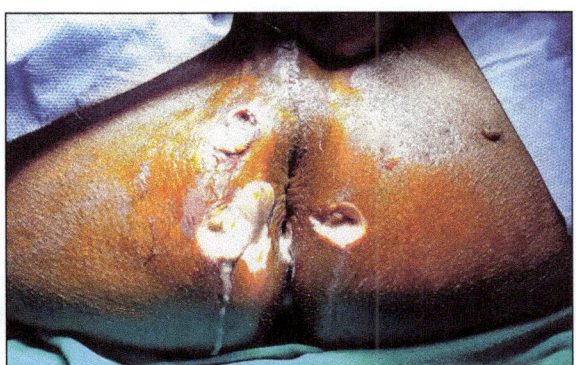

Figure 10.4: Peri-anal Crohn's disease.

- Rest systemic examination
- Remember:
  - Look for central line and if any parenteral nutrition is ongoing.
  - In super speciality exams it is possible to get cases who have completed their surgical treatment and now are presenting with recurrent symptoms due to pouchitis.
  - Patients with Crohn's disease may present with intestinal obstruction (most probably subacute, if kept in examinations) (small bowel obstruction is much more common than large bowel obstruction). In such patients with small bowel SAIO, look for clinical findings such as abdominal distension, step ladder pattern of peristalsis, hyperperistaltic bowel sounds. On general examination also check for tachycardia and dehydration. Alternatively they may present with lump in abdomen due to phlegmon formation (less commonly abscess). In such patients there may be tachycardia and fever on general examination. On abdominal examination mention the following characteristic of the lump:

- Site
- Size
- Shape,
- Surface
- Margins
- Tenderness
- Warmth
- Consistency
- Mobility
- Movement with respiration
- Plane: intraperitoneal or retroperitoneal

EXAMPLE CASE

History

- My patient Mr XYZ, is a 24-year-old unmarried gentleman hailing from Mumbai, is a 3rd year engineering student.
- He presented with chief complaints of on and off passage of bloody stools since 4 months.
- Patient's history dates back to 4 months back when he started passing blood mixed stools which was non foul smelling, small in quantity, semisolid in consistency, 2-3 times per day. Over time the frequency has increased such that he passes blood mixed stools around 4–5 times per day.
- It is associated with mild intermittent crampy left lower quadrant abdominal pain since last 3.5 months, which is insidious in onset and relieved on passing stools.
- It is also associated with occasional low-grade fever, not associated with chills which resolves with medications.
- There is no:
  - History of sensation of incomplete evacuation, tenesmus, urgency; spurious diarrhea; nocturnal defecation.
  - History of perianal pain; discharge; mass coming out per rectum; incontinence
  - History of nausea, vomiting, abdominal distension, ball rolling sensation, borborygmi

- o   History of food intolerance
- o   History of joint pain; skin lesion, tender nodule or ulcers on leg or trunk; and red/watery eyes
- o   History of pruritus, fatigue, jaundice
- o   History of weight loss, Loss of appetite
- o   History of smoking, appendicectomy
- o   History of recent travel or outside food intake
- For these symptoms patient had consumed some over the counter medications 3 months back, following which symptoms temporarily reduced only to relapse again.
- He seeked medical care for these symptoms last week following which he was evaluated with colonoscopy and biopsy.
- No history of any other comorbid illness, TB or surgery
- No history of smoking, alcohol or red meat consumption,
- Patient is unmarried
- There is no history of IBD or cancer in first degree relatives
- Patient is not able to perform strenuous activities but is able to perform all daily self care

Examination

- My patient is a young gentleman, who is averagely built, averagely nourished, with a height of 160 cm, weight of 55 kg and BMI being 21.5 kg/m^2
- He is conscious, co-operative, well oriented to time, place and person; Lying comfortably in bed; well hydrated and afebrile.
- Pulse is 80/min, BP is 110/70 mm Hg
- There is no pallor, jaundice, cyanosis, clubbing, generalized or localized lymphadenopathy. There is no palpable left supraclavicular lymph node; pedal or dependent edema, arthritic joints, red eye, skin lesions or scratch marks
- Examination of oral cavity reveals adequate oral hygiene with no obvious mucosal lesions
- Examination of the abdomen:
  - o   On inspection: Abdomen is flat, umbilicus is central, inverted. All quadrants are moving equally with respiration. There is no visible lump, scar, sinus, engorged veins, pulsations, peristalsis or cough impulse.

- o Inspection of groin hernial sites reveals no swelling or cough impulse and Inspection of genitalia is unremarkable. Inspection of renal angles reveals no fullness
- o On Palpation: Abdomen is soft and non-tender. Liver and spleen are not palpable. There isn't any other palpable lump.
- o There is no palpable cough impulse over groin hernia sites and examination of genitals is unremarkable. There is no tenderness in renal angles. Examination of back and spine is essentially normal.
- o On percussion, upper border of liver dullness is in the 5th intercostal space in midclavicular line with liver span being 14 cm. Rest of the abdomen is tympanitic with no evidence of free fluid.
- o On auscultation normal bowel sounds are heard. There is no bruit, hum or rub
- Examination of perianal area reveals no fissure, skin tag, external hemorrhoids, external opening of fistula in ano, perianal abscess, sinus, growth, prolapse or perianal excoriation.
- On digital rectal examination, tone is normal, squeeze pressure is good. There is no palpable growth
- Proctoscopic examination reveals erythematous, granular appearing rectal mucosa.
- Rest systemic examination is essentially normal

To Summarize

- My patient is a 24 year old male with no co-morbid illness with WHO 1 performance status, presents with 4 months history of frequent passage of blood mixed semisolid stools, associated with crampy left lower quadrant abdominal pain and low grade fever
- Proctoscopic evaluation reveals erythematous granular mucosa. Otherwise general and abdominal examination is unremarkable

The most probable diagnosis in my patient is inflammatory bowel disease, most likely ulcerative colitis

How to Proceed: (Sequence and justification)

- Review available medical records
- Routine blood investigations (Hemogram, Liver Function Test, Renal Function Test, Serum Electrolyte, INR).
  - o LFT needs to be done to look for features of primary sclerosing cholangitis (raised bilirubin and alkaline phosphatase levels)

- Additional blood tests: ESR, CRP, ASCA testing
  - CRP has an important role in the evaluation of IBD patients. Higher the level, more the local and systemic inflammation
- Stool tests:
  - Stool routine microscopy and stool culture to rule out infectious colitis; clostridium difficile toxin assay to rule out pseudomembranous colitis;
  - Fecal calprotectin: levels rise in case of intestinal mucosal inflammation. Higher the levels more the mucosal damage.
- X-ray chest as a routine
- X-ray abdomen: in case obstruction, perforation or toxic megacolon is clinically suspected. In case of obstruction multiple air fluid levels will be seen. In case of perforation free gas under diaphragm may be seen. In toxic megacolon grossly distended colon will be noted.
- Colonoscopy:
  - For the endoscopic diagnosis of IBD by looking for inflamed colonic mucosa
  - To see for site, extent and severity of inflammation (Mayo Endoscopic Score)
  - To look for complications such as stricture, DALM (dysplasia associated lesion or mass), adenoma or carcinoma
  - To examine the ileum for presence of inflammation which would suggest either Crohn's disease or backwash ileitis in UC
  - To obtain biopsy for histopathological confirmation
  - Ulcerative colitis:
    - In UC there will be contiguous, circumferential symmetric involvement from the rectum proximally. Rectum is almost always involved. Perianal involvement is rare
    - Typical endoscopic findings include: edema, erythema, loss of vascular markings, granularity, pseudo-polyp, mucosal friability, erosions and bleed on touch. Ulcers and strictures are less common
    - It is important to know the extent of the disease involvement to classify the disease as per the Montreal Classification.

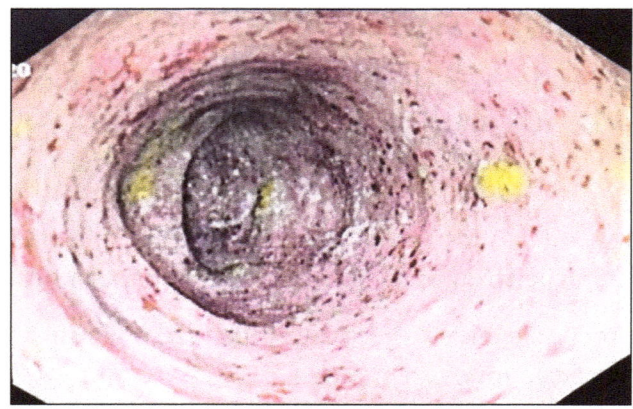

Figure 10.5: Colonoscopic findings in UC.

\multicolumn{3}{l}{Table 10.3: Mayo Endoscopic Score}
Score	Disease activity	Endoscopic features
0	Normal	None
1	Mild	Erythema, Decreased vascular pattern, Mild friability
2	Moderate	Marked Erythema, Absent vascular pattern, Friability, Erosions
3	Severe	Spontaneous bleeding, Ulceration

Table 10.4: Montreal classification for Ulcerative colitis

- Extent of colitis:
  - E1: ulcerative proctitis: limited to rectum; proximal extent being recto-sigmoid junction
  - E2: left sided colitis: disease limited to the left colon: proximal extent being splenic flexure.
  - E3: extensive colitis: disease extends proximal to the splenic flexure. It includes pancolitis and backwash ileitis.
- Severity of disease:
  - S0: Clinical remission
  - S1: Mild disease as per True Love and Witts criteria (discussed previously)
  - S2: moderate disease as per True Love and Witts criteria
  - S3: severe disease as per True Love and Witts criteria

- o Crohn's disease
    - Rectum is generally spared. Skip lesions are characteristic. Perianal involvement is common
    - Typical endoscopic findings include: edema, erythema, cobble-stoning, erosions and apthous ulcers. Ulcers and strictures are more common
    - See Montreal Classification of Crohn's disease which has been previously discussed
- Upper GI endoscopy: to rule out proximal GI involvement in case of CD.
- Cross sectional imaging:
    - o It has a more important role in evaluation of Crohn's disease as compared to UC.
    - o Importance lies in its ability to identify small bowel involvement, which if present suggests diagnosis of CD over UC.
    - o It also helps in the evaluation of complications of IBD
    - o Penetrating pattern of CD may result in internal and/or external fistula, abscess, mass, perforation, all of which are best evaluated with cross sectional imaging.
    - o Stricturing pattern of CD may result in features of intestinal obstruction which again is better evaluated using cross sectional imaging.
    - o Additionally evaluation of liver and biliary system is possible which will help to rule out PSC
    - o USG (A+P): It is an extension of bed side clinical evaluation, it's cheap, non invasive and easily available
        - May be performed
            - To examine the liver if PSC is clinically suspected
            - To look for collection/abscess
    - o CT: including CECT (A+P) with oral, rectal and IV contrast, CT enterography (oral administration of contrast), CT enteroclysis (administration of contrast via naso-jejunal tube):
        - For the radiographic diagnosis of IBD
        - To identify site, extent and pattern disease
        - To look for complications: obstruction, perforation, phlegmon, abscess, fistula, cancer
        - Findings suggestive of IBD include:
            - Bowel wall thickening

- Mucosal hyperenhancement
- Halo sign
- Comb sign
- Loss of haustrations of colon

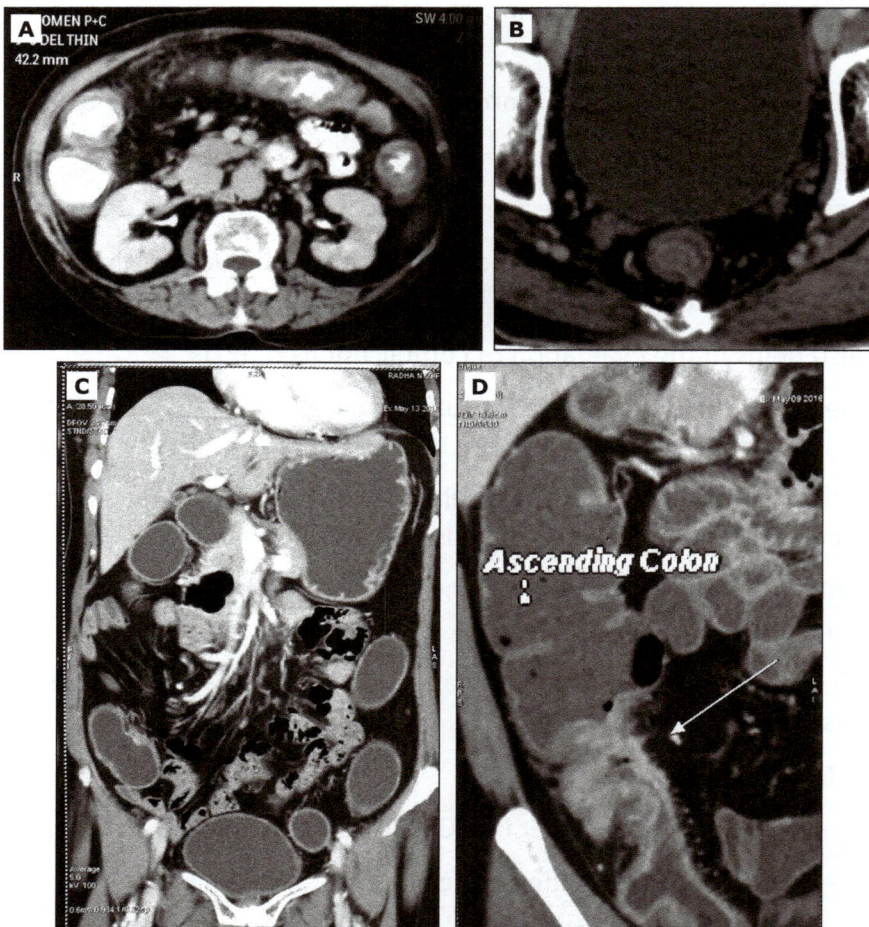

Figure 10.6: CT findings suggestive of IBD: Wall thickening (A), Mucosal hyperenhancement with submucosal hypo-enhancement (B), Comb sign (C) and Stricture (D).

- o MRI: including MRI (A+P) with oral, rectal and IV contrast, MRI enterography (oral administration of contrast), MRI enteroclysis (administration of contrast via naso-jejunal tube):
    - Role is similar to CT.
    - Additionally, MRI pelvis is used for evaluation of perianal CD
    - And it provides cholangiogram to help rule out PSC

- Advantage:
  - No ionizing radiation
  - May be performed in patients with deranged renal functions
- Disadvantage:
  - Long acquisition time
  - Expensive
  - Not easily available
  - Risk of contrast associated nephrogenic systemic fibrosis

• Additional investigations:
  o Capsule endoscopy: To rule out small bowel involvement

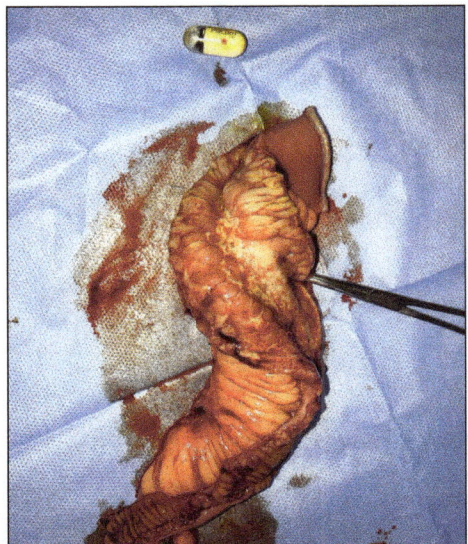

Figure 10.7: Bowel stricture causing retention of capsule. This may be prevented by trial administration of degradable patency capsule.

  o Enteroscopy: To rule out small bowel involvement
    - Push enteroscopy
    - Single or double balloon enteroscopy
    - Spiral enteroscopy
  o Barium meal follow through
  o Enteroclysis

- Principles of treatment of CD
  - Treatment is primarily medical with surgical modality being used selectively. This is because CD can affect any part of GIT from mouth to anus and it will be impossible to extirpate all the involved bowel.
  - Aim is to achieve and maintain remission while preventing relapse
  - Medical treatment options
    - 5-aminosalycilic acid, mesalamine
    - Azathioprine
    - Steroids: hydrocortisone, prednisolone
    - Biological: infliximab, adalimumab
  - Induction is usually done with steroids and maintenance with 5-ASA or azathioprine
  - Alternatively biological may be used for both induction and maintenance. Azathioprine is usually administered with biological to prevent formation of anti-drug antibodies.
  - Surgery:
    - Indications
      - Obstruction
      - Perforation
      - Un-resolving phlegmon/abscess
      - Intractable disease
      - Internal or external fistula
      - Growth retardation
      - Bleeding
      - Malignancy
    - Options:
      - Resection and anastomosis
      - Resection and stoma creation
      - Stricturoplasty

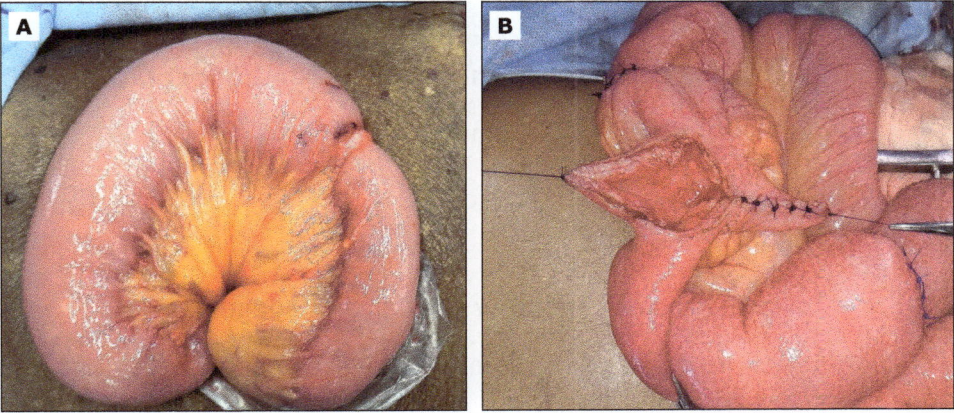

Figure 10.8: Heineke Mikulicz stricturoplasty.

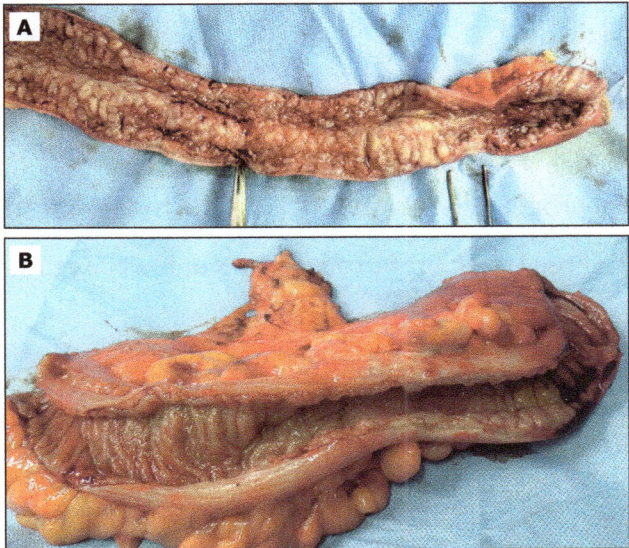

Figure 10.9: Segmental intestinal resection specimens showing features of Crohn's disease: Bowel wall thickening, mucosal ulceration, cobble-stoning, mesenteric fat creeping.

- Principles of treatment of UC
    - As UC is restricted to colon (except in rare cases of backwash ileitis) surgery with extirpation of entire colon and rectum is potentially curative
    - However trial at remission by medical management is generally recommended. This is because majority of the patients are young with many social and academic obligations and who have not completed their family (surgery may lead to infertility).
    - Medical treatment options
        - 5-aminosalycilic acid, mesalamine: oral and/or per rectal

- Azathioprine
- Steroids: hydrocortisone, prednisolone: oral and/or per rectal
- Biological: infliximab, adalimumab
- Surgery:
  - Indications
    - Toxic megacolon refractory to medical management
    - Severe acute colitis refractory to medical management
    - Bleeding
    - Perforation
    - Malignancy
    - Intractable disease
  - Options:
    - Total proctocolectomy with ileal pouch-anal anastomosis (IPAA)
      - Three stage: preferred in cases of toxic megacolon or severe acute colitis
        - 1st stage: colectomy with end ileostomy
        - 2nd stage: completion proctectomy with IPAA and diversion loop ileostomy
        - 3rd stage: stoma reversal
      - Two stage: preferred in elective cases
        - 1st stage: total procto-colectomy with IPAA and loop ileostomy
        - 2nd stage: stoma reversal
      - Modified two stage:
        - 1st stage: colectomy with end ileostomy
        - 2nd stage: completion proctectomy with IPAA
      - Single stage: least preferred
        - Whole surgery performed in a single stage

CHAPTER 10: CASE OF INFLAMMATORY BOWEL DISEASE   237

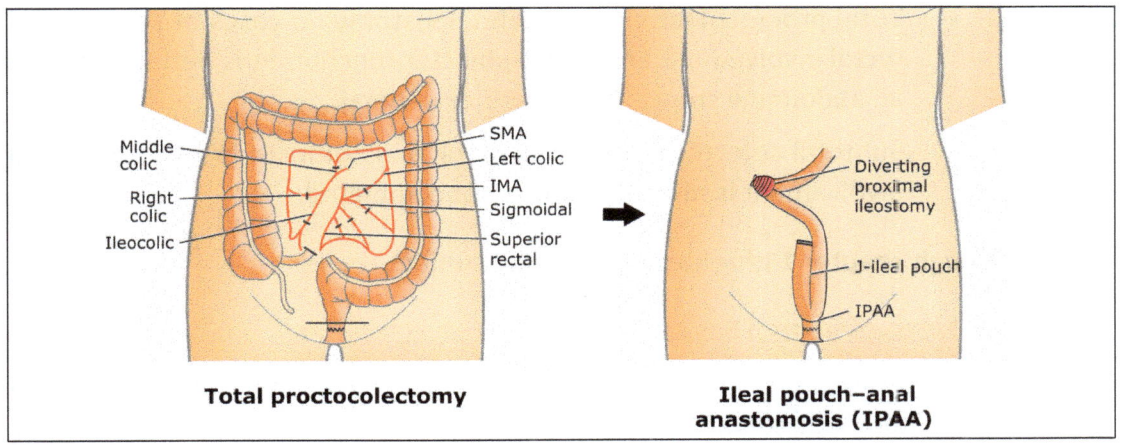

Figure 10.10: Total proctocolectomy with IPAA.

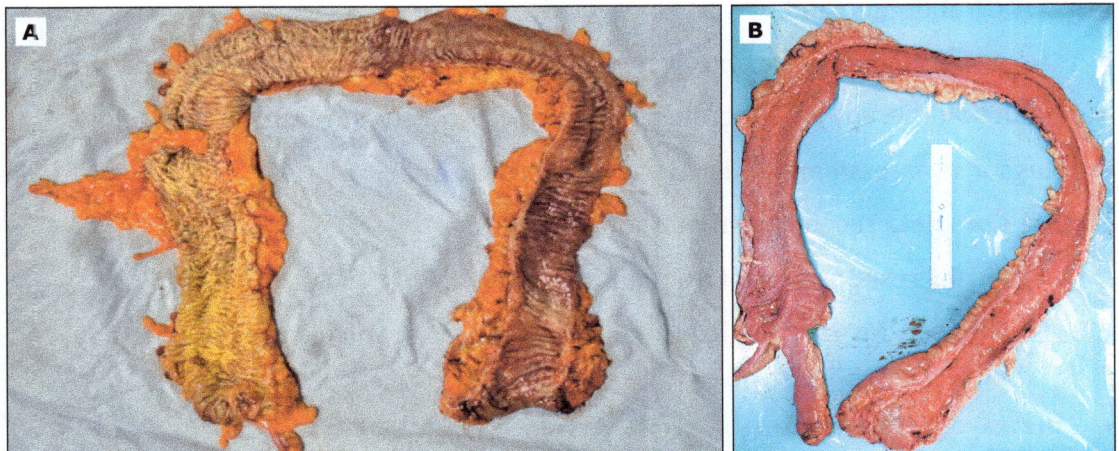

Figure 10.11: Total proctocolectomy specimen.
(A) proximal extent being mid-transverse colon, (B) Pan-Colitis.

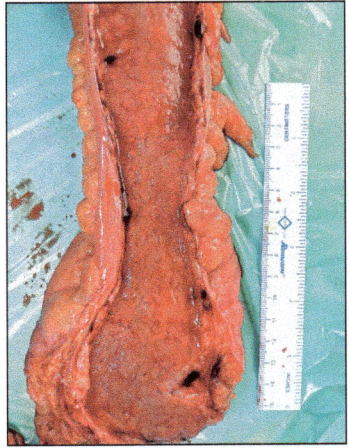

Figure 10.12: Surgical specimen in Ulcerative Colitis revealing a finely granular, erythematous, friable mucosa.

- Total proctocolectomy with end ileostomy: in cases of severe ano-rectal involvement and poor sphincter function (it is better to create an abdominal stoma than a perineal stoma)
- Subtotal colectomy with ileo-rectal anastomosis: in case the rectal involvement is mild or family is not completed.

- **Go through chapter 13 for literature on the subject.**

Principle of Management of Severe Acute Colitis

- Blood tests (including CRP), Stool tests (to rule out infectious colitis and pseudomembranous colitis)
- X-ray abdomen to rule out perforation, toxic megacolon
- SOS CT abdomen and pelvis
- Un-prepared limited flexible sigmoidoscopy for confirmation of diagnosis
- Induction therapy with steroids: IV hydrocortisone or IV methyl prednisolone
- Response assessment at day 3 using Oxford criteria
    - Complete response: stool frequency < 3/day
    - Partial response: stool frequency 3–8/day, CRP < 45 mg/l
    - No response: stool frequency > 8/day or stool frequency 3–8/day and CRP > 45 mg/l
- In case of no response:
    - Initiate second line medical rescue therapy: infliximab or cyclosporine
    - Reassess at day 5 of first initiation of treatment: in case of no response: consider emergent surgery
- Response present: continue steroids and reassess on day 5–7.
- **Go through chapter 13 for literature on the subject.**

11 Case of Rectal & Left Colonic Carcinoma

Format for History Taking

- History of bleeding per rectum (PR):
  - Painful or painless
  - Passage of fresh bright red blood or altered blood
  - With or without blood clots
  - Quantity
  - Separate from stools or mixed with it
- History of alteration in bowel habits:
  - Constipation/obstipation or diarrhea
  - Onset: Insidious or sudden
  - Duration
  - Progression
  - History of laxative use
  - History of straining at stools
- What does he pass:
  - Stool quantity
  - Stool frequency
  - Stool consistency: loose/soft/semisolid/hard
  - Color
  - Odor
  - Mucus is present or not
- History of rectal symptoms:
  - Sensation of incomplete evacuation
  - Urgency
  - Tenesmus
  - Spurious diarrhea

- History of perianal symptoms:
  - Perianal pain
  - Discharge
  - Mass per rectum
  - Incontinence
- History of urinary symptoms: dysuria, hematuria, fecaluria
- History of abdominal pain, abdominal distension, nausea, vomiting, ball rolling sensation, borborygmi
- History of fever with chills
- History of postural dizziness, syncope, fatigue, shortness of breath, need for blood transfusion
- History of loss of weight, loss of appetite
- History of jaundice, respiratory distress, back/bone pain
- Treatment history:
  - Evaluation with cross-sectional imaging, colonoscopy with/without biopsy.
  - Whether chemotherapy and/or radiotherapy was initiated, when was it initiated, duration of therapy received, time of completion, time since completion
  - History of adverse events during chemo-radiotherapy, Post CRT course
- Past history
- Personal history
- Family history: history of colo-rectal cancer in first and second degree family
- Performance history

Justification for Each Component in History

- History of bleeding per rectum (PR):
  - Whether the PR bleed was painful or painless: PR bleed in Colorectal cancer is painless. Hemorrhoids can also cause painless bleed PR. Painful bleed suggests fissure in ano, thrombosed hemorrhoids or inflammatory bowel disease.
  - History of passage of fresh bright red blood or altered blood: fresh bright red bleed suggests bleed from pathology in anus or mid/lower rectum. Whereas bleed from a more proximal site results in passage of altered dark blood.
  - Blood clots: presence of blood clots suggests significant bleed

- Quantity: Quantifying the amount of bleed by inquiring regarding the quantity of blood passed is important
- Blood separate from stools or mixed with stools: Blood separate from stools suggests that the possible site of bleed is in anus, lower or mid rectum. Whereas passage of blood mixed stools suggest bleed from a more proximal site. This is because peristalsis causes mixing of blood with stools in these sites. Hemorrhoidal disease causes drip bleed, whereas in fissure in ano there is streaking of blood over stools.

- History of alteration in bowel habits: carcinoma rectum and left colon usually causes gradually increasing constipation. Alternatively, there may be alternating bouts of constipation and diarrhea in a patient with left colonic growth; hold up of stools proximal to site of block by tumor will lead to stercoral inflammation/colitis which in turn will cause diarrhea. Alternatively patient with constipation due to carcinoma may consume laxative resulting in diarrhea.
- Take detailed history of alteration in bowel habits and narrate a detailed account of what he actually passes: stool quantity; stool frequency; stool consistency (loose/soft/semisolid/hard); color, mucus is present or not.
- History of straining at stools: this symptom is not specific to carcinoma rectum, but is one of the components of Rome definition for constipation, hence to be inquired for.
- History of sensation of incomplete evacuation in an elderly patient is an important pointer towards rectal malignancy
- Urgency and tenesmus are irritative rectal symptoms. It could be suggestive of an inflammatory disease process in rectum (e.g. Inflammatory bowel disease) or rectal malignancy. Tenesmus has been variably defined as "the sensation of incomplete defecation" or "a repeated painful urge to defecate without excreting stool". Urgency refers to the urgent urge to pass stools.
- History of spurious diarrhea: (spurious=not real) it is a condition in which patient attempts to empty rectum several times a day, often passing just flatus and a small amount of blood-stained mucus or liquid mucus mixed feces. It is seen in carcinoma rectum and fecal impaction.
- History of perianal pain: it suggests fissure in ano
- History of perianal discharge: it suggests fistula in ano
- History of mass per rectum: it could suggest either tumor, prolapsed (grade 4) internal hemorrhoids, external hemorrhoids or rectal prolapse. To differentiate: inquire if it is soft(benign) or firm (neoplastic), prolapsing with straining (hemorrhoids/rectal prolapse) or not, reducible (hemorrhoids/rectal prolapse) or not.

- History of urinary symptoms, especially fecaluria, if present, suggests recto-urinary/colo-urinary fistula.
- History of abdominal pain, abdominal distension, nausea, vomiting, ball rolling sensation, borborygmic: These symptoms are suggestive of associated intestinal obstruction.
- History of postural dizziness, syncope, fatigue, shortness of breath, need for blood transfusion: to quantify the blood loss. The presence of these symptoms suggests anemia.
- History of loss of weight, loss of appetite: alarming symptoms, suggestive of malignancy
- History of jaundice, respiratory distress, back/bone pain: symptoms to suggest metastatic disease.
- Treatment history: Evaluation with cross-sectional imaging, colonoscopy with or without biopsy. History of colonoscopy with biopsy, helps the student by hinting him towards the clinical diagnosis of a luminal pathology, in this case malignancy.
- Whether chemotherapy and/or radiotherapy was initiated, when was it initiated, duration of therapy received, time of completion, time since completion, history of adverse events during chemo-radiotherapy, post CRT course. Although such history confirms clinical diagnosis, it is best to mention this history briefly, and not elaborate on the same. Some examiners may not like it.
- Family history: history of colo-rectal cancer in first and second degree family: colorectal cancer is more common in patients with family history of colo-rectal cancer. Such history is also important to rule out colorectal cancer syndrome such as:
    - Lynch syndrome: due to mismatch repair gene (MLH 1, MSH2, PMS 2) mutation
    - FAP (familial adenomatous polyposis): due to APC (adenomatous polyposis coli) gene mutation
    - Peutz Jeghers syndrome: due to STK11 gene mutation
    - Juvenile polyposis syndrome: due to SMAD4, BMPR1A gene mutation
    - Cowden syndrome: due to PTEN gene mutation
- Performance history: to assess whether patient can withstand required treatment including chemotherapy, radiotherapy and surgery.

Format for Examination
- What is the appearance of the patient: young/middle-aged/elderly, lady/gentleman

- Whether the patient is clinically
  - Poorly/averagely/well built
  - Poorly/averagely/well nourished
- Measure height, weight, BMI
- Whether the patient is clinically
  - Conscious/stuporous
  - Co-operative/unco-operative
  - Well/poorly oriented to time, place and person
  - Lying comfortably in bed/in discomfort/in pain(rolling in pain)
  - Well hydrated/dehydrated
  - Febrile/Afebrile.
- Mention Pulse, BP
- Look for
  - Pallor, jaundice, cyanosis, clubbing
  - Generalized or localized lymphadenopathy
  - Palpable left supraclavicular lymph node
  - Pedal or dependent edema
  - Skin lesions: look for skin lesions like epidermoid cyst which may be seen in Gardner syndrome, keratocanthomas and sebaceous tumors which may be seen in Muir-Torre syndrome.
- Examination of oral cavity: look for oral hygiene, any obvious mucosal lesions. Do not miss pigmented macules on lips or oral mucosa which is seen in Peutz Jeghers syndrome

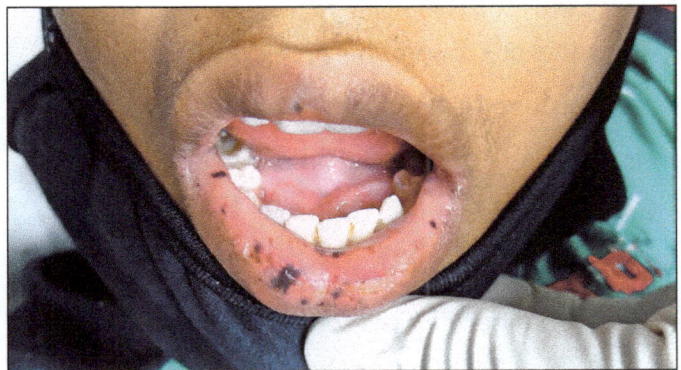

Figure 11.1: Pigmented macules seen on lips and oral mucosa in a patient with Peutz Jeghers syndrome.

- Examination of the abdomen:
  - On Inspection: See if:
    - Abdomen is flat/distended/scaphoid
    - Umbilicus is central/displaced (upwards/downwards/sideways) inverted/everted/flat.
    - All quadrants are moving equally with respiration or not (there may be localized or generalized restriction to abdominal wall movement with respiration in case of localized or generalized peritonitis)
    - See if there is any visible lump
    - Look for visible scar, sinus, engorged veins, pulsations, peristalsis or cough impulse.
    - Don't forget to inspect the groin hernial sites (to look for swelling or cough impulse i.e. hernia) and genitalia.
    - Inspection of renal angles to look for fullness
  - On Palpation: See if:
    - Abdomen is soft and non-tender (Alternatively abdomen could be rigid and/or tender)
    - Liver is palpable or not; hepatomegaly may be present in case of colorectal cancer, liver metastasis
      - If yes, measure from costal margin in midclavicular line in cm or finger width,
      - See if:
        - It is tender/nontender;
        - Surface is smooth/nodular
        - Borders are round/sharp, regular/irregular,
        - Consistency is soft/firm/hard
    - Spleen is enlarged or not
    - Any other palpable lump.
    - Do not forget to:
      - Palpate groin hernia sites to look for cough impulse
      - Examine genitals

- Look for tenderness in renal angles
- Examine back and spine for tenderness/gibbus.
- On Percussion:
  - Look for upper border of liver dullness (generally in the 5th intercostal space) in midclavicular line.
  - Note the liver span (normal being 12–14 cm)
  - Note in the rest of the abdomen (generally tympanitic)
  - Tests for free fluid
- On auscultation:
  - Auscultate for bowel sounds. Hear for hyperperistaltic bowel sounds if there is clinical suspicion of intestinal obstruction
  - Auscultate for bruit, hum and rub

- Per rectal examination: It is the most important part of clinical examination in case of carcinoma rectum. The format is as follows:
  - Examination of perianal area for: Look for fissure, skin tag, external hemorrhoids, external opening of fistula in ano, perianal abscess, sinus, growth or prolapse, skin excoriation
  - Digital rectal examination: with a gloved finger:
    - To note the anal tone and squeeze pressure
    - To palpate for any mucosal lesion. If present, note:
      - The distance of the growth from anal verge.
      - The longitudinal extent in cm
      - Circumferential extent to be mentioned as extending from ... 'O' clock to ... 'O' clock
      - Proximal extent of the growth
      - Consistency: soft/firm/hard
      - Form: ulcerative/proliferative/ulcero-proliferative/polypoidal
      - Fixity: fixed or not
      - Also note what is seen on the gloved finger: normal stool/blood/mucus/pus.
  - In a clinical case of rectal prolapse: if it is not clinically obvious, ask the patient to squat and strain. This will help manifest an occult prolapse. If present:

- Measure the length of prolapse.
- Whether it is spontaneously reducing or not.
- What is the orientation of mucosal folds i.e. whether it is circumferential (rectal prolapse) or radial (prolapsed hemorrhoids).
- Note whether there is any mucosal erosion or ulcer.

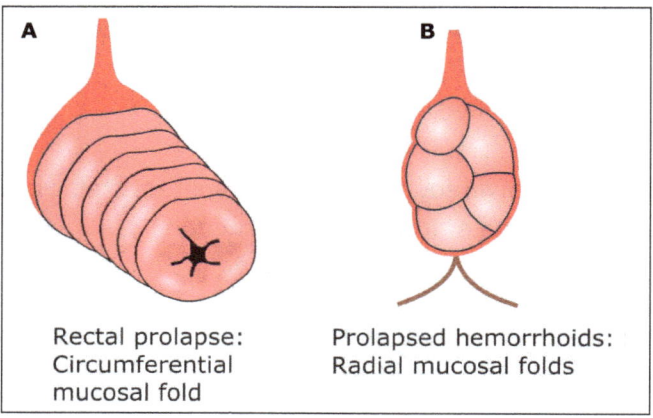

Figure 11.2: Rectal prolase (A) versus Prolapsed hemorrhoid (B).

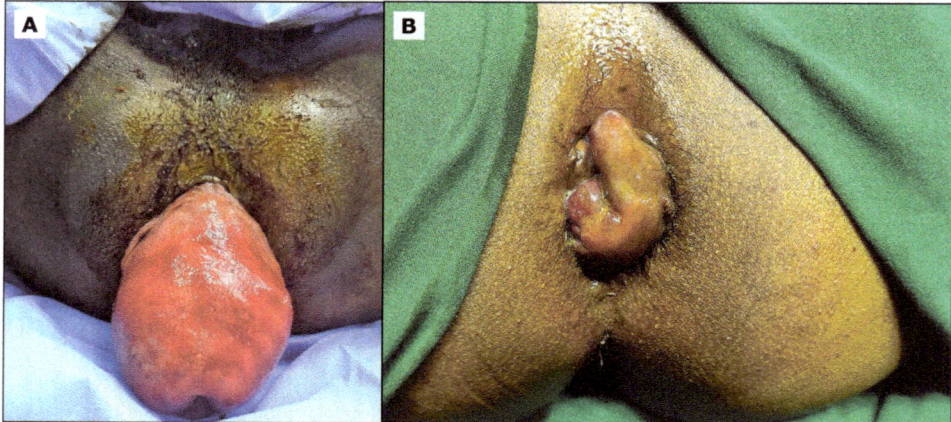

Figure 11.3: (A) Rectal Prolapse, (B) Hemorrhoids.

○ Do not forget:
- To note if patient is using any kind of diaper or pad
- To look for excoriation of perianal skin due to feces in a patient with incontinence or in a patient using diaper.
- To note tone and squeeze pressure and mention it as first point in DRE. This is of importance in operative planning. If the sphincter function is poor in

a patient with low rectal cancer, sphincter salvage may just not be possible (i.e. abdomino-perineal resection [Miles surgery/APR] becomes necessary).
  - Perform proctoscopy, if available
- Rest systemic examination

EXAMPLE CASE

History

- My patient Mrs XYZ, is a 54-year-old lady hailing from Mumbai, is a homemaker.
- She presented with chief complaints of passing blood per rectum since last one month.
- She was apparently alright 1 month back, when she noticed blood in stools. The per rectal bleed was painless, small in quantity, bright red in color and separate from stools.
- It is associated with constipation, which is insidious in onset, gradually increasing in severity over last one month. Previously she used to pass well formed stools once or twice daily but recently she is passing small quantity of hard stools once in three days along with blood as previously described.
- There is also sensation of incomplete evacuation
- There is no history of:
  - Urgency, tenesmus, spurious diarrhea
  - Perianal pain, discharge, mass, or history suggestive of incontinence
  - Abdominal pain, abdominal distension, nausea, vomiting, ball rolling sensation or borborygmi
  - Fever with chills
  - Postural dizziness, syncope, fatigue, shortness of breath or need for blood transfusion
  - Loss of weight, loss of appetite
  - Jaundice, respiratory distress, back/bone pain
- She sought medical care for these symptoms for which she was evaluated with colonoscopy and biopsy.
- There is no previous history of diabetes, hypertension, ischemic heart disease or TB.
- She has not undergone any major surgery in the past.

- There is no history of alcohol consumption or smoking
- She is post menopausal,
- There is no history of colo-rectal cancer in first and second degree family members
- She is able to perform all her daily routine activity without any difficulty

Examination

- My patient is an elderly lady, who is averagely built, averagely nourished, with a height of 160 cm, weight of 55 kg and BMI being 21.5 kg/m^2
- She is conscious, Co-operative, well oriented to time, place and person; Lying comfortably in bed; well hydrated and afebrile.
- Pulse is 72/min, BP is 110/70 mm Hg
- There is no pallor, jaundice, cyanosis, clubbing, generalized or localized lymphadenopathy. There is no palpable left supraclavicular lymph node; pedal or dependent edema or skin lesions
- Examination of oral cavity reveals adequate oral hygiene with no obvious mucosal lesions
- Examination of the abdomen:
  - On inspection: Abdomen is flat, umbilicus is central, inverted. All quadrants are moving equally with respiration. There is no visible lump, scar, sinus, engorged veins, pulsations, peristalsis or cough impulse.
  - Inspection of groin hernial sites reveals no swelling or cough impulse and Inspection of genitalia is unremarkable. Inspection of renal angles reveals no fullness
  - On Palpation: Abdomen is soft and non-tender. Liver and spleen is not palpable. There isn't any other palpable lump.
  - There is no palpable cough impulse over groin hernia sites and examination of genitals is unremarkable. There is no tenderness in renal angles. Examination of back and spine is essentially normal.
  - On Percussion, upper border of liver dullness is in the 5th intercostal space in midclavicular line with liver span being 14 cm. Rest of the abdomen is tympanitic with no evidence of free fluid.
  - On auscultation normal bowel sounds are heard. There is no bruit, hum or rub
- Examination of perianal area reveals no fissure, skin tag, external hemorrhoids, external opening of fistula in ano, perianal abscess, sinus, growth, prolapse or perianal excoriation.

- On digital rectal examination, tone is normal, squeeze pressure is good. A firm, non-tender, proliferative growth is palpable at 7 cm from anal verge, proximal extent could not be reached (or could not be appreciated; alternatively if the proximal extent could be appreciated mention it along with the longitudinal extent of the tumor). The growth extends from 2 'O' clock to 6 'O' clock and is not fixed. The gloved finger is stained with blood.
- Rest systemic examination is essentially normal

To Summarize
- My patient is a 54-year-old female with no comorbid illness and ECOG 1 performance status presents with 1-month history of painless passage of fresh bright red blood per rectum, separate from stools, associated with progressive constipation and sensation of incomplete evacuation
- On examination: On digital rectal examination a firm growth is palpable 7 cm from anal verge, sphincter tone is good. General and abdominal examination is otherwise unremarkable

The most probable diagnosis in my patient is Carcinoma rectum

How to Proceed: (Sequence and Justification)
- Review of available medical records
- Proctoscopy and punch biopsy in the outpatient clinic itself, if it is a case of rectal growth felt on DRE
- Routine blood investigations (Hemogram, Liver Function Test, Renal Function Test, Serum Electrolyte, INR)
- X-ray chest: to look for lung metastasis.
- X-ray Abdomen if intestinal obstruction is clinically suspected
- USG (A+P):
  - It is an extension of bed side clinical evaluation, it's cheap, non invasive and easily available
  - To look for liver metastasis, ascites, omental/peritoneal metastasis.
- **Please note**:
  - Presence of isolated limited liver metastasis, isolated limited lung metastasis, isolated limited peritoneal metastasis and synchronous limited liver and lung metastasis is not a contraindication to curative intent treatment in colo-rectal

cancer, unlike in Ca esophagus, stomach, pancreas where palliative intent treatment would have been initiated. Hence even if lung or liver metastasis is detected on X-ray chest or USG abdomen further evaluation with CT or PET-CT is still justified to further stage and characterize the disease. Further management plan in such situation should then be planned in a tumor board/multi-disciplinary team (MDT) meeting after thorough deliberation.
    o In this chapter we shall only discuss management of non metastatic left colonic and rectal cancers. Management of CRCLM (colorectal cancer liver metastasis) is very complex and is out of scope of this book. This topic however needs to be thoroughly studied by sub-speciality surgical gastroenterology/oncology residents.
- Colonoscopy:
    o Primary role in carcinoma rectum (which can be evaluated on proctoscopy itself) is to rule out synchronous pathology (malignancy, polyp, IBD) in proximal rectum and colon.
    o If no growth is felt on DRE then scopy is performed to confirm the presence of a neoplastic growth in the proximal rectum or colon; if present note:
        - Note the site and size
        - Note the longitudinal and circumferential extent
        - Morphology: proliferative/ulcerative/ulcero-proliferative/infiltrative
        - Whether passable or not
        - Presence of synchronous lesion: Malignancy, polyp, IBD
        - Biopsy: 6-8 in number

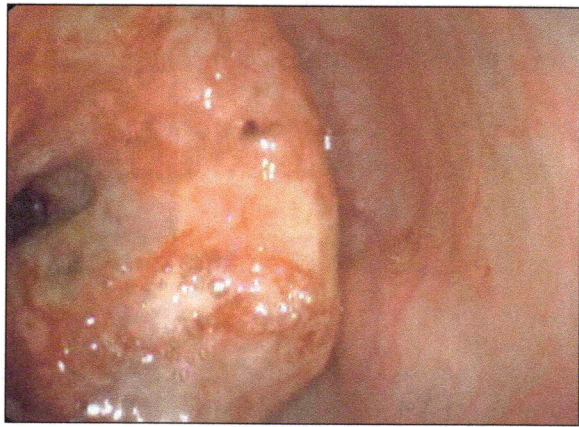

Figure 11.4: Colonoscopy image showing proliferative lumen occluding growth in recto-sigmoid junction.

- Blood CEA level:
  - It is tumor marker used in the evaluation of colo-rectal cancer.
  - Normal level: < 4 ng/ml
  - Levels are raised in smokers
  - Role:
    - Diagnosis
    - Staging
    - Prognostification
    - Response assessment: post neoadjuvant therapy, post surgery, post adjuvant
    - Surveillance
- CECT of the chest, abdomen and pelvis: to stage the disease: local and distant staging.
  - To evaluate the site, size, extent of growth
  - Involvement of adjacent organs/vessels
  - To look for lymph nodes
  - To look for distant metastasis: liver metastasis, omental/peritoneal metastasis, Krukenberg tumor, ascites, lung metastasis, pleural effusion.

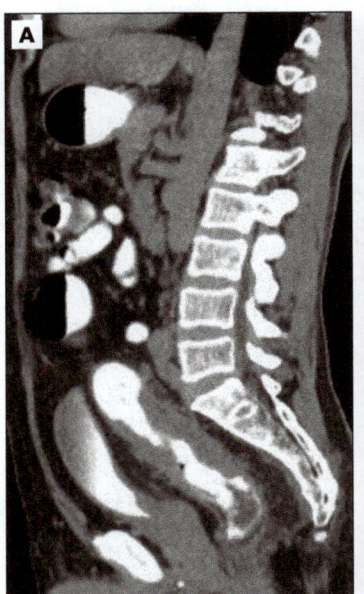 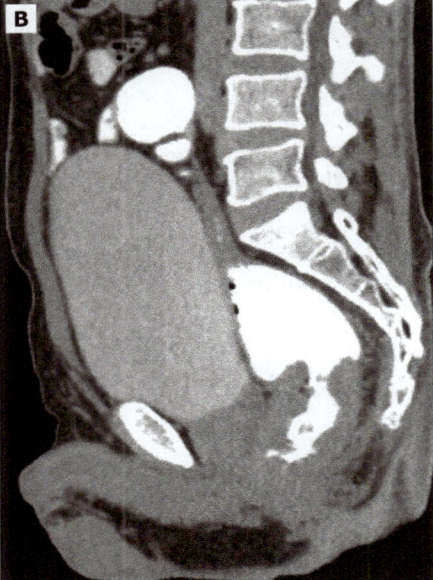

Figure 11.5: CT showing rectal carcinoma.

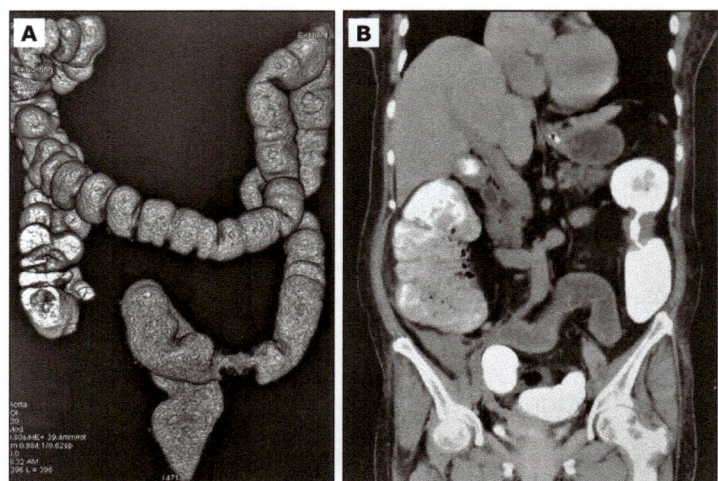

Figure 11.6: CT showing napkin ring like growth in sigmoid colon (A) and descending colon (B).

- MRI pelvis, rectal protocol: it is the modality of choice for local staging of rectal cancer. Images are obtained in T1 and T2 phase in oblique axial, coronal and sagittal sections with or without IV contrast.

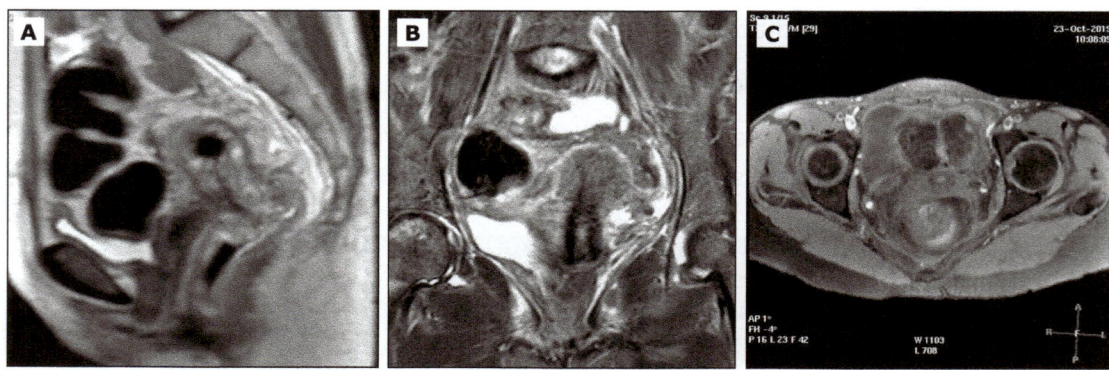

Figure 11.7: MRI-rectal protocol: sagittal (A), coronal (B) and oblique axial views (C). Initially the sagittal sections are reviewed to note the length of tumor, relation of tumor to the peritoneal reflection, involvement of anterior and posterior organs and to prepare oblique axial sections. In coronal sections relation of the tumor to levator ani, sphincters and pelvic side walls is noted. Finally in oblique axial views the exact T and N stage is noted. T3 tumors are then further subclassified based on the depth of mesorectal invasion into T3a (< 1 mm), T3b (1-5 mm), T3c (5-15 mm) and T3d (> 15 mm). Also CRM is noted

- Points to be noted
  - T stage:
    - Most importantly, to note the extent of mesorectal infiltration in case of T3 tumors
    - Involvement of levator ani, sphincter

- Adjacent organ involvement: prostate, seminal vesical, urinary bladder, ureter, uterus, vagina, cervix, sacrum, pelvic side wall
  - N stage: number of enlarged nodes and their levels
  - CRM (circumferential radial margin) threatened or not
  - Presence of extra mural vascular invasion (EMVI)
- FDG-PET-CT: PET is done primarily to rule out distant metastasis which may have not been picked up on CECT.

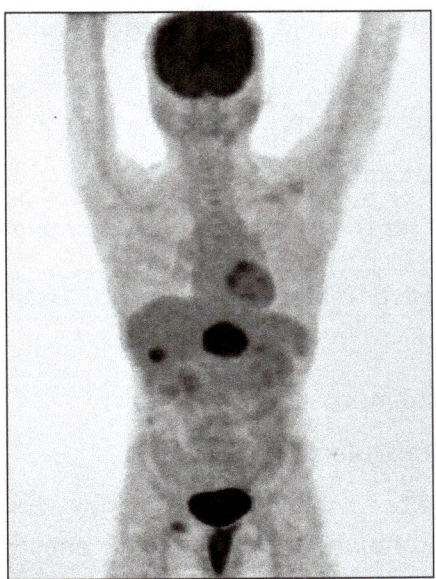

Figure 11.8: FDG PET scan showing FDG avid rectal tumor and liver metastasis.

- Staging laparoscopy. Done to look for peritoneal metastasis/occult liver metastasis which may be missed on pre-op. imaging
- Optional staging investigation:
  - EUS: endoscopic ultrasound: useful modality for T and N staging. Guided fine needle aspiration (FNA) and/or core biopsy is possible with EUS
  - EMR: endoscopic mucosal resection: It is considered for clinically early stage T1 cancers. It is potentially therapeutic.
  - ESD: endoscopic submucosal dissection: It is considered for clinically early stage T1 cancers. It is potentially therapeutic.
  - TRUS: Transrectal ultrasound
  - Determination of tumor MMR (mismatch repair gene) or MSI (microsatellite

instability) status. It helps in prognostification and determining if adjuvant chemotherapy is required or not in stage 2 cancers. MSI-H (high) tumors have better prognosis than MSI-L (low) or MSS (microsatellite stable) tumors. Adjuvant chemotherapy is indicated in stage 2 cancers which are MSI-H.

- o KRAS mutation analysis: It is considered in cases of metastatic colorectal cancer. Anti-EGFR therapy is considered only in cases with wild type KRAS. Anti EGFR therapy is ineffective in cases with mutated KRAS.
- o BRAF V600E mutation testing: It is considered in cases of metastatic colorectal cancer. it helps in prognostification. Tumors with this mutations usually have poor tumor biology and demonstrate resistance to conventional chemotherapy.

- At the end of the staging work up, classify whether the disease is:
  - o Locally resectable or not
  - o If metastatic, whether the metastases is resectable or not

Table 11.1: Colo-Rectal cancer is staged as per AJCC-TNM staging system

- T stage:
  - T1: Tumor invades submucosa
  - T2: Tumor invades muscularis propria
  - T3: Tumor invades subserosal connective tissue without penetrating through serosa (visceral peritoneum) or invading adjacent structures
  - T4: Tumor penetrating through serosa +/- invading adjacent structures
- N stage:
  - N1: Metastasis to 1-3 lymph nodes (LN)
  - N2: Metastasis to 4 or more LN
- M stage:
  - M0: No distant metastasis
  - M1: Distant metastasis present
- Stage:
  - Stage I: T1, T2
  - Stage II: T3, T4
  - Stage III: N1, N2
  - Stage IV: M1

- Management principles:
  - Principles of management of non metastatic Ca colon differs from that of Ca rectum.
    - In Ca colon: treatment would include upfront surgery followed by adjuvant chemotherapy (if indicated). There is no role for radiotherapy. More recently neo-adjuvant chemotherapy has been used in locally unresectable T4b tumors.
    - In Ca Rectum: treatment would include Neoadjuvant therapy (including radiation) (if indicated) followed by surgery followed by adjuvant therapy (if indicated)
- Neoadjuvant therapy for Rectal Cancer:
  - For disease with clinical stage =/> 2 i.e. =/> T3, N+
  - Advantage:
    - To downstage/downsize the tumor
    - To evaluate tumor biology i.e. if the cancer progresses on therapy then it suggests aggressive tumor biology and such patients would not benefit from aggressive surgery. On the contrary good response to therapy suggests good tumor biology hence better prognosis.
    - Therapy is given to tissues with intact vascularity and which are well oxygenated
    - Radiated tissues will be removed at surgery
    - Systemic micro-metastasis is dealt with by the systemic chemotherapy
    - Higher proportion of patients will receive chemotherapy and/or radiation
  - Disadvantage:
    - Loss of window of opportunity in case the disease progresses
  - Options:
    - Neo-adjuvant Long Course Chemoradiation:
      - 5-FU or capecitabine based CRT
      - 45-50.4 gray RT given in 25-28 divided fractions (with 1.8 gray being given in each fraction) over a period of 6 weeks
      - This is followed by restaging and surgery after 6 weeks followed by adjuvant chemotherapy later
      - Its role was established by German rectal cancer study group trial

- Neo-adjuvant Short Course Radiation:
  - 25 gray RT given in 5 divided fractions (with 5 gray being given in each fraction) over a period of 5 days
  - In this regimen chemotherapy is not given concurrently along with radiation
  - This is followed by surgery after 7-10 days followed by adjuvant chemotherapy later
  - Short course RT is not used for T4 tumors
  - Its role was established by Swedish trial and Dutch trial
- Total neoadjuvant therapy:
  - Chemotherapy followed by chemoradiation followed by surgery with no adjuvant therapy:
  - CAPE-OX or FOLFOX or 5-FU/leucovorin or capecitabine (Chemotherapy) followed by capecitabine or 5-FU (infusional 5-FU preferred over bolus) based radiation (Chemoradiation) followed by surgery
- Response assessment
  - Proctoscopy/colonoscopy
  - MRI pelvis rectal protocol
  - CECT/PET-CT to rule out new distant metastasis
- Habr-Gama approach or Wait and watch policy:
  - It involves following a non-operative approach in patients with clinically complete response following neoadjuvant chemoradiation.
  - Instead of surgery, patients with clinically complete response are put under a strict surveillance protocol including timely DRE, CEA, proctoscopy/colonoscopy, imaging (MRI pelvis rectal protocol, CECT).
- Surgery for left colonic and rectal cancer:
  - Trans anal excision
    - TEMS: Trans anal endoscopic microsurgery
    - TEO: Trans anal endoscopic operation
    - TAMIS: Trans anal minimally invasive surgery
  - Trans abdominal resection:
    - Left hemicolectomy
    - Sigmoidectomy
    - Anterior resection: rectum transected above level of peritoneal reflection

- Low anterior resection: rectum transected below level of peritoneal reflection
- Ultra low anterior resection: rectum transected at level of levator ani
- Inter-sphincteric resection: rectum transected below level of levator ani with dissection in the inter-sphincteric plane
- Hartmanns procedure
- Abdomino-perineal resection
    - Classical APR
    - Extra-levator Abdomino-perineal excision

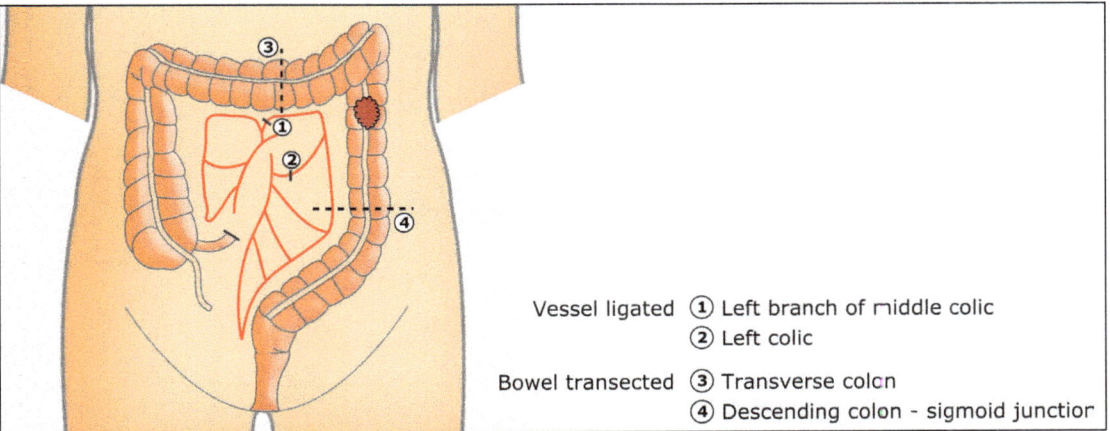

Vessel ligated ① Left branch of middle colic
② Left colic
Bowel transected ③ Transverse colon
④ Descending colon - sigmoid junction

Figure 11.9: Left hemicolectomy.

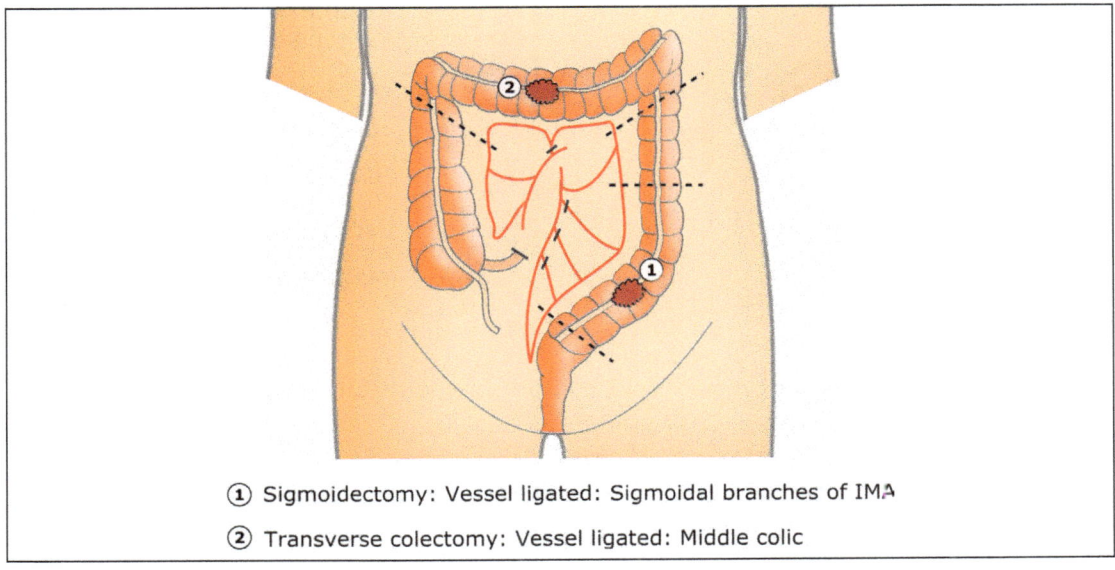

① Sigmoidectomy: Vessel ligated: Sigmoidal branches of IMA
② Transverse colectomy: Vessel ligated: Middle colic

Figure 11.10: Sigmoidectomy/Transverse colectomy.

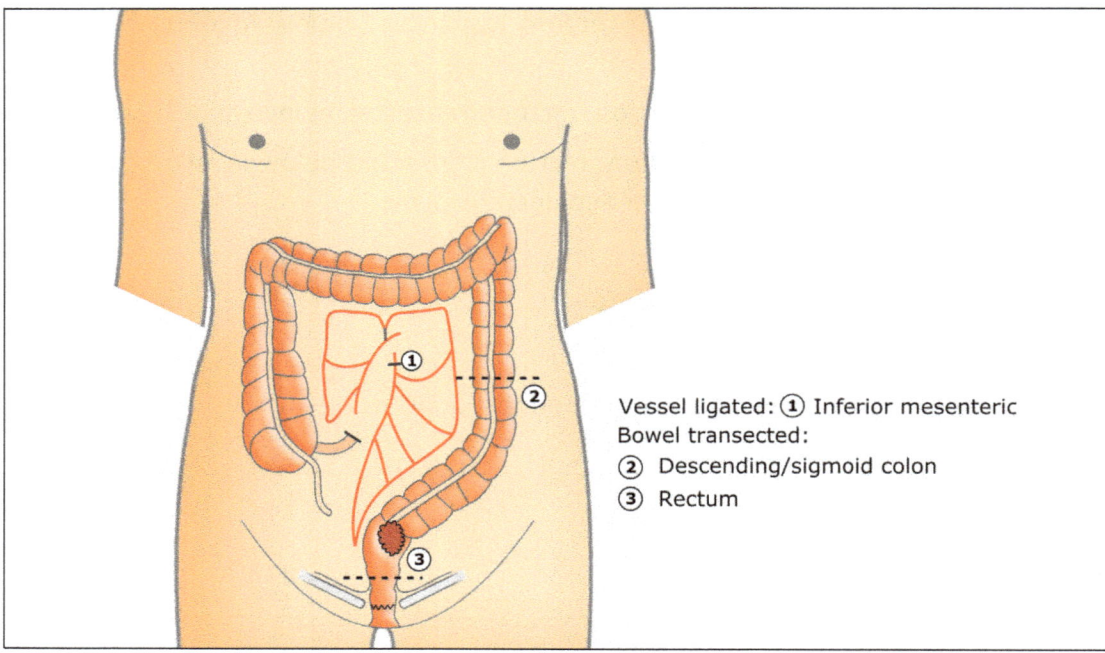

Figure 11.11: Anterior resection.

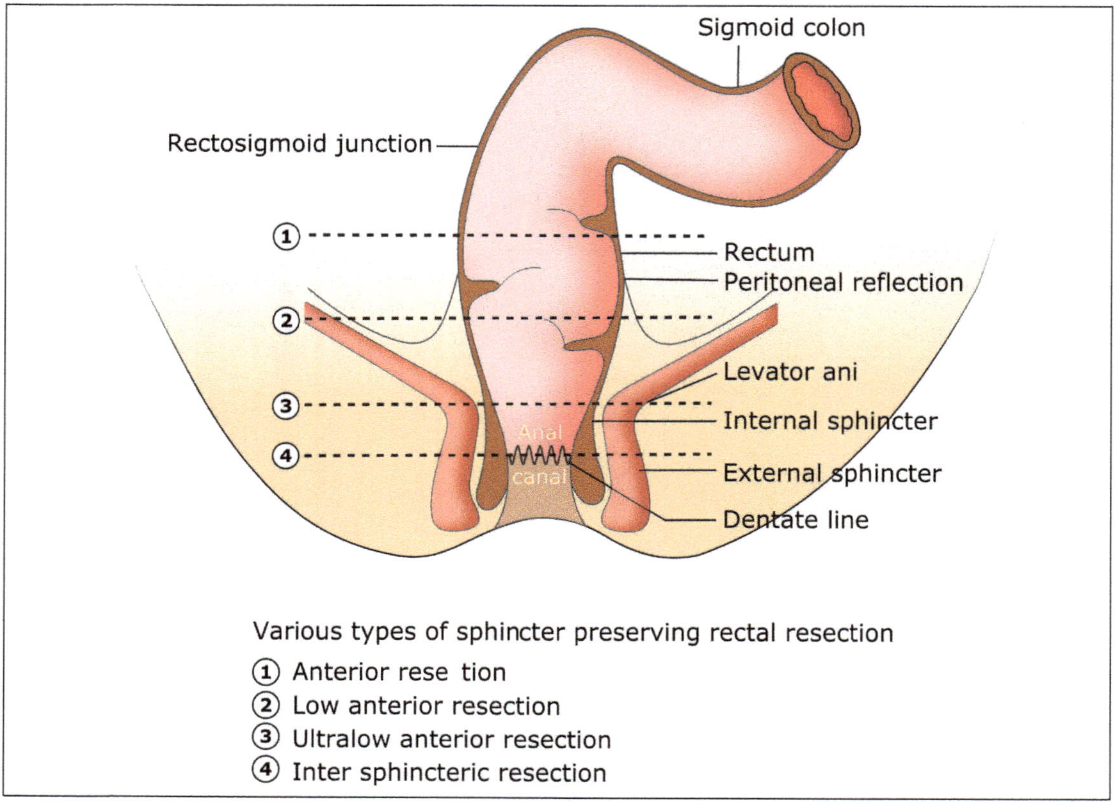

Figure 11.12: Types of sphincter sparing rectal resection.

CHAPTER 11: CASE OF RECTAL & LEFT COLONIC CARCINOMA   259

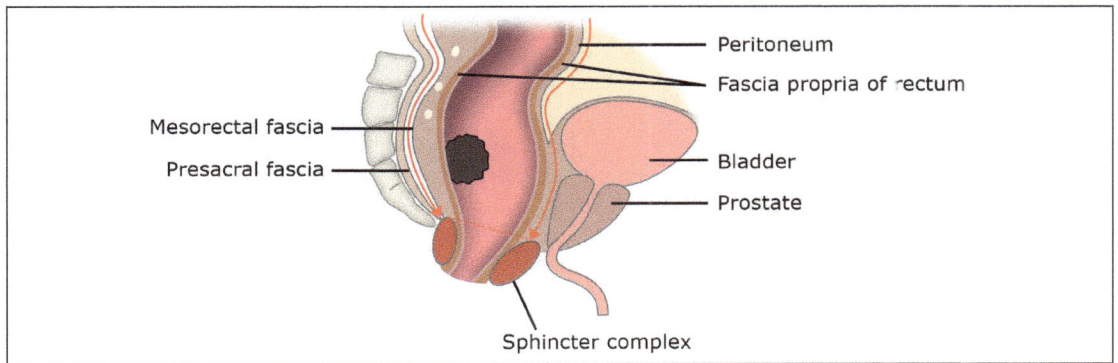

Figure 11.13: Concept of Total Mesorectal excision (TME). The dissection plane posteriorly is in the holy plane of Heald between the Presacral and Mesorectal fascia, Anteriorly once the peritoneal reflection is opened up the dissection is carried between the Fascia Propria of rectum and prostatic capsule through the Denovilliers Fascia.

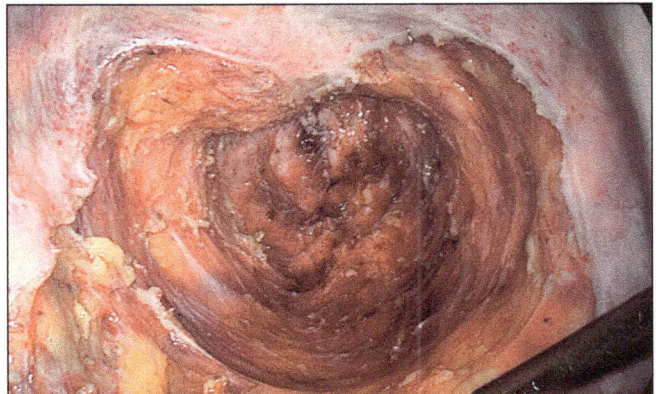

Figure 11.14: TME plane also called as Holy plane of Heald.

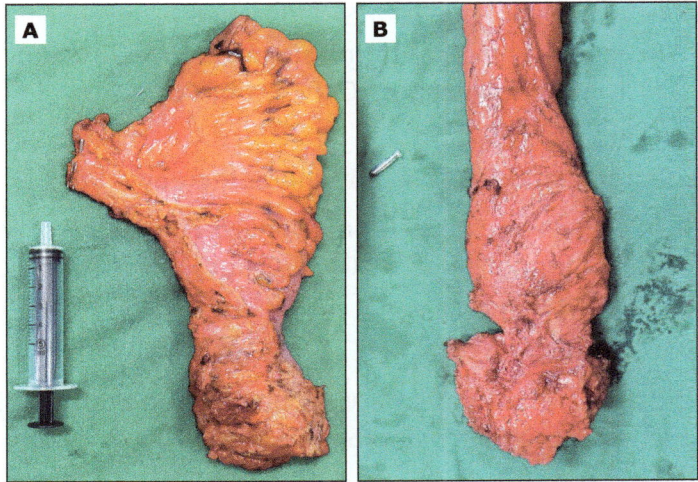

Figure 11.15: (A) Ultra Low AR specimen (note the IMA pedicle) (B) ELAPE specimen (note the rim of levator muscle).

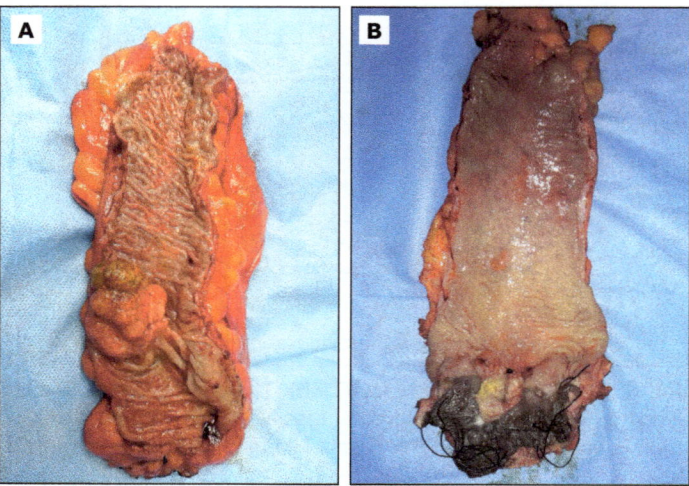

Figure 11.16: Anterior resection specimen (A), APR specimen (B).

- Read about
  - Concepts of TME: total mesorectal excision for surgery in rectal cancer
  - Concepts of CME: complete mesocolic excision for surgery in colonic cancer
  - Both have been discussed in chapter 13
- Adjuvant therapy for rectal cancer:
  - Adjuvant Chemoradiation: in case neoadjuvant radiation was not given for rectal cancers (for disease with pathological stage =/> 2 i.e =/> T3, N+
    - Options:
      - Sandwich therapy: Chemotherapy followed by chemoradiation followed by chemotherapy:
        - CAPE-OX or FOLFOX or 5-FU/leucovorin or capecitabine followed by capecitabine or 5-FU (infusional 5-FU preferred over bolus) based radiation followed by CAPE-OX or FOLFOX or 5-FU/leucovorin or capecitabine
      - Chemoradiation followed by chemotherapy
        - Capecitabine or 5-FU (infusional 5-FU preferred over bolus) based radiation followed by CAPE-OX or FOLFOX or 5-FU/leucovorin or capecitabine
  - Adjuvant chemotherapy:
    - It is indicated in all patients who have received neoadjuvant therapy irrespective of the final pathological stage
    - Options:
      - FOLFOX: leucovorine, 5-FU and oxaliplatin. 2 weekly for 6 months.

- CAPEOX: Capecitabine and oxaliplatin. 3 weekly for 6 months.
- 5-FU or capecitabine
- FOLFIRI: Leucovorine, 5-FU and irinotecan

- Adjuvant chemotherapy for colonic cancers

Table 11.2: Indications for adjuvant chemotherapy in colonic cancer

- T4
- N+
- T3 with high risk features:
  - Obstruction or perforation
  - LVI: Lymphovascular invasion
  - PNI: Perineural invasion
  - < 12 lymph nodes sampled
  - MSI-high (microsatellite instability); MMR-deficient (mismatch repair gene); MSS (microsatellite stable)

  - Options:
    - FOLFOX: leucovorine, 5-FU and oxaliplatin. 2 weekly for 6 months.
    - CAPEOX: Capecitabine and oxaliplatin. 3 weekly for 6 months.
    - 5-FU or capecitabine
    - FOLFIRI: leucovorine, 5-FU and irinotecan
- Surveillance
  - Modality used:
    - History and physical examination
    - Blood CEA levels
    - USG abdomen and pelvis
    - CECT chest, abdomen and pelvis
    - Colonoscopy
- Go through chapter 13 for literature on the subject.
- Also read about management of Anal carcinoma

12 Case of Lump in Abdomen & How to Proceed in a Case of HCC, Ileo-Cecal TB and Right Colonic Malignancy

Introduction

In this chapter we will be discussing:

- The general format of history taking and examination in a patient with lump in abdomen
- How to formulate the list of differential diagnosis (D/D) based on the location of the lump (right upper quadrant, epigastrium, left upper quadrant, right lower quadrant, left lower quadrant)
- What specific history and examination findings are to be looked for, in some common GI diagnoses
- How to proceed in a case of
    - Hepatocellular carcinoma
    - Ileo-cecal tuberculosis
    - Right colonic malignancy

General Format for History Taking

- History of Lump:
    - Onset (that is, how was it noticed): insidious or sudden
    - Duration
    - Progression: stable in size/increasing in size/decreasing in size.
- Associated symptoms:
    - Pain in abdomen,
    - Nausea, vomiting
    - Fever, chills
    - Jaundice
    - Loss of weight, loss of appetite,
    - Abdominal distension, fullness
- History to identify etiology

- Treatment history
- Past history
- Personal history
- Family history
- Performance history.

On Examination

- Note the following points about the lump
    - Site
    - Size
    - Shape
    - Surface
    - Margins
    - Tenderness
    - Consistency
    - Mobility
    - Movement with respiration
    - Plane:
        - Whether the lump is intraperitoneal or not: by performing leg raising test
        - Whether the lump is retroperitoneal or not: by asking the patient to assume lateral decubitus position and palpating if the lump falls forward or not. A retroperitoneal mass won't fall ahead.

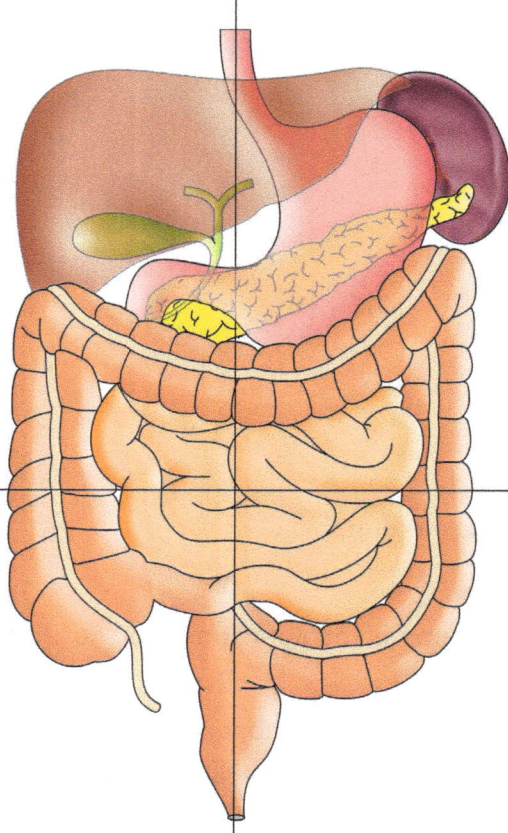

Figure 12.1: Quadrant wise organ distribution

Lump in Right Upper Quadrant (RUQ) of Abdomen

- Remember: organs in RUQ include: liver, gall bladder, hepatic flexure of colon, distal ascending colon, proximal transverse colon, head of pancreas, Distal stomach, right adrenal gland, right kidney, retroperitoneum

So the Possible Differential Diagnosis are:

- Gall bladder lesion
    - Mucocele of the gall bladder
    - Empyema of the gall bladder
    - Xanthogranulomatous cholecystitis
    - Carcinoma gall bladder
    - Malignant obstructive jaundice
        - Peri-ampullary malignancy
        - Carcinoma head of pancreas
        - Distal Cholangiocarcinoma
- Liver lesion
    - Reidel's lobe
    - Hemangioma
    - Hydatid cyst
    - Simple hepatic cyst
    - Adult polycystic liver disease
    - Focal Nodular hyperplasia
    - Adenoma
    - Regenerating nodule/dysplastic nodule
    - MCN-B (mucinous cystic neoplasm- Biliary), IPMN (intraductal papillary neoplasm)
    - Hepatocellular carcinoma
    - Hepatic metastasis
- Colonic lesion:
    - Carcinoma hepatic flexure of colon,
    - Carcinoma proximal transverse colon,
    - Carcinoma distal descending colon.

- Gastric lesion- pyloric malignancy:
  - Adenocarcinoma
  - Lymphoma
  - GIST
- Pancreatic lesion
  - Pancreatic Neoplasm:
    - Adenocarcinoma
    - Serous cystadenoma
    - IPMN: Intraductal papillary mucinous neoplasm
  - Pancreatic pseudocyst
- Adrenal Mass
- Renal Mass
- Retroperitoneal mass

Specific History/Examination Findings for the Common GI D/D:

- Mucocele of the gall bladder:
  - History: Patient may be asymptomatic or may have dull right upper quadrant abdominal pain precipitated by a fatty meal.
  - On abdominal palpation: Pear shaped, non tender, smooth distended gallbladder will be palpable in the right hypochondrium with side to side mobility which moves with respiration. Lateral medial and lower margins will be well defined and the upper portion goes under the rib cage. On percussion dull note over the GB is continuous with that of liver.
- Empyema gall bladder: In history in addition to pain there will be fever and on abdominal palpation the GB will be tender.
- Xanthogranulomatous cholecystitis (XGC):
  - Patient may present with symptoms of cholecystitis (chronic > acute) (pain, nausea, vomiting). Additionally patient may give history of lump in abdomen. The inflammatory process may extend into the liver and/or surrounding organs causing obstructive jaundice, GOO.
  - On examination a firm to hard, tender/non-tender lump will be palpable in the right hypochondrium, moving with respiration but having no intrinsic mobility. Lateral medial and lower margins will be palpable, the upper portion goes under the rib cage. On percussion dull note over the GB is continuous with that of liver.

- It may mimic carcinoma GB in all aspects. However remember patients with XGC are usually well preserved unlike Ca GB. Symptoms of loss of weight and loss of appetite are also uncommon

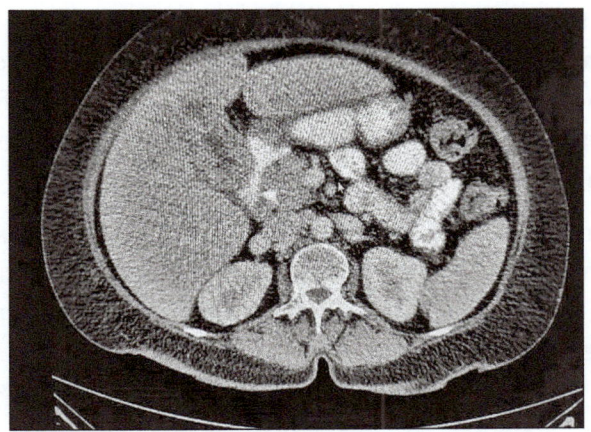

Figure 12.2: CT showing thick walled GB as seen in XGC.

- Carcinoma gall bladder & Malignant obstructive jaundice: discussed in detail in chapter 6.

- Hepatic Hemangioma:
    - There is no specific history. It is usually asymptomatic and is to be considered as a differential diagnosis in any young patient with lump in RUQ. Occasionally patient may have giant hemangioma (> 10 cm), in which case patient may have stretching type of pain in RUQ. Complications like Kasabach Merritt syndrome and cardiac failure may be rarely seen.
    - On palpation a soft to firm, rounded, compressible, non tender lump may be felt in the RUQ which is continuous with the liver, going under the rib cage. It will not have side to side mobility but will move cranio-caudally with respiration.
    - On auscultation, bruit may be heard over it

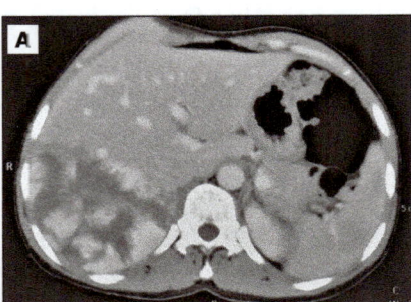
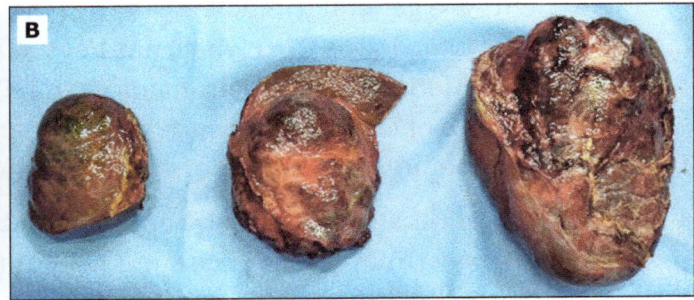

Figure 12.3: Hepatic hemangioma.

- Hydatid cyst:
  - Patient may be asymptomatic, or he/she may have RUQ abdominal pain/discomfort/heaviness. History of contact with a pet animal could be present. Fever could be present which would suggest secondary cyst infection or cysto-biliary communication. In case of cysto-biliary communication patient could additionally develop cholangitis (Charcot's triad: pain, fever and jaundice). This is another differential diagnosis which needs to be considered in a young patient with lump in RUQ
  - On palpation a firm, rounded, tender/non tender lump may be felt in the RUQ which is continuous with the liver, going under the rib cage. It will not have side to side mobility but will move cranio-caudally with respiration. Hydatid thrill may be present

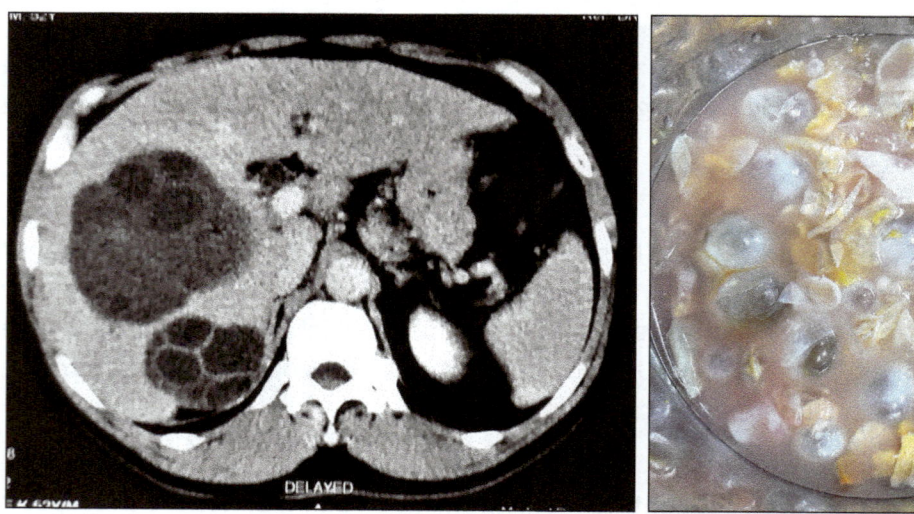

Figure 12.4: Hydatid cyst.

- Simple Hepatic cyst:
  - Patients are generally middle-aged with the only presenting feature being a painless lump in the RUQ which has been gradually increasing in size over a long duration of time (usually many years). Presence of pain should suggest occurrence of complication such as secondary infection (in which case fever will also be present) or hemorrhage into the cyst
  - On palpation a soft to firm, rounded, non tender lump may be felt in the RUQ/epigastrium which is continuous with the liver, going under the rib cage. It will not have side to side mobility but will move cranio-caudally with respiration.

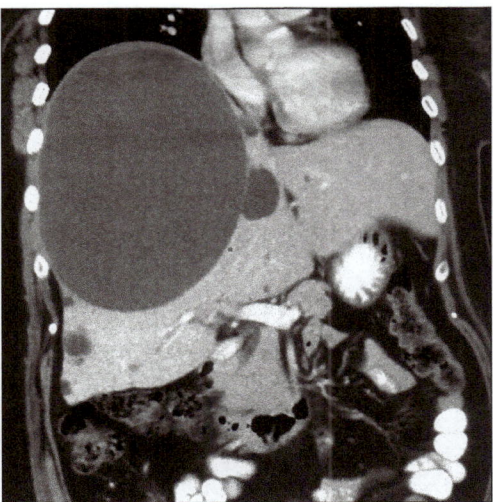

Figure 12.5: Simple hepatic cyst.

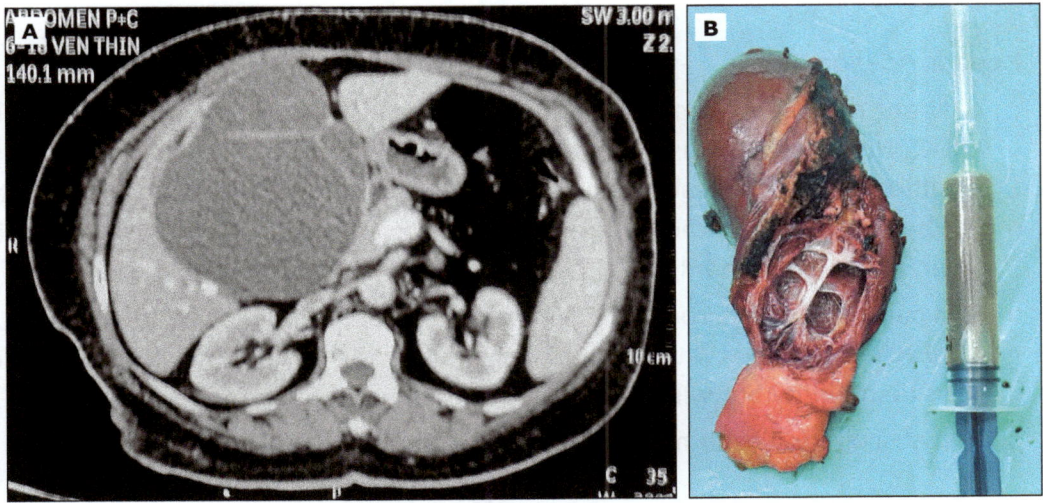

Figure 12.6: (A) Hepatic Cystadenoma,
(B) Surgical specimen of a Hepatic Cystadenoma (note the septations).

- Hepatic abscess:
  - There will be history of RUQ abdominal pain, fever, chills. There may be jaundice. Amebic liver abscess usually develops in young alcoholic males. Pyogenic abscess commonly develops in the elderly in the setting of cholangitis (right upper quadrant abdominal pain, fever, jaundice) due to choledocholithiasis or malignant obstructive jaundice; or alternatively in the setting of diverticulitis (constipation, straining at stools, left lower quadrant abdominal pain, fever, GI bleed) or any other intra-abdominal infectious pathology which may drain to the liver via the portal venous system
  - On examination, one may expect to find tender hepatomegaly. Additionally there may be intercostal tenderness.

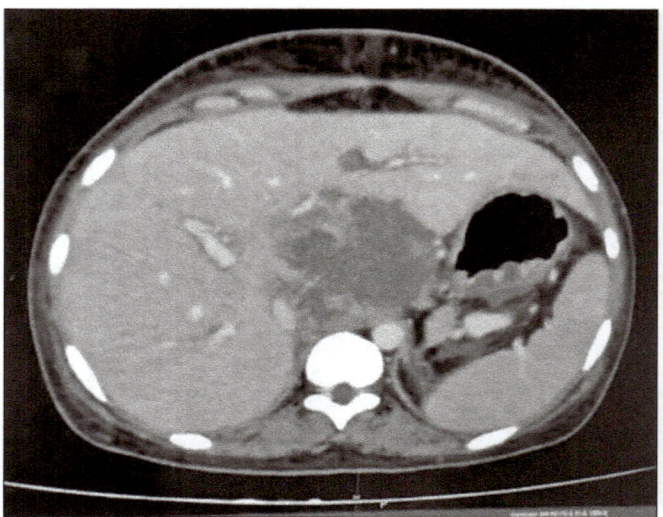
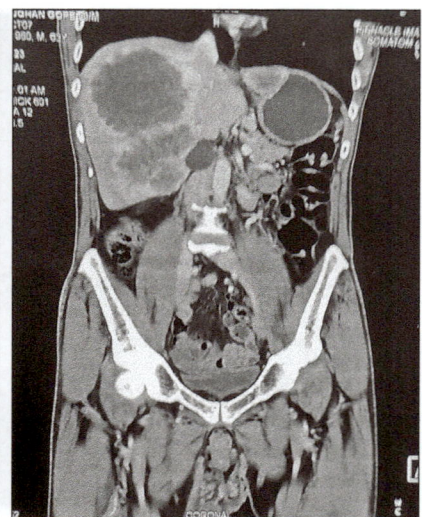

Figure 12.7: Liver abscess.

- Hepatic Adenoma:
  - Patient may be asymptomatic or may have history of pain and lump in the RUQ. History of OCP use in females and anabolic steroid use in males is to be inquired for. Complications include bleed and malignant transformation. It is to be considered in the differential diagnosis of a young female patient with pain and lump in the RUQ.
  - On palpation a firm, rounded, tender/non tender lump may be felt in the RUQ which is continuous with the liver, going under the rib cage. It will not have side to side mobility but will move cranio-caudally with respiration.
  - On auscultation bruit may be heard over the lump

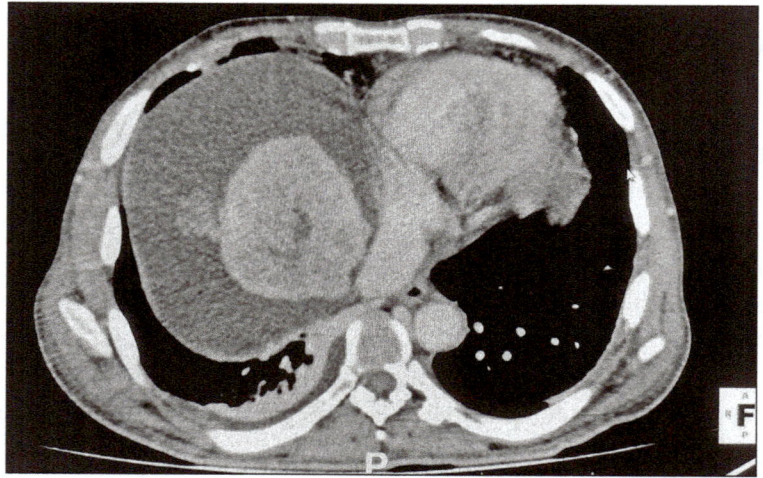

Figure 12.8: Bleeding Hepatic Adenoma; note the spurt.

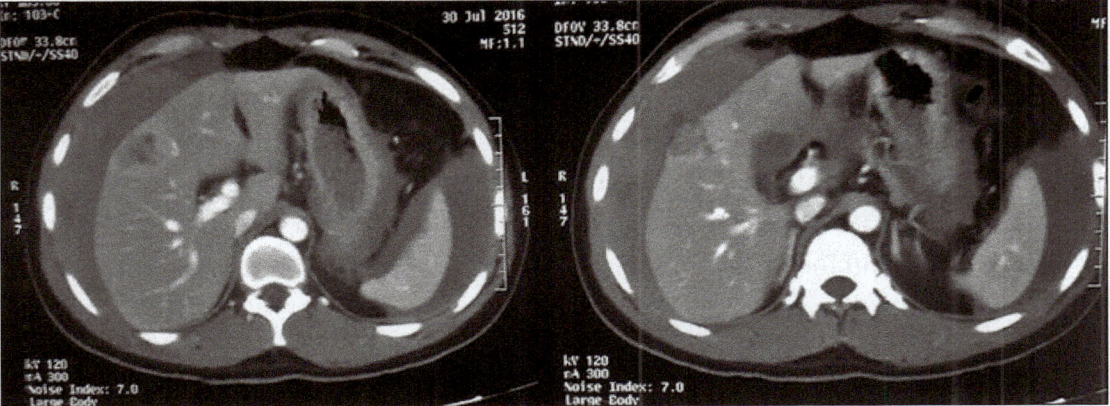

Figure 12.9: Ruptured hepatic adenoma.

- Focal Nodular hyperplasia: It is another differential diagnosis which need to be considered in a young female with lump in RUQ.
  - Abdominal examination finding similar to hepatic adenoma may be observed
- Hepatocellular carcinoma (HCC):
  - Patients are usually middle-aged or elderly. It usually develops in patients with cirrhotic liver, so there may be history to suggest the same, as in history of:
    - Abdominal distension due to ascites
    - Jaundice due to hepatic decompensation
    - GI bleed due to variceal bleed
    - Altered sensorium due to hepatic encephalopathy
    - Reduced urine output due to hepatorenal syndrome
    - History to suggest hypersplenism
  - Ask for history of alcohol consumption, history of recurring jaundice (hepatitis), previous blood transfusion, high risk sexual behavior, IV drug abuse.
  - Ask for history of loss of weight; loss of appetite: both of which are pointers towards malignancy
  - Ask for history of abdominal distension; respiratory discomfort; hemoptysis; Bony pain; back pain; blackout; seizures: history which is suggestive of malignant dissemination
  - On examination look for icterus, peripheral signs of CLD
  - On palpation a firm to hard, rounded, tender/non tender lump with smooth/

nodular may be felt in the right hypochondrium or/and epigastrium which is continuous with the liver, going under the rib cage. It will not have side to side mobility but will move cranio-caudally with respiration. Bruit may be heard on auscultation.
- Additionally features of CLD such as abdominal distension due to ascites, dilated engorged periumbilical veins and splenomegaly should be looked out for.
- You can find further discussion on this topic ahead in this Chapter.

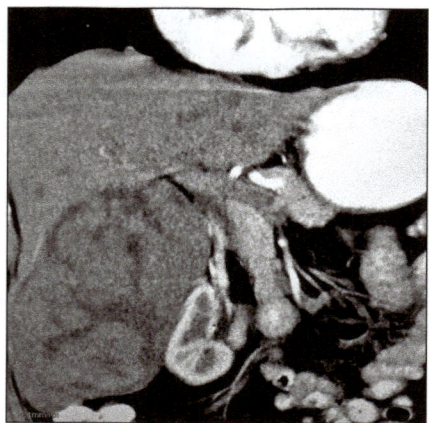

Figure 12.10: Hepatocellular carcinoma.

- Hepatic metastasis:
  - Metastasis could be from a primary in abdomen (colo-rectum, stomach, small intestine, pancreas, gall bladder, adrenal or kidney) or out side (lung, breast).
  - Think of Hepatic metastasis if there is any history or physical examination finding of any such primary along with lump in right upper quadrant. In this condition the liver gets enlarged irregularly and nodules of various size becomes palpable. Umbilication of the nodules due to a soft necrotic centre is a characteristic feature.

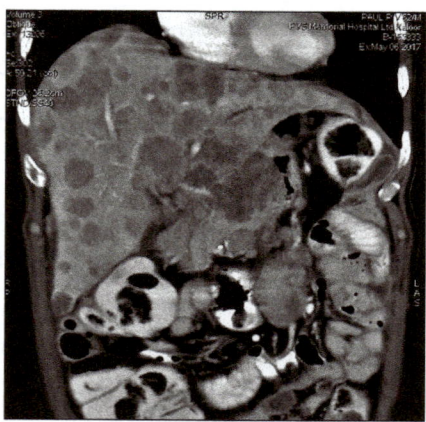

Figure 12.11: Hepatic metastasis.

- Colonic carcinoma of hepatic flexure of colon, proximal transverse colon, distal Ascending colon:
  - Patients present with alteration in bowel habits and bleed per rectum. Patients may pass black or dark red stools. Less commonly patient may develop features of intestinal obstruction (colicky abdominal pain, nausea, vomiting, constipation, obstipation, abdominal distension). Patient may give history of colonoscopy and biopsy.
  - Ask for history of loss of weight; loss of appetite: pointers towards malignancy
  - Ask for history of abdominal distension; respiratory discomfort; hemoptysis; Bony pain; back pain; blackout; seizures: history suggestive of malignant dissemination
  - On abdominal palpation one may find a firm to hard rounded, non tender lump with a smooth/nodular surface with margins felt all around, non continuous from the liver not going under the rib cage i.e. one can insinuate fingers between mass and ribcage. It may be mobile but will not move with respiration.
  - You can find further discussion on this topic ahead in this Chapter.
- Pyloric malignancy:
  - Patients present with features of gastric outlet obstruction: post prandial fullness, post prandial, non bilious voluminous vomiting containing partially digested food which was previously eaten. Patient may give history of sensation of early satiety. Patient may have GI bleed in form of hematemesis, melena. Patient will have loss of weight and loss of appetite and may give history suggestive of malignant dissemination (abdominal distension; respiratory discomfort; hemoptysis; Bony pain; back pain; blackout; seizures). Patient may give history of upper GI endoscopy and biopsy.
  - On abdominal palpation one may find a firm to hard rounded, non tender lump with a smooth/nodular surface with margins felt all around, non continuous from the liver not going under the rib cage i.e. one can insinuate fingers between mass and ribcage. It may be mobile but will not move with respiration
  - Additionally on examination look for poor nutritional status, visible gastric peristalsis and succussion splash. Also perform ausculto-percussion test to demarcate gastric outline.
  - You can find further discussion on this topic in Chapter 5.
- Pancreatic lesion: discussed in detail in chapter 6.

How to Proceed in a case of HCC: (Sequence and justification)

- Review available medical records
- Hemogram, LFT, INR and other routine blood investigations (Renal Function Test, Serum Electrolyte).

- o Hemogram to look for anemia, leucopenia and thrombocytopenia
- o LFT to look for bilirubin levels, albumin levels and liver enzyme levels (SGOT/AST, SGPT/ALT, ALP).
- o INR to look for coagulopathy
- o RFT to look for raised creatinine which would suggest hepato-renal syndrome
- o SE to look for hyponatremia
- o Bilirubin level, albumin level and INR is required for calculation of Child Pugh score. Creatinine, bilirubin and INR is required for calculation of MELD score. Creatinine, bilirubin, INR and sodium level is required for calculation of MELD-Na score. All three of these are used for grading the severity of the cirrhotic liver disease.

Table 12.1: Child Turcot Pugh score

- Parameters:
  - Bilirubin:
    - 1 point: < 2 mg/dl
    - 2 point: 2-3 mg/dl
    - 3 point: > 3 mg/dl
  - Albumin:
    - 1 point: > 3.5 g/dl
    - 2 point: 2.8-3.5 g/dl
    - 3 point: < 2.8 g/dl
  - INR:
    - 1 point: < 1.7
    - 2 point: 1.7-2.3
    - 3 point: > 2.3
  - Ascites:
    - 1 point: absent
    - 2 point: controlled with medication
    - 3 point: refractory
  - Hepatic encephalopathy:
    - 1 point: none
    - 2 point: grade 1-2
    - 3 point: grade 3-4
- CTP A: score 5-6
- CTP B: score 7-9
- CTP C: score 10-15

- Additional blood tests:
  - Serum ammonia: in case patient has clinical features of hepatic encephalopathy
  - ABG (arterial blood gas) and serum lactate levels
  - TEG: thrombo-elastography.
    - Cirrhotics are in a state of rebalanced hemostasis i.e. they have both pro and anti thrombotic tendency. Hence even if INR is raised patient may still have a pro-thrombotic tendency.
    - In such cases TEG provides reliable information about rate and strength of clot formation, clot stability and fibrinolysis
    - It thus facilitates targeted and goal directed therapy of coagulopathy
- Hepatitis panel:
  - Hepatitis B: first HBsAg is performed, if positive then perform HBeAg, HBeAb, HBcAb and quantitative HBV DNA levels
  - Hepatitis C: Hepatitis C antibody is checked for first, if positive then perform quantitative HCV RNA levels and HCV genotyping
- X-ray chest: to look for lung metastasis, pleural effusion (hepato pulmonary syndrome)
- USG (A+P):
  - It is an extension of bed side clinical evaluation, it's cheap, non invasive and easily available
  - USG has multifold role in management of HCC, it includes:
    - Diagnosis of cirrhosis
    - Screening of cirrhotic patients for HCC
    - Diagnosis of HCC
    - Guided therapy: RFA, MWA (discussed later)
    - Surveillance following treatment
  - Features to suggest cirrhosis:
    - Shrunken liver
    - Altered echotexture
    - Nodular surface
    - Dilated portal vein, increased flow velocity, reversal of flow

- Venous collaterals
- Splenomegaly
- Ascites

○ Since cirrhotic (and also non cirrhotic hepatitis B positive patients) are at high risk for HCC, 6 monthly screening is recommended in them. Modality used for screening is USG with or without AFP levels

- If no nodule or mass seen: continue 6 monthly screening
- If nodule less than 1 cm in size is seen: repeat USG at 3 month interval to see if the nodule is stable or enlarging over time. If stable over 18-24 months then return to standard screening protocol. If enlarging, then evaluate further
- If nodule more than 1 cm in size is seen: further evaluate with a 4 phase CT and/or MRI with or without biopsy

○ Findings to suggest HCC: hypoechoic (or less often hyperechoic) nodule more than 1 cm in size in a cirrhotic liver should raise suspicion of HCC.

○ In case a suspicious nodule is seen, also look for:

- Portal vein thrombosis
- Enlarged lymph nodes
- Ascites
- Metastasis elsewhere: peritoneal, omental

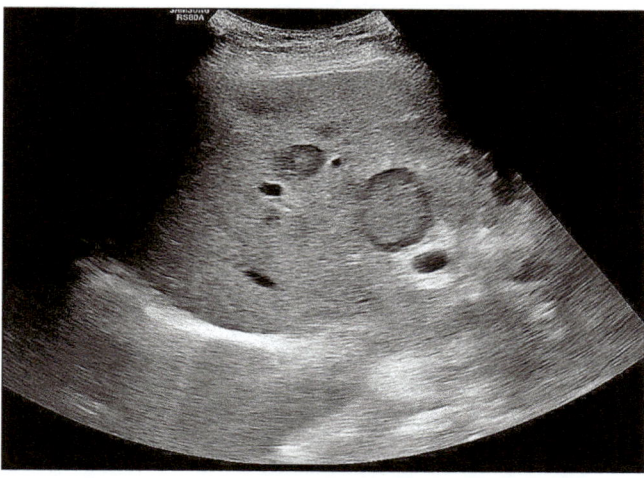

Figure 12.12: USG showing hetero-echoic HCC.

- Serum AFP level: AFP stands for Alfa Feto Protein
  - Normal: 10 ng/ml
  - Role:
    - Screening
    - Diagnosis of HCC
    - Assessing resectability
    - Assessing feasibility for liver transplant. Levels > 1000 ng/ml predict poor outcome following liver transplant
    - Prognostification
    - Response assessment
    - Surveillance
- DCP (des-gamma carboxy prothrombin) also known as PIVKA (protein induced by vitamin K absence) is another important tumor marker used in the evaluation of HCC. Levels < 100 mAU/ml suggests good prognosis
- Upper GI endoscopy: to look for varices and if present treat them using variceal band ligation or sclerotherapy
- CECT of the chest, abdomen and pelvis:
  - A 4 phase CECT is performed for the evaluation of liver lesions
    - Early arterial phase (at 18 seconds)
    - Late arterial or early portal venous phase (at 35 seconds)
    - Late portal venous phase (at 75 seconds)
    - Equilibrium phase (between 3-10 minutes)
  - Role:
    - To confirm the diagnosis
    - To stage the disease
  - Imaging feature suggestive of HCC include:
    - Arterial phase hyperenhancement (as HCC is primarily fed by hepatic artery)
    - Venous or Delayed phase washout
    - Appearance of capsule
    - Threshold growth

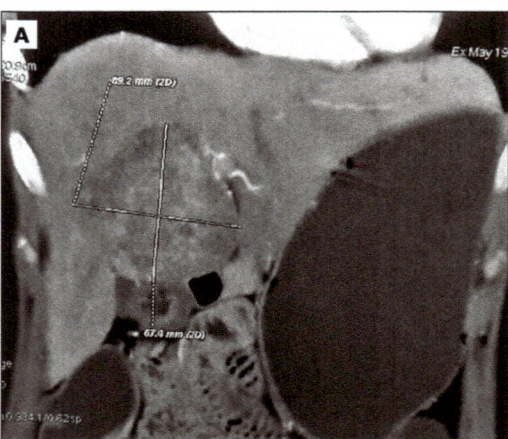 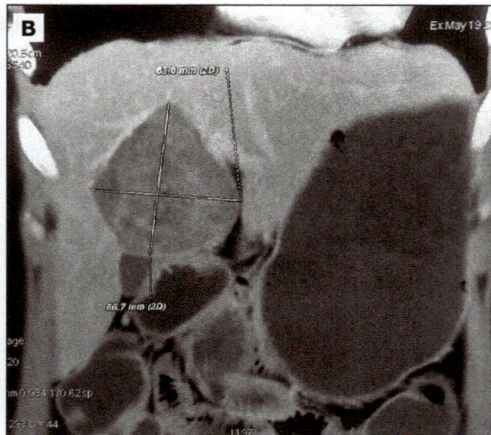

Figure 12.13: CT showing HCC with hyperenhancement in arterial phase (A) and washout in delayed phase (B).

- o If a lesion with such characteristics is seen in a cirrhotic liver, diagnosis of HCC may be affirmatively assumed without need for biopsy confirmation
- o However, if a similar lesion is seen in a non-cirrhotic liver or lesion without these characteristic features is seen in a cirrhotic liver: then biopsy confirmation may be needed prior to further treatment planning. The treatment algorithm in such cases are best formulated in the setting of a multi-disciplinary team (MDT) meeting
- o Staging:
    - Note the total number of lesions
    - Note the size and location of each lesion
    - Look for vascular involvement (portal and hepatic veins)
    - Look for tumor thrombosis
    - Look for lymph nodes
    - Look for ascites, omental, peritoneal and adrenal metastasis
    - Look for lung and bone metastasis
- Contrast enhanced dynamic MRI:
  - o Role similar to CECT
  - o It is especially useful a in cirrhotic liver where there is diagnostic dilemma on USG and CT. It is useful in differentiating an HCC from a regenerating or dysplastic nodule in a cirrhotic liver

- HCC is generally hypointense on T1 phase and hyperintense on T2 phase. The capsule surrounding the tumor is also well visualized.
- CEUS: contrast enhanced ultrasound.
    - It's a wonderful investigative tool for evaluation of liver lesions
    - In this, a special contrast agent consisting of gas filled micro-bubbles is intravenously administered.
    - Shell of the micro-bubble is made up of galactose or albumin and the gas core consists of either air, nitrogen or perfluorocarbon
    - Phases of examination include:
        - Arterial phase
        - Venous phase and
        - Post vascular Kupffer phase, during which the microbubbles are taken up by Kupffer cells. In this phase tumor appears as a contrast defect as most tumors are devoid of Kupffer cells
    - CEUS provides accurate information to help in the detection and characterization of liver lesions

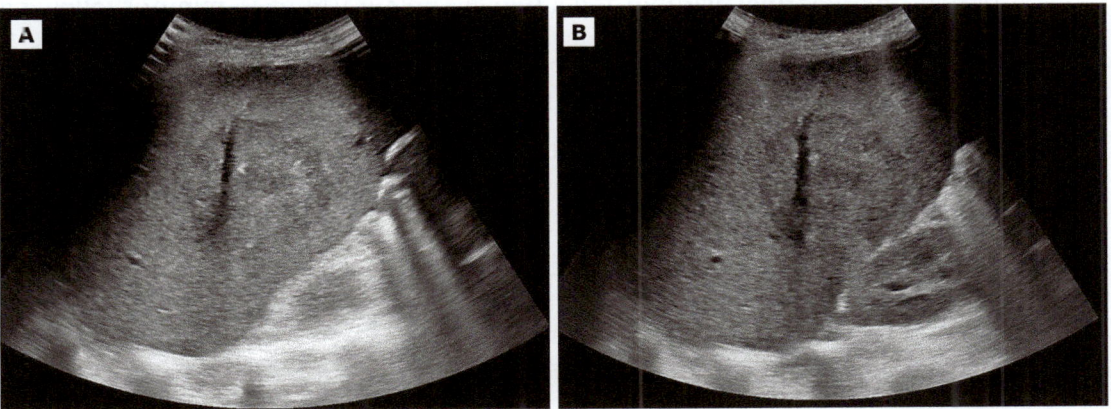

Figure 12.14: CEUS showing space occupying lesion in liver with arterial phase enhancement (A) and venous phase washout (B)

- Bone scan:
    - Done to rule out bony metastasis
    - It is performed selectively in patients with skeletal symptoms
- FDG-PET-CT:
    - Not routinely recommended, as most well differentiated HCC are poorly FDG avid

- o FDG avidity in case of HCC suggests poor differentiation with aggressive tumor biology. It predicts poor response to therapy
- Interventional radiology:
  - o Image guided percutaneous trans-hepatic biopsy of the liver lesion: if deemed necessary by MDT as discussed previously
  - o Percutaneous or Transjugular Liver biopsy: to grade the severity of liver fibrosis/cirrhosis
  - o Measurement of Hepatic venous pressure gradient (HVPG) to grade the severity of portal hypertension
- ICG (indocyanine green) clearance test.
  - o It is used to assess functional reserve of the liver
  - o In normal circumstances ICG is rapidly excreted by the liver. So, if the liver is diseased then its capacity to excrete ICG will also be hampered.
  - o ICG clearance test involves measurement of amount of ICG retained in blood (in form of percentage) 15 minutes following ICG administration. Normally it is less than 10%
  - o As per Makuuchi protocol, major liver resection should be considered only in patients with normal bilirubin and ICG levels below 10% at 15 minutes following ICG administration
- Other parameters to assess functional reserve of liver:
  - o Child Turcot Pugh score: CTP A patient may tolerate major hepatic resection. CTP B patient may tolerate limited resection. No surgery is advised in CTP C patient
  - o MELD score: patient with score more than 8 are at higher risk of surgical morbidity and mortality
- Optional investigation: Fibroscan, transient elastography
- Based on the above workup the stage of the cancer is determined. Barcelona Clinic liver cancer (BCLC) staging system is commonly used.
- Other staging systems include:
  - o Hong Kong liver cancer (HKLC) staging system
  - o TNM
  - o Okuda
  - o CLIP: Cancer of Liver Italian Program
  - o CUPI: Chinese University Prognostic Index

Table 12.2: BCLC staging system

- Very early stage (0): single tumor < 2 cm, CTP A, performance status (PS) 0
- Early stage (A): 1-3 nodule each less than 3 cm, CTP A/B, PS 0
- Intermediate stage (B): multinodular, unresectable, CTP A/B, PS 0
- Advanced stage (C): portal vein invasion, extrahepatic spread (nodal and/or distant), CTP A/B, PS 1-2
- Terminal stage (D): CTP C, PS 3-4

- Therapeutic options include:
    - Surgery:
        - Liver resection
        - Liver transplant
            - Live donor Liver transplant
            - Diseased donor Liver transplant

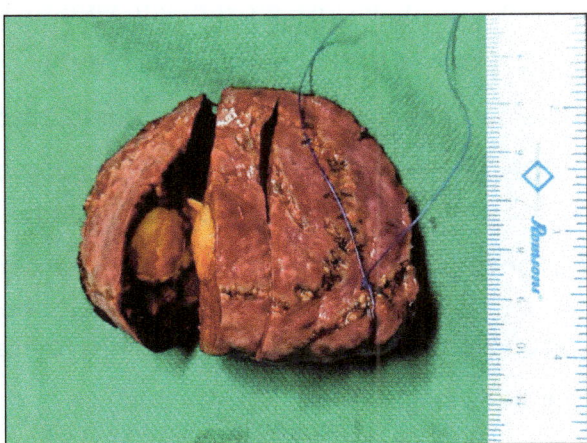

Figure 12.15: Surgical Specimen of Liver resection; cut section revealing the HCC.

    - Non-surgical options:
        - Trans arterial embolization:
            - TACE: Trans arterial chemoembolization. Doxorubicin is the commonly used chemotherapeutic agent
            - TARE: Trans arterial radio embolization. Yttrium-90 is the commonly used radio-nuclide. Rhenium 188 is a cheaper alternative

- Percutaneous therapy:
  - Thermal ablation
    - RFA: Radio frequency ablation. Preferred modality
    - MWA: Microwave ablation. Preferred
    - Cryoablation
    - Laser ablation
  - Chemical ablation
    - PEI: Percutaneous ethanol injection
    - Percutaneous acetic acid injection
  - Nonthermal - Non-chemical
    - IRE: Irreversible electroporation
    - High intensity focus ultrasound (HIFU)
  - Generally RFA is used for HCC < 3 cm in size away from major vessels/structures. MWA is used for peri-vascular HCC between 3-5 cm in size. IRE is used for HCC in close proximity to vital structures.
- Radiotherapy: External beam radiotherapy (EBRT)
- Systemic chemotherapy: Sorafenib, Regorafenib, Nivolumab

- Management of HCC is very complex and the treatment algorithm in such cases is best formulated in the setting of a multi-disciplinary team meeting.
- Also remember, prior to proceeding with definitive management of HCC, liver function needs to be optimized. Hepatology consult should be sought for. Abstinence from alcohol and smoking is of utmost importance.
- Management as per BCLC stage:
  - 0: resection or ablation
  - A: resection and/or ablation. Alternatively, transplant may be considered
  - B: TACE, TARE
  - C: Sorafenib
  - D: best supportive/palliative care
- Criteria for liver transplantation:
  - These criteria have been set so as to select patients with CLD and HCC who would achieve favorable long term prognosis with a liver transplant

- o Milan criteria:
  - ▪ Single tumor less than or equal to 5 cm in diameter or 1-3 tumor, each less than or equal to 3 cm.
- o Expanded criteria include:
  - ▪ UCSF criteria: Single tumor less than or equal to 6.5 cm in diameter or 1-3 tumor, with the largest lesion being less than or equal to 4.5 cm and total diameter of all lesions combined being less than 8.
  - ▪ Up-to-7 criteria: sum of total number of tumor and size of the largest tumor in cm being less than 7
  - ▪ Tokyo criteria: 5-5 rule: less than 5 tumors with none individually being more than 5 cm in size
- Also remember:
  - o RFA, MWA, TACE, TARE, EBRT may be used as bridging therapy in a patient who fulfils transplant criteria, to prevent disease progression while he/she is waiting for a transplant
  - o Alternatively, these modalities may be used for downstaging an HCC which is currently outside transplant criteria

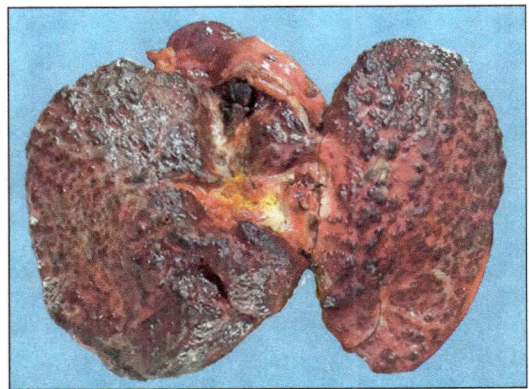

Figure 12.16: Liver transplant specimen: Explanted cirrhotic liver with HCC.

- Surveillance
  - o Modality used:
    - ▪ History and examination
    - ▪ CBC, LFT, AFP
    - ▪ USG
    - ▪ CT
- **Go through chapter 13 for literature on the subject.**

Lump in Epigastrium

- Remember: organs in epigastrium include: left lobe of liver, transverse Colon, body of Pancreas, stomach, omentum, retroperitoneum.

So the possible Differential Diagnosis are:

- Liver lesion
    - Hemangioma
    - Hydatid cyst
    - Simple liver cyst
    - Adult polycystic liver disease
    - Abscess: pyogenic/amebic
    - Adenoma
    - Focal Nodular hyperplasia
    - Regenerating nodule/dysplastic nodule
    - MCN-B (mucinous cystic neoplasm-Biliary), IPMN (intraductal papillary mucinous neoplasm)
    - Hepatocellular carcinoma
    - Hepatic metastasis
- Gastric lesion-
    - Gastric adenocarcinoma
    - Gastric lymphoma
    - Gastric GIST
- Pancreatic lesion
    - Pancreatic neoplasm
        - Adenocarcinoma
        - Mucinous cystic neoplasm
        - IPMN: Intraductal papillary mucinous neoplasm
        - SPEN: Solid pseudopapillary epithelial neoplasm
    - Pancreatic pseudocyst
- Transverse colic malignancy
- Omental lesion: omental cyst, tuberculous involvement, metastasis.
- Para-aortic lymhnodes: lymphoma/metastasis (especially from testis: hence always examine the testis)
- Retroperitoneal mass

Specific History/Examination Findings for the Common GI D/D:

- Most of them have been discussed previously

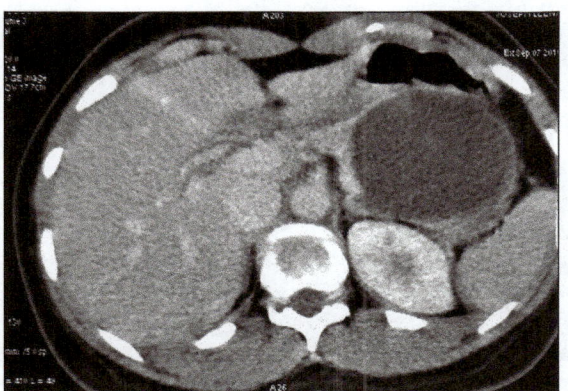

Figure 12.17: Pancreatic pseudocyst.

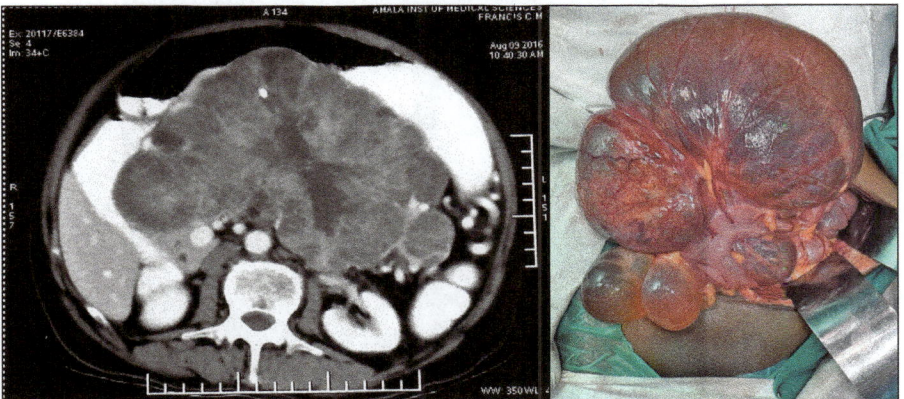

Figure 12.18: Pancreatic serous cystadenoma.

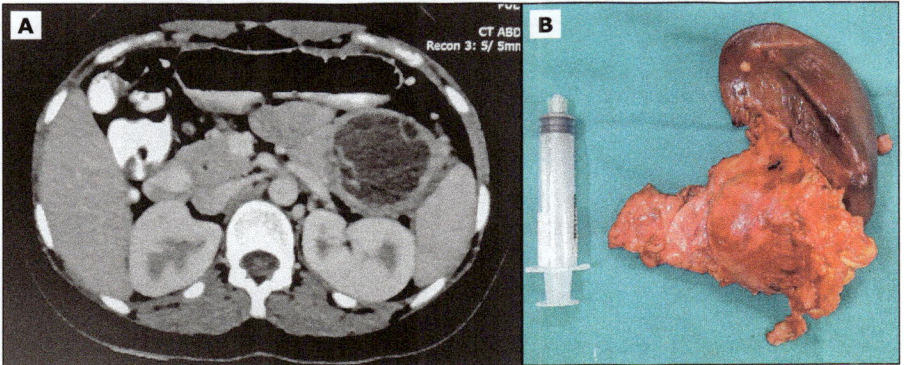

Figure 12.19: Pancreatic mucinous cystic neoplasm.
(A) Note the enhancing septation,
(B) surgical specimen of Laparoscopic Distal Pancreatico-Splenectomy performed for a MCN.

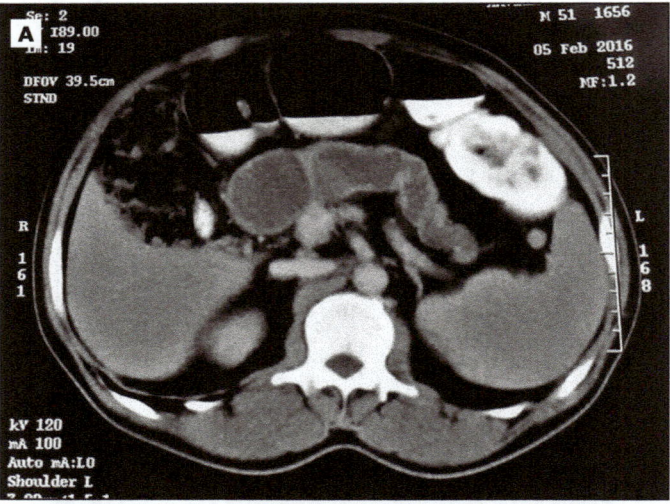

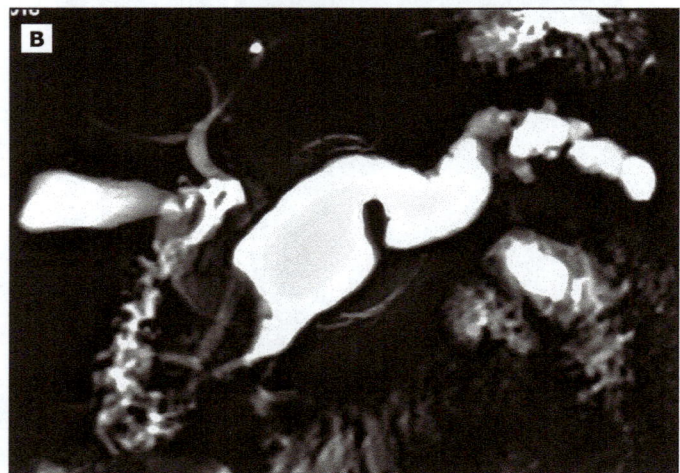

Figure 12.20: Main duct IPMN.

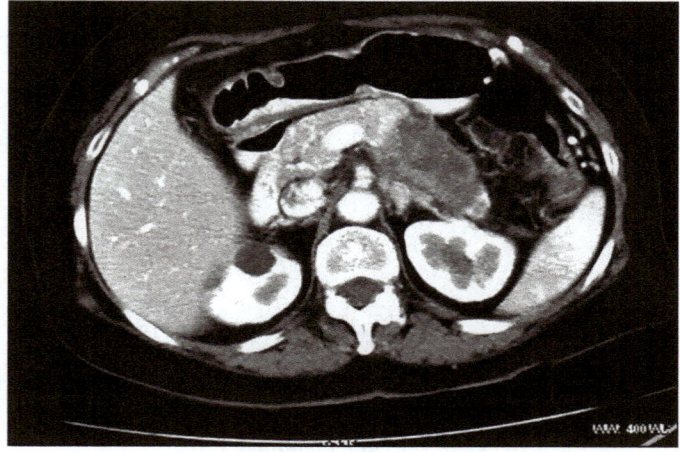

Figure 12.21: Adenocarcinoma body of pancreas

Lump in Left Upper Quadrant of Abdomen:

- Remember: organs in Left upper quadrant of abdomen include: spleen, distal transverse Colon, splenic flexure, proximal descending colon, tail of Pancreas, greater curve of stomach, left kidney, left adrenal gland, retroperitoneum.

So the possible Differential Diagnosis are:

- Splenomegaly: common causes (which would be kept in exams):
    - Portal hypertension
    - Malignancy: Lymphoma, leukemia
    - Hereditary spherocytosis
    - Idiopathic thrombocytopenic purpura
    - Splenic cyst: parasitic cyst (hydatid cyst) (most common), pseudocyst, true cyst
    - Splenic abscess
    - Infection: malaria, kala-azar, typhoid, CMV, EBV, TB
    - Tropical splenomegaly
    - Felty syndrome
    - Sarcoidosis
    - Storage disorder
- Gastric lesion-
    - Gastric adenocarcinoma
    - Gastric lymphoma
    - Gastric GIST
- Pancreatic lesion
    - Pancreatic neoplasm
        - Adenocarcinoma
        - Mucinous cystic neoplasm
        - IPMN: Intraductal papillary mucinous neoplasm
        - SPEN: Solid pseudopapillary epithelial neoplasm
    - Pancreatic pseudocyst
- Colonic malignancy
- Adrenal Mass
- Renal Mass
- Retroperitoneal mass

Specific History/Examination Findings for the Common GI D/D

- Portal hypertension: discussed in detail in chapter 8.

- Lymphoma:
  - Spleen may be affected as a part of a generalized disease or alternatively patient may have primary splenic lymphoma.
  - It generally affects the young. Patient may present with swellings in the neck, axilla and inguinal regions. B symptoms like weight loss, periodically recurring fever (Pel-Ebstein fever) and night sweats may be present.
  - Abdominal symptoms include left upper quadrant pain, discomfort, heaviness.
  - History suggestive of hypersplenism may be present:
    - Anemia: History of shortness of breath, fatigue
    - Leukopenia: History of repeated fever or infection
    - Thrombocytopenia: History of gum bleed, epistaxis, easy bruisability, hematuria, menorrhagia
  - Patient may have bone/back pain due to bone marrow infiltration.
  - On examination one may find generalized lymphadenopathy. Lymph nodes are discrete, firm rubbery in consistency and not fixed to its surroundings
  - Moderate to severe splenomegaly will be present
- Hereditary spherocytosis:
  - It is a type of hemolytic anemia. Patients are young and present with features of anemia (History of fatigue, shortness of breath, postural dizziness or syncope, need for blood transfusion) and jaundice. However, urine won't be high colored as in obstructive jaundice (acholuric jaundice). Family history may be present. Patients tend to develop pigmented gall stones causing biliary colic, cholecystitis, choledocholithiasis, cholangitis and biliary pancreatitis. Hence when gall stones are identified in a young patient, one must rule out hemolytic anemia.
  - On examination look for pallor and moderate splenomegaly

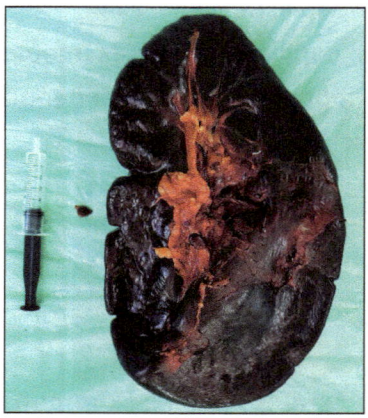

Figure 12.22: Surgical specimen of a Splenectomy performed for Hereditary Spherocytosis, note the splenunculus which has to be sought for and excised.

- Idiopathic thrombocytopenic purpura
  - It affects the young. Presents with features of thrombocytopenia such as history of gum bleed, epistaxis, easy bruisability, hematuria, menorrhagia. Patient characteristically develops cutaneous and mucous membrane purpuras.
  - On examination look for purpuras. Mild splenomegaly will be present. Tourniquet test may be elicited: when a sphygmomanometer cuff is applied to the arm and inflated beyond systolic blood pressure, petechial hemorrhages develop in the arm distal to the cuff.
- Tropical Splenomegaly:
  - It occurs due to immunological over stimulation in response to repeated attacks of malarial infection over a long period of time
  - Inquire regarding history of malarial infection. History suggestive of hypersplenism may be present
  - On examination massive splenomegaly will be present
- Felty syndrome: consists of chronic rheumatoid arthritis, leucopenia and splenomegaly
- Most of the other differential diagnoses have already been discussed previously

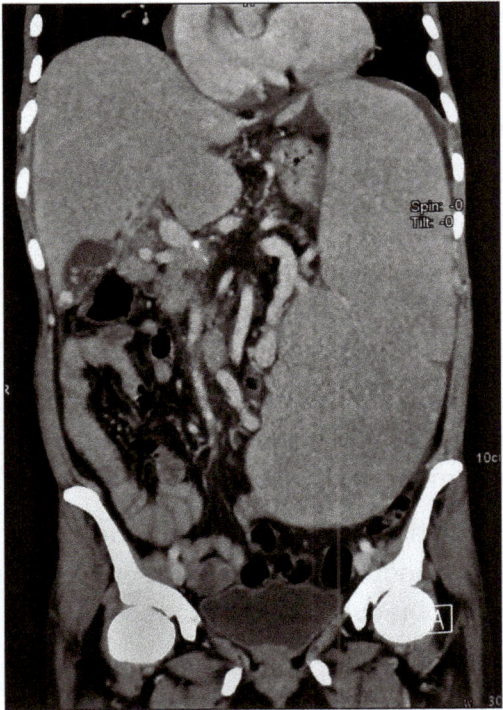

Figure 12.23: Splenomegaly.

Lump in Right Lower Quadrant of the Abdomen

- Remember: organs in right lower quadrant include: terminal ileum, cecum, ascending colon, appendix, retroperitoneum, mesentery, lower pole of right kidney, ectopic right kidney, undescended right testis, right tubo-ovarian structures

So the possible Differential Diagnosis are:

- Ileo-cecal tuberculosis
- Ileo-cecal Crohn's
- Colonic malignancy: cecum/ascending colon; adenocarcinoma/lymphoma
- Appendiceal mucocele
- Appendiceal mass/abscess
- Appendiceal malignancy
- Amebic typhlitis
- Actinomycosis
- Lymph node mass: TB, lymphoma
- Retroperitoneal mass
- Renal lower pole mass
- Ectopic kidney
- Undescended testis
- Right tubo-ovarian lesion: cyst, malignancy

Specific History/Examination Findings for Common GI D/D

- Ileo-cecal tuberculosis:
  - Patients present with lump and/or dull to crampy pain in RLQ. Patients are generally young. They may have cough with expectoration, evening rise in temperature, anorexia, weight loss and weakness. They may also have loose stools. Patient may develop features of intestinal obstruction (colicky abdominal pain, nausea, vomiting, constipation, obstipation, abdominal distension, ball rolling sensation and borborygmi). Patient may give history of colonoscopy and biopsy and history of treatment with AKT (anti tuberculous/Koch's treatment)
  - On abdominal palpation one may find a firm to hard rounded, tender/non tender lump with a smooth/nodular surface with margins felt all around. It may be mobile but will not move with respiration.
  - Also look for generalized lymphadenopathy.
  - You can find further discussion on this topic ahead in this Chapter.

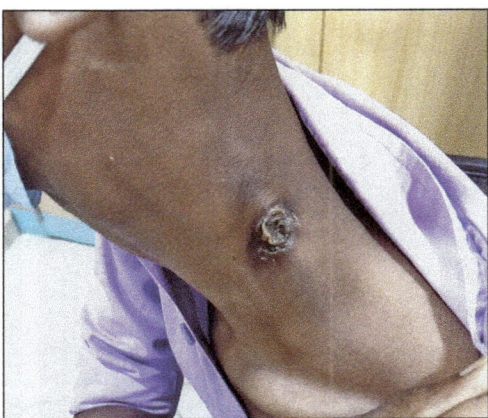

Figure 12.24: Findings on cervical examination like Cervical Lymph nodes and Tuberculous sinus (as in this picture) should not be missed.

- Ileo-cecal Crohn's: (also discussed separately in chapter 10).
  - Lump may form due to inflammatory ileo-cecal thickening, phlegmon formation or abscess formation
  - They present with pain, fever, altered bowel habits, blood in stools. In case of stricturing pattern of disease they may develop features of obstruction: pain, nausea, vomiting, distension, ball rolling sensation, borborygmi. Ask for perianal symptoms, features of extra intestinal manifestations and primary sclerosing cholangitis.
  - On examination look for poor nutritional status, scars of previous surgery, perianal Crohn's disease and extraintestinal manifestations.
  - On abdominal palpation one may find a firm to hard rounded, tender/non tender lump with a smooth/nodular surface with margins felt all around. It may be mobile but will not move with respiration.

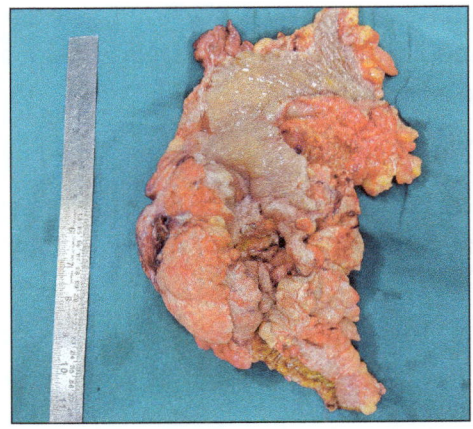

Figure 12.25: Ileo-cecal Phlegmon in a patient with Crohn's disease presenting with an RIF mass.

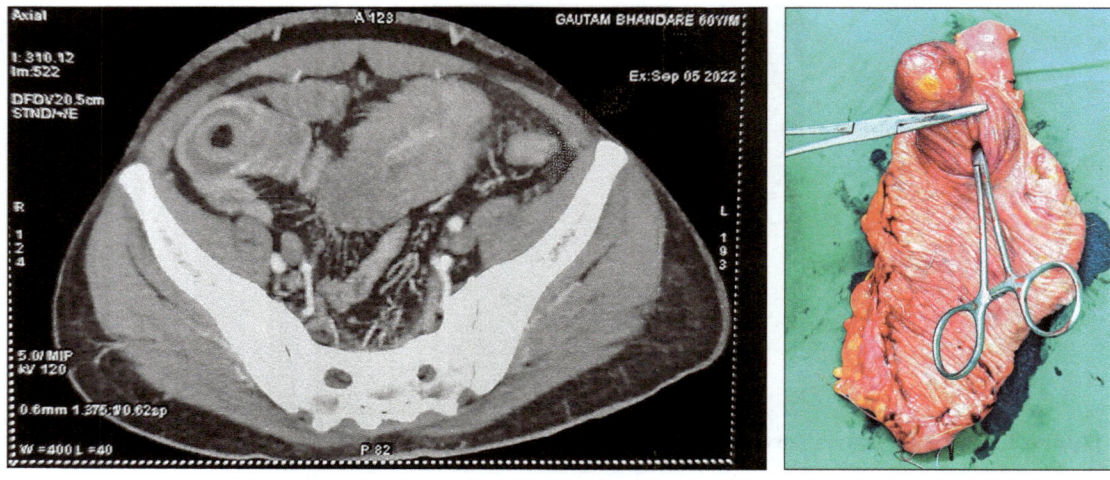

Figure 12.26: Ileo-cecal Intussusception due to lead points like lipoma, polyps or lymphoma can also result in an RIF mass.

- Colonic malignancy:
    - Patients are generally middle-aged or elderly. They usually present with passage of melena or reddish stools, anemia, anorexia and weight loss. They may have pain and alteration of bowel habits. Right sided lesions less commonly cause obstructive symptoms because it is more capacious. This is in contrast to left sided lesions which usually present with obstructive symptoms and passage of bright red blood per anum.
    - Ask for history of loss of weight; loss of appetite: pointers towards malignancy
    - Ask for history of abdominal distension; respiratory discomfort; hemoptysis; Bony pain; back pain; blackout; seizures: history suggestive of malignant dissemination
    - On abdominal palpation one may find a firm to hard rounded, non tender lump with a smooth/nodular surface with margins felt all around. It may be mobile but will not move with respiration.
    - You can find further discussion on this topic ahead in this Chapter.
- Appendiceal mucocele: there is no specific history or physical examination finding except for a well defined lump in RLQ. If it ruptures it may result in pseudomyxoma peritonie

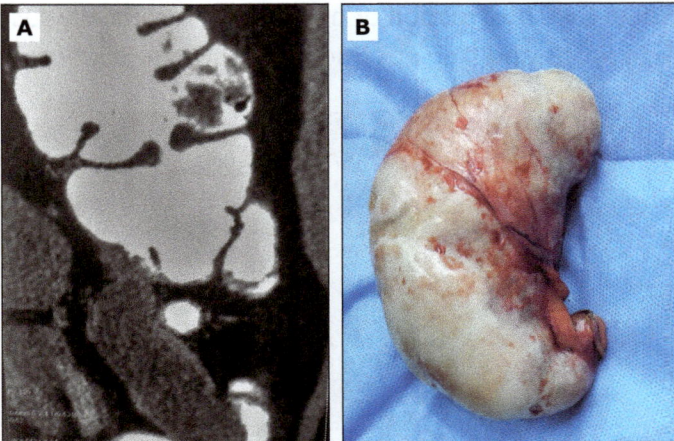

Figure 12.27: Appendiceal mucocele.

- Appendiceal mass/abscess:
  - Patient will have features of appendicitis: pain, nausea, vomiting, fever, loose stools.
  - On examination apart from mass there will be tenderness in Mc Burney's point.
- Appendiceal malignancy: presentation is similar to that of right colonic malignancy. GI bleed, however, is less common.

How to Proceed in a Case of Ileo-cecal Tuberculosis: (Sequence and justification)

- Review available medical records
- Routine blood investigations (Hemogram, Liver Function Test, Renal Function Test, Serum Electrolyte, INR).
- Additional blood tests: ESR, CRP
- Stool routine microscopy and stool culture, if patient complains of loose stools
- X-ray chest to look for features of pulmonary tuberculosis:
  - Pulmonary infiltrates or consolidation
  - Cavitary lesions
  - Pleural effusion
  - Hilar or mediastinal lymphadenopathy
  - Discrete fibrotic scar
- Sputum sample for Ziehl Neelsen (ZN) staining to look for acid fast bacilli (AFB) +/- Gene Xpert: in case X-ray chest shows features of TB or patient complains of productive cough. Two samples are collected: one spot and one early morning.

- X-ray abdomen: in case obstruction or perforation is clinically suspected to look for multiple air-fluid levels and free gas under diaphragm respectively.

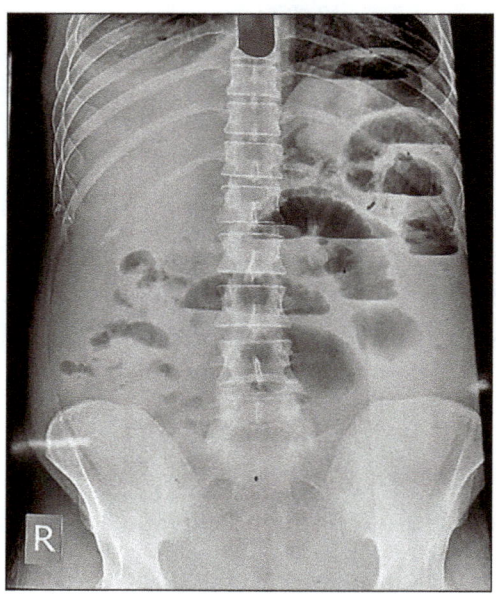

Figure 12.28: X-ray showing Step ladder pattern of air-fluid levels suggesting Intestinal obstruction.

- USG abdomen and pelvis: It is an extension of bed side clinical evaluation, its cheap, non invasive and easily available.
  - It is used to characterize the right iliac fossa mass which in this case is ileo-cecal tuberculosis.
  - Findings to expect in a case of abdominal TB:
    - Thickening of terminal ileum and cecum
    - Mesenteric lymphadenopathy. They may be discrete or conglomerated. There may be central hypoechoic area due to central necrosis
    - Ascites: free or loculated. Ascitic fluid loculated between two loops of bowel gives rise to Club Sandwich sign.
    - Peritoneal, omental and mesenteric nodularity and thickening
    - Omental caking
- CT: including CECT (A+P) with oral, rectal and IV contrast, CT enterography (oral administration of contrast), CT enteroclysis (administration of contrast via naso-jejunal tube):
  - To confirm the findings seen on USG and further characterize the disease

- Findings to expect:
  - Thickening of terminal ileum and cecum with mucosal hyperenhancement with engorged Vasa recta
  - Pulled up cecum with deformed IC valve
  - Terminal ileal, cecal and/or ascending colon strictures
  - Matting of small bowel loops with or without cocoon formation
  - Mesenteric lymphadenopathy. They may be discrete or conglomerated. There may be central hypointense area due to central necrosis
  - Ascites: free or loculated. The Hounsfeild unit is relatively higher compared to water as the ascitic fluid is exudative in nature
  - Peritoneal, omental and mesenteric nodularity and thickening
  - Omental caking

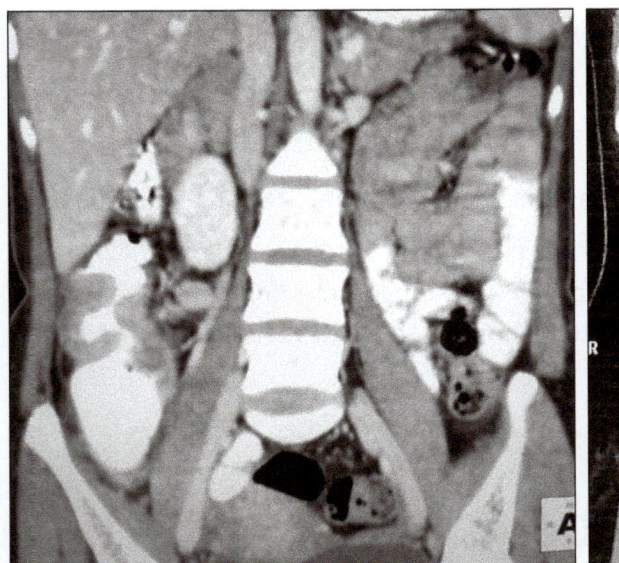 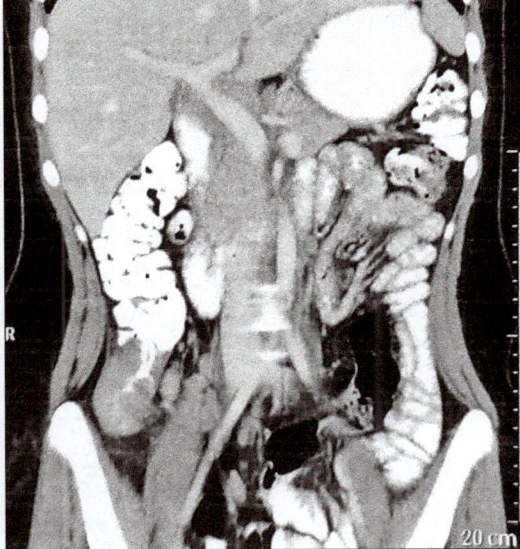

Figure 12.29: CT showing hyperplastic cecal TB.

- Additionally it helps:
  - To examine the rest of the bowel for disease involvement
  - To look for complications: obstruction, perforation, phlegmon formation, abscess formation, fistula

- ▪ To characterize the pulmonary disease
- MRI: including MRI (A+P) with oral, rectal and IV contrast, MRI enterography (oral administration of contrast), MRI enteroclysis (administration of contrast via naso-jejunal tube):
  - ○ Role is similar to CT.
- Colonoscopy:
  - ○ To examine the right colon and terminal ileum.
  - ○ To see for site, extent and severity of the inflammatory process
  - ○ To note the morphology:
    - ▪ Hypertrophic
    - ▪ Ulcerative
    - ▪ Ulcero- Hypertrophic
  - ○ To rule out cancer
  - ○ Main role is to obtain biopsy for:
    - ▪ Histopathological examination
    - ▪ Gram and ZN staining
    - ▪ Gene-Xpert: it's a cartridge based nucleic acid amplification test. It provides rapid diagnosis and antibiotic sensitivity pattern too.
    - ▪ Culture using solid media (Lowenstein-Jensen medium) or liquid media (Mycobacterial growth indicator tube). It is the gold standard test. However, it is time consuming.

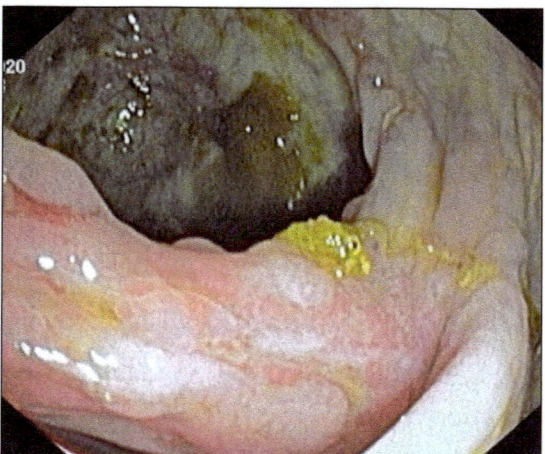

Figure 12.30: Colonoscopy showing Cecal tuberculosis.

- Ascitic fluid study:
  - Routine examination and microscopy: In TB the ascitic fluid is generally low SAAG (Serum ascites albumin gradient < 1.1), with low glucose levels, high protein level and lymphocyte predominant leukocytosis on microscopy.
  - Fluid ADA (adenosine deaminase) levels: it is raised in TB
  - Culture and Gene-Xpert
- Additional investigations:
  - Capsule endoscopy: to look for small bowel involvement
  - Enteroscopy: to look for small bowel involvement
    - Push enteroscopy
    - Single or double balloon enteroscopy
    - Spiral enteroscopy
  - Barium meal follow through: findings include:
    - Accelerated transit time
    - Pulled up cecum
    - Fleischner or inverted umbrella sign: due to narrowing of terminal ileum with thickening and/or wide gaping of the IC valve
    - Goose neck deformity: due to loss of normal angle of the IC junction
    - Stierlin sign: narrowing of terminal ileum with rapid emptying of its contents
    - String sign: persistent narrow steam of contrast in distal ileum
  - Enteroclysis
  - Fecal calprotectin: levels rise in case of active intestinal mucosal inflammation. It's an optional investigation

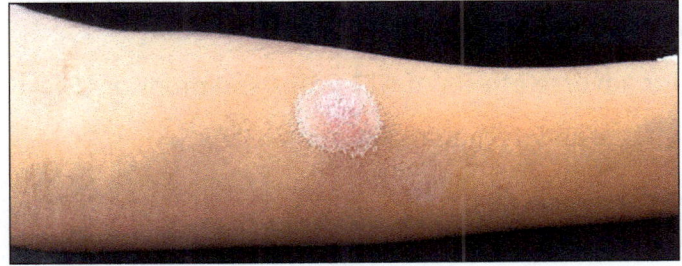

Figure 12.31: Occasionally a Mantoux test may be performed. A strongly positive test result as seen in the image is significant.

- Medical management:
  - It is the primary modality of treatment
  - It consists of administration of category 1 Anti Tuberculosis Therapy (ATT) as per the RNTCP act. It is as follows:
    - Intensive phase: it consists of 2 months of Isoniazid (H), Rifampicin (R), Pyrazinamide (Z) and Ethambutol (E) in daily dosages as per 4 weight band categories.
    - Continuation phase: it consists of 4 months of Isoniazid, Rifampicin and Ethambutol in daily dosages as per 4 weight band categories.
    - That is: 2 month HZRE followed by 4 month HRE
    - Some physicians continue ATT for 9-12 months, however advantage of prolonged therapy over 6-month regimen has not been proven.
  - In case the patient has been previously been treated with ATT (or is a case of relapse, treatment failure or treatment defaulter), then category 2 ATT as per RNTCP act is administered. It consists of:
    - Intensive phase: It consists of 2 months of daily H, R, Z, E and Streptomycin (S) followed by one month of daily H, R, Z and E
    - Continuation phase: It consists of 5 months of daily H, R and E
    - That is: 2 month HZRES followed by 1 month HRZE followed by 5 month HRE
  - Monitoring of patients while on ATT:
    - History and physical examination: to look for resolution of symptoms and to watch for persistence or reappearance of symptoms
    - Weight charting: Patients tend to gain weight which they have previously lost. Lack of gain weight is a sign of disease persistence/recurrence
    - Explain the patient that he/she may pass orange or red colored urine due to rifampicin administration. Patient should be reassured that it is nothing to be worried about.
    - Watch for adverse effects of ATT drugs and monitor LFT.
  - Major side effects and its management:
    - Jaundice, hepatitis, acute liver failure:
      - It may occur as a side effect of H, R and Z. In addition, R may cause asymptomatic jaundice without hepatitis. Hence it is important to regularly monitor patient's LFT.

- Advise of an expert needs to be sought.
- Once DILI (drug induced liver injury) has occurred, then all ATT drugs should be stopped. However, it is considered unsafe to stop ATT then a non hepatotoxic regimen consisting of S, E and a fluoroquinolone should be started.
- Once the drug induced hepatitis or DILI has resolved, the drugs are re-introduced one at a time. If symptoms recur or LFTs become abnormal as the drugs are re-introduced, the last drug added should be stopped.
- The usual order in which the drugs are re-introduced are: R followed by H followed by Z.
- In case of non-resolution of hepatitis, non hepatotoxic regimen consisting of S, E and a fluoroquinolone should be started or continued

- Skin rashes with or without itching: It may occur as a side effect of H, R, Z and S. If patient develops itching without rash one may try symptomatic management in the form of anti-histaminic and moisturizing cream. Development of rash however necessitates stoppage of ATT and referral to an expert.
- Visual impairment: It may occur as a side effect of E. It may necessitate stoppage of E.
- Deafness, Dizziness/vertigo, decreased urine output: It may occur as a side effect of S. It may necessitate stoppage of S.
- Shock, purpura, acute renal failure: It may occur as a side effect of R. It may necessitate stoppage of R.

o Minor side effects and its management:
- Gastro-intestinal symptoms: nausea, abdominal pain, anorexia: It may occur as a side effect of H, R and Z. To reduce these symptoms, patient may be advised to consume the medication with small meals or just before bedtime.
- Joint pains: It may occur as a side effect of Z. PCM or NSAIDs may be prescribed to achieve symptomatic relief.
- Burning numbness or tingling sensation in hands and/or feet: It may occur as a side effect of H. Pyridoxine should be given along with ATT to prevent this side-effect.
- Drowsiness: It may occur as a side effect of H. Reassure the patient and advise him/her to take the medication just before bedtime.

- Flu syndrome (fever, chills, malaise, headache, bone pain): It is seen with intermittent dosing of R. If it occurs change from intermittent dosing to daily administration of R.
- Surgical management:
  - Medical management usually suffices in most cases.
  - Indications for surgery are:
    - Unresolving obstruction
    - Perforation
    - Unresolving phlegmon/abscess
    - Unresolving symptomatic disease
    - Internal or external fistula
    - Inability to differentiate from malignancy
  - Options:
    - Ileo-cecal resection with ileo-ascending anastomosis or stoma
    - Right hemicolectomy with ileo-transverse anastomosis with or without proximal loop ileostomy
  - ATT need to be initiated in the post-operative period
- Surveillance

How to Proceed in a case of Right Colonic Carcinoma: (Sequence and justification)

- Review available medical records
- Routine blood investigations (Hemogram, Liver Function Test, Renal Function Test, Serum Electrolyte, INR)
- X-ray chest: to look for lung metastasis.
- X-ray abdomen: if intestinal obstruction is clinically suspected
- USG (A+P):
  - It is an extension of bed side clinical evaluation, it's cheap, non invasive and easily available
  - It is used to characterize the right iliac fossa mass which in this case is Right colonic malignancy.
  - If malignancy is suspected: look for liver metastasis, ascites, omental/peritoneal metastasis.

- **Please note**:
  - Presence of isolated limited liver metastasis, isolated limited lung metastasis, isolated limited peritoneal metastasis and synchronous limited liver and lung metastasis is not a contraindication to curative intent treatment in colo-rectal cancer, unlike in Ca esophagus, stomach, pancreas where palliative intent treatment would have been initiated. Hence even if lung or liver metastasis is detected on X-ray chest or USG abdomen further evaluation with CT or PET-CT is still justified to further stage and characterize the disease. Further management plan in such situation should then be planned in a tumor board/multi-disciplinary team (MDT) meeting after thorough deliberation.
- Colonoscopy:
  - Performed to confirm the presence of a neoplastic growth in the colon; if present note:
    - Note the site and size
    - Note the longitudinal and circumferential Extent
    - Morphology: proliferative/ulcerative/ulcero-proliferative/infiltrative
    - Whether passable or not
    - Presence of synchronous lesion: malignancy, polyp, IBD
    - Biopsy: 6–8 in number

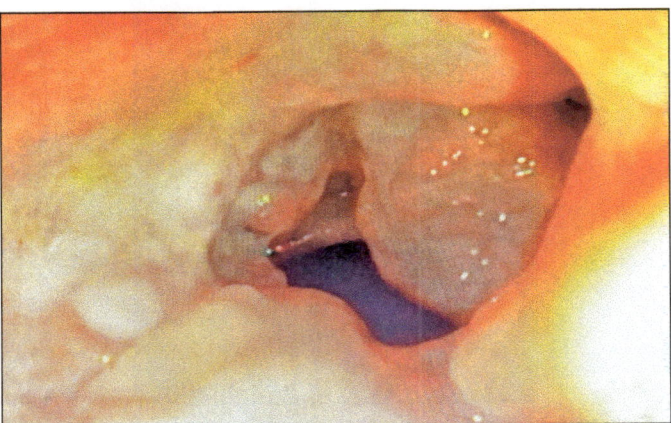

Figure 12.32: Colonoscopy showing carcinoma colon.

- Blood CEA level:
  - It is tumor marker used in the evaluation of colo-rectal cancer.
  - Normal level: < 4 ng/ml

- - - Levels are raised in smokers
  - Role:
    - Diagnosis
    - Staging
    - Prognostification
    - Response assessment: post surgery, post adjuvant therapy
    - Surveillance
- CECT of the chest, abdomen and pelvis: to stage the disease: local and distant staging.
  - To evaluate the site, size, extent of growth
  - Involvement of adjacent organs/vessels
  - To look for lymph nodes
  - To look for distant metastasis: liver metastasis, omental/peritoneal metastasis, krukenberg tumor, ascites, lung metastasis, pleural effusion.

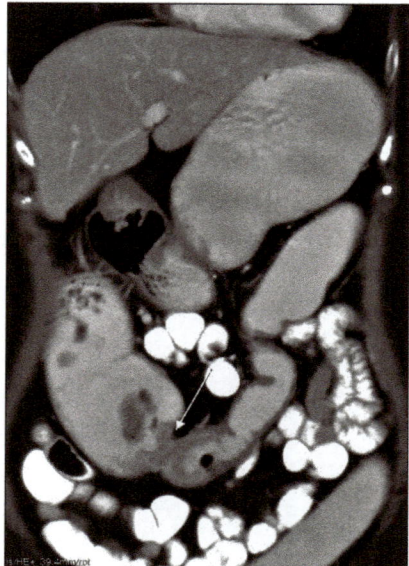

Figure 12.33: CT image showing right colonic malignancy.

- FDG-PET-CT: PET is done primarily to rule out distant metastasis which may have not been picked up on CECT.
- Staging laparoscopy. Done to look for peritoneal metastasis/occult liver metastasis which may be missed on pre-operative imaging

- Optional investigation:
  - Determination of tumor MMR (mismatch repair gene) or MSI (microsatellite instability) status. It helps in prognostification and determining if adjuvant chemotherapy is required or not in stage 2 cancers. MSI-H (high) tumors have better prognosis than MSI-L (low) or MSS (microsatellite stable) tumors. Adjuvant chemotherapy is indicated in stage 2 cancers which are MSI-H.
  - KRAS mutation analysis: It is considered in cases of metastatic colorectal cancer. Anti-EGFR therapy is considered only in cases with wild type KRAS. Anti EGFR therapy is ineffective in cases with mutated KRAS.
  - BRAF V600E mutation testing: It is considered in cases of metastatic colorectal cancer. It helps in prognostification. Tumors with this mutations usually have poor tumor biology and demonstrate resistance to conventional chemotherapy.
- At the end of the work up, the tumor is staged as per AJCC-TNM staging system

Table 12.3: AJCC-TNM staging system for Colorectal cancer

- T stage:
  - T1: Tumor invades submucosa
  - T2: Tumor invades muscularis propria
  - T3: Tumor invades subserosal connective tissue without penetrating through serosa (visceral peritoneum) or invading adjacent structures
  - T4: Tumor penetrating through serosa +/- invading adjacent structures
- N stage:
  - N1: Metastasis to 1-3 lymph nodes (LN)
  - N2: Metastasis to 4 or more LN
- M stage:
  - M0: No distant metastasis
  - M1: Distant metastasis present
- Stage:
  - Stage I: T1, T2
  - Stage II: T3, T4
  - Stage III: N1, N2
  - Stage IV: M1

- Management principles:
  - Treatment would include upfront surgery followed by adjuvant chemotherapy (if indicated).

- o There is no role for radiotherapy.
- o More recently neo-adjuvant chemotherapy has been used in locally unresectable T4b tumors.
- Surgery for right colonic cancer:
- o Right hemicolectomy
- o Extended Right hemicolectomy

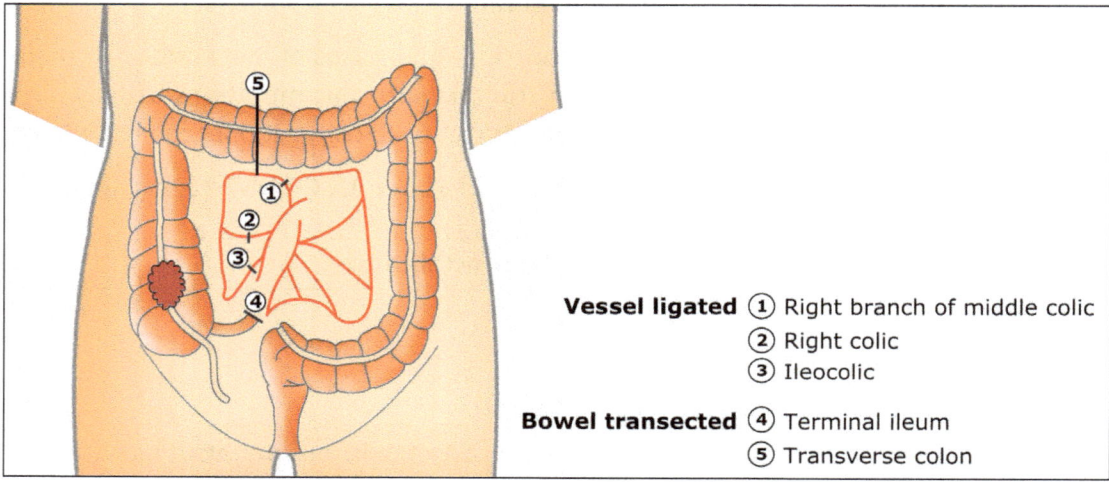

Figure 12.34: Right hemicolectomy.

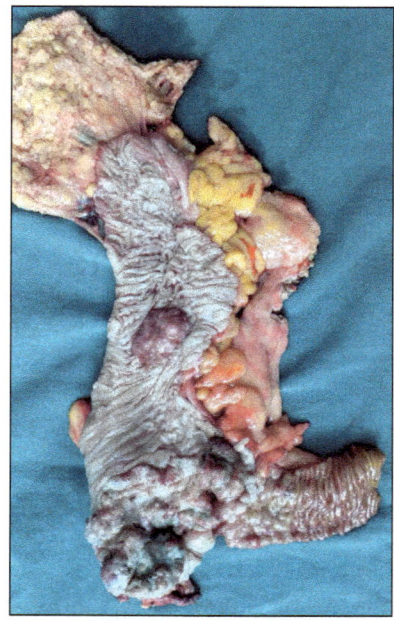

Figure 12.35: Radical right hemicolectomy specimen showing 2 synchronous malignancies.

- Adjuvant chemotherapy
  - Indications:
    - T4
    - N+
    - T3 with high risk features:
      - Obstruction or perforation
      - LVI: Lymphovascular invasion
      - PNI: Perineural invasion
      - < 12 lymph nodes sampled
      - MSI-high (microsatellite instability); MMR-deficient (mismatch repair gene); MSS (microsatellite stable)
  - Options:
    - FOLFOX: leucovorine, 5-FU and oxaliplatin. 2 weekly for 6 months.
    - CAPEOX: Capecitabine and oxaliplatin. 3 weekly for 6 months.
    - 5-FU or capecitabine
    - FOLFIRI: leucovorine, 5-FU and irinotecan
- Surveillance
  - Modality used:
    - History and physical examination
    - Blood CEA levels
    - USG abdomen and pelvis
    - CECT chest, abdomen and pelvis
    - Colonoscopy
- **Go through chapter 13 for literature on the subject.**

Lump in Left Lower Quadrant of Abdomen

- Remember: organs in left lower quadrant include: descending colon, sigmoid colon, retroperitoneum, mesentery, lower pole of left kidney, ectopic left kidney, undescended left testis, left tubo-ovarian structures

So the possible Differential Diagnosis are:
- Colonic malignancy
- Sigmoid diverticulitis
- Retroperitoneal mass
- Renal lower pole mass
- Ectopic kidney
- Undescended testis
- Left tubo-ovarian lesion: cyst, malignancy

Specific History/Examination Findings for Common GI D/D

- Diverticulitis:
  - Patients are generally obese elderly males presenting with constipation, straining at stools, left lower quadrant abdominal pain, fever, and fresh bright red lower GI bleed.
  - On abdominal palpation one may find a firm to hard rounded, tender/non tender lump with a smooth/nodular surface with margins felt all around. It may be mobile but will not move with respiration.

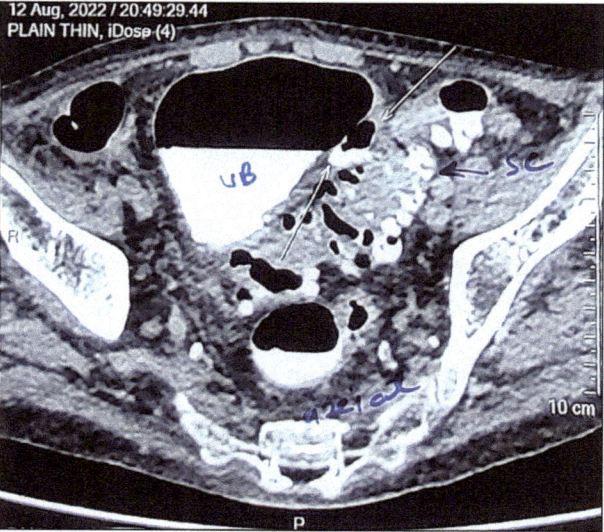

Figure 12.36: Diverticular phlegmon with colo-vesical fistula presenting with an LIF mass.

- Colonic malignancy: discussed separately

13 Literature/Trials in GI Surgery which an Exam-Going Resident Must Know

INTRODUCTION

- In this chapter we have attempted to compile all the important trials and studies which are of importance in the field of GI surgery/GI oncology. We have also tried to touch upon controversial topics where there are two or more approaches/options; here we have discussed the pros and cons of each option and provided a general consensus/recommendation.
- This knowledge is of importance to super-speciality residents preparing for final exams and broad speciality residents preparing for competitive entrance exams.
- We have mentioned the names of the important studies and only briefly described the study methodology and results. The reader is requested to further read it in detail as required.
- The important outcome parameters in oncology trials are: overall survival (OS), 1 year, 3 year and 5 year survival, progression free survival (PFS), disease free survival (DFS), recurrence free survival (RFS), local recurrence (LR).
- Abbreviations used in this chapter:
    - PS: performance status
    - LN: lymph node
    - Ca: carcinoma
    - AC: adenocarcinoma
    - SCC: squamous cell carcinoma
    - CT: chemotherapy
    - RT: radiotherapy
    - CRT: chemoradiation
    - NA: neo-adjuvant
    - MA: meta-analysis

ESOPHAGEAL & GEJ CANCER

- MRC/OE2: It found pre-op CT with 5-FU and cisplatin to be efficacious in esophageal cancer compared to surgery alone
- **CROSS trial**: It studied regimen consisting of carboplatin + paclitaxel + 41.4 gray RT in esophageal SCC, esophageal and gastro-esophageal junction (GEJ) AC compared to surgery alone. Overall pathological complete response rate was 29% (49% for SCC and 23% for AC). It found the regimen to be efficacious compared to surgery alone. It is a landmark trial which established role of NA-CRT in esophageal and GEJ cancer.
- **MAGIC trial**: It studied regimen consisting of 3 cycles of ECF (epirubicin, cisplatin and 5-Fluorouracil) before and after surgery (i.e. peri-operative chemotherapy) in esophageal, GEJ and gastric AC compared to surgery alone. It found the regimen to be efficacious compared to surgery alone. It is a landmark trial which established role of peri-op CT in esophageal, GEJ and gastric AC.
- Neo-AEGIS trial: This trial compared CROSS regimen vs MAGIC regimen in esophageal and GEJ AC. The trial found both the regimens to be equivalent and resulted in similar overall survival.
- RTOG trial and INT-0123 trial: These trials established the role of definitive CRT in esophageal SCC
- In general:
    - NA-CRT is advocated for mid or lower esophageal SCC.
    - Definitive CRT is advocated for cervical and proximal esophageal SCC. It is also advocated in patients with poor PS who would not tolerate surgery.
    - Peri-operative CT is generally advocated in cases of esophageal/GEJ AC. However, NA-CRT may be considered in cases where R0 resection seems difficult.
- MUNICON I & II trial: It studied the role of FDG-PET-CT in response to assessment following NA treatment. Both trials showed that the continuation of neoadjuvant chemotherapy in metabolic responders resulted in a favourable outcome. However, the poor prognosis of metabolic non-responders could not be improved by Immediate surgery (MUNICON I) or addition of neoadjuvant radiation therapy (MUNICONII) Indicating dismal tumor biology of these tumors.
- ESOPRESSO trial: It investigated the role of esophagectomy after clinical complete response (cCR) to NA-CRT for esophageal SCC. It concluded that close observation with salvage surgery might be a reasonable option in patients achieving cCR after NA-CRT. The concept is similar to Habr-Gama approach for rectal cancer.

- SANO trial, ESOSTRATE trial: These trials are studying the concept of Surgery As Needed in Esophageal cancer. These are ongoing trials attempting to compare NA-CRT followed by surgery vs active surveillance (i.e. a non-surgical approach) in patients who have achieved a clinically complete response following NA-CRT. Concept is similar to Habr-Gama approach for rectal cancer.
- Extent of lymphadenectomy:
  - Dutch trial: It suggested extensive lymphadenectomy to be beneficial if < 8 lymph nodes (LN) are positive for metastasis.
  - Akiyama et al: Their study found 3 field lymphadenectomy to be better than 2 field for esophageal Ca
  - Rizk et al using WECC (world esophageal cancer collaboration) data: Their study suggested removal of atleast 10 LN for T1 esophageal tumor, 20 LN for T2 esophageal tumor and 30 LN for T3/T4 esophageal tumor
  - Overall Japanese studies found 3 field lymphadenectomy to be better whereas western data suggests 2 field lymphadenectomy to be better.
  - General consensus is to perform standard 2 field lymphadenectomy for distal esophageal cancers, extended or total 2 field lymphadenectomy for mid esophageal cancers and 3 field lymphadenectomy for proximal esophageal cancers.

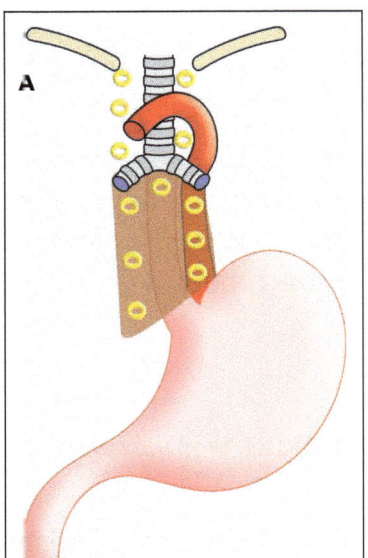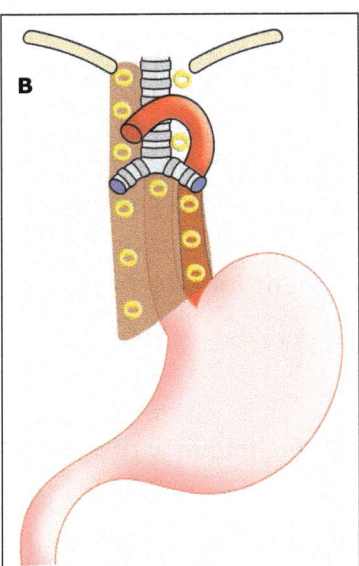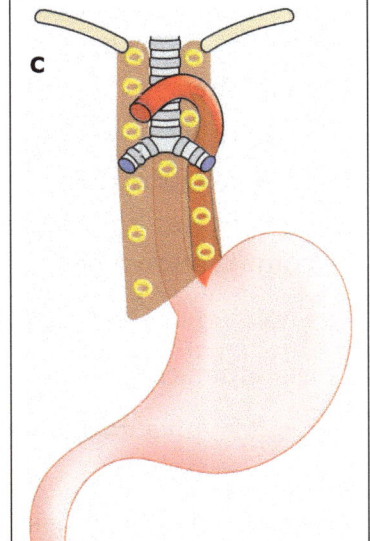

Figure 13.1: Extent of 2 Field Lymphadenectomy for esophageal cancer;
(A) Standard: lymphadenectomy up to the subcarinal lymph nodes,
(B) Extended: Standard + lymphadenectomy of right Paratracheal and right recurrent nerve lymph nodes,
(C) Total: Standard + lymphadenectomy of right & left paratracheal and right & left recurrent nerve lymph nodes.

- HIVEX trial: It compared trans-thoracic esophagectomy (TTE) vs trans-hiatal esophagectomy (THE) for esophageal cancers. They found TTE to be better for esophageal Ca and THE for GEJ Ca.
    - In general, the consensus is to perform THE for GEJ and lower esophageal AC; TTE for esophageal SCC. THE may also be considered in patients with poor PS or poor respiratory reserve.
- ICAN trial: It compared cervical vs intrathoracic anastomosis following esophagectomy for esophageal cancer post neo-adjuvant NA-CRT. Each was found to have its pros and cons.
    - Cervical anastomosis: The risk of leak is higher compared to intrathoracic anastomosis. However, the leak can be easily managed with less morbidity and less chances of mediastinitis. Also the radicality of the surgery is better as more esophagus is removed.
    - Intrathoracic anastomosis: The risk of leak is lower compared to cervical anastomosis due to less tension on the anastomosis and relatively better vascularity. However, if the anastomosis leaks it can lead to mediastinitis which is difficult to manage and can even be lethal.
    - In general, most surgical units prefer a cervical anastomosis.
- TIME trial: it compared minimally invasive surgery (MIS) vs open surgery for esophageal cancers. MIS was found to be associated with better short term recovery outcomes (less blood loss, less pain, less pulmonary morbidity, shorter length of hospital stay) with equivalent long term oncological outcomes.
- ROBOT trial: It compared robotic vs open esophagectomy for resectable esophageal cancer. Robotic esophagectomy was found to be associated with better short term recovery outcomes (less pain, less post-operative complications) with equivalent long term oncological outcomes.
- Choice of conduit: stomach vs colon
    - Stomach:
        - Advantages: Simpler technique with single anastomosis, well vascularized, mobile
        - Dis-advantages: Risk of reflux, aspiration, function deteriorates with time
    - Colon:
        - Advantages: Versatile, long length, good blood supply, acid resistant, function improves with time

- Dis-advantages: Complex with at least 3 anastomosis, longer operation time, higher ischemia rates, colonic redundancy may become a problem
  - In general stomach is the preferred choice of conduit for esophageal replacement in malignant cases and colon is preferred in benign cases.

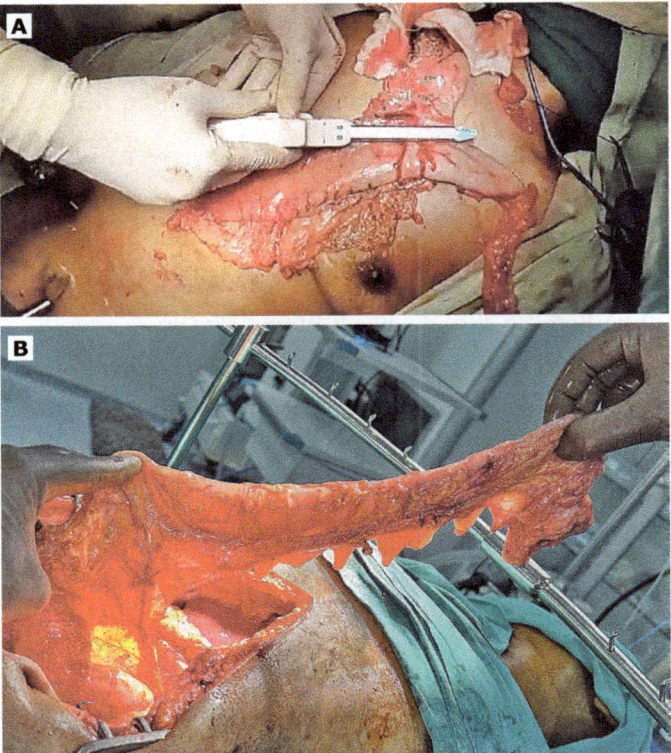

Figure 13.2: (A) Tubularised Gastric Conduit, (B) Colonic Conduit

- Route of conduit: Posterior mediastinum vs substernal: posterior mediastinum is generally preferred due to its shorter length. Also angulation of the conduit is minimal.
- Technique of anastomosis: Hand sewn vs stapled: Stapled anastomosis has been found to be associated with less risk of stricture formation
- Performance of gastric drainage procedure (pyloroplasty/pyloromyotomy/digitoclasty/botulinum toxin injection)
  - Advantages: Improves gastric emptying, decreases the risk of aspiration
  - Dis-advantages: Increased risk of alkaline reflux and dumping syndrome
  - It is not routinely recommended.

GASTRIC CANCER

- ACCORD trial: it found pre-op CT to be efficacious in gastric cancer compared to surgery alone

- CROSS trial: it studied regimen consisting of carboplatin + paclitaxel + 41.4 gray radiation in esophageal SCC, esophageal and GEJ AC compared to surgery alone. Overall pathological complete response rate was 29% (49% for SCC and 23% for AC). It found the regimen to be efficacious compared to surgery alone. It is a landmark trial which established role of NA-CRT in esophageal and GEJ cancer.

- **MAGIC trial:** it studied regimen consisting of 3 cycles of ECF (epirubicin, cisplatin and 5-Fluorouracil) before and after surgery (i.e. peri-operative chemotherapy) in esophageal, GEJ and gastric AC compared to surgery alone. It found the regimen to be efficacious compared to surgery alone. It is landmark trial which established role of peri-op. CT in esophageal, GEJ and gastric AC.

- Neo-AEGIS trial: This trial compared CROSS regimen vs MAGIC regimen in esophageal and GEJ AC. The trial found both the regimens to be equivalent and resulted in similar overall survival..

- V-325 trial: it studied regimen consisting of 3 cycles of DCF (Docetaxel, cisplatin and 5-Fluorouracil) before and after surgery (i.e. peri-operative chemotherapy) in gastric AC compared to regimen consisting of cisplatin and 5-FU. It found the regimen to be efficacious compared to the control.

- AIO/FLOT-4 trial: it studied regimen consisting of 4 cycles of FLOT (5-FU, leucovorine, oxalilatin and docetaxel) before and after surgery (i.e. peri-operative chemotherapy) in gastric AC compared to regimen consisting of epirubicin, cisplatin and 5-FU. It found the regimen to be efficacious compared to the control. However, the toxicity was higher in the FLOT group. Hence FLOT is generally recommended in young patients with good PS.

- CLASSIC trial: it studied role of adjuvant CT in gastric AC following D2 gastrectomy compared to D2 gastrectomy alone. Regimen consisted of Cape-OX (capecitabine + oxaliplatin). It found the regimen to be efficacious compared to D2 gastrectomy alone.

- Intergroup (INT) 0116/SWOG trial: it studied role of adjuvant 5-FU based CRT in gastric AC compared to surgery alone. It found the regimen to be efficacious compared to surgery alone.

- ARTIST trial: it compared adjuvant CT vs CRT in gastric cancer. It found the adjuvant CRT to be of advantage in case where D1 gastrectomy was performed

- In general:
  - Peri-operative CT is the preferred approach
  - In case no pre-operative CT was administered then adjuvant therapy is usually indicated.
  - Adjuvant CT is the preferred adjuvant therapy in case a D2 gastrectomy is performed (CLASSIC trial). Whereas CRT may be advised in case a D1 gastrectomy is performed (ARTIST trial).
- Seiwert, Stein et al described the classification system used to classify GEJ Ca.

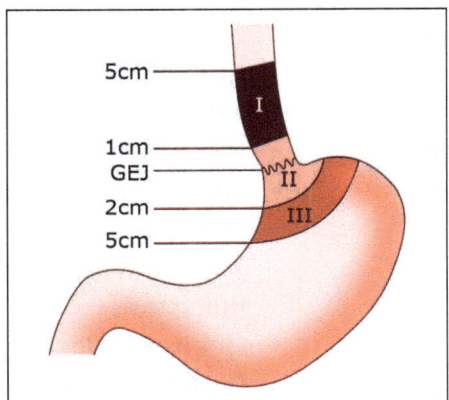

Figure 13.3: Siewert-Stein classification of GEJ adenocarcinoma.

- Bormann et al described classification system to classify gastric tumors based on their morphology

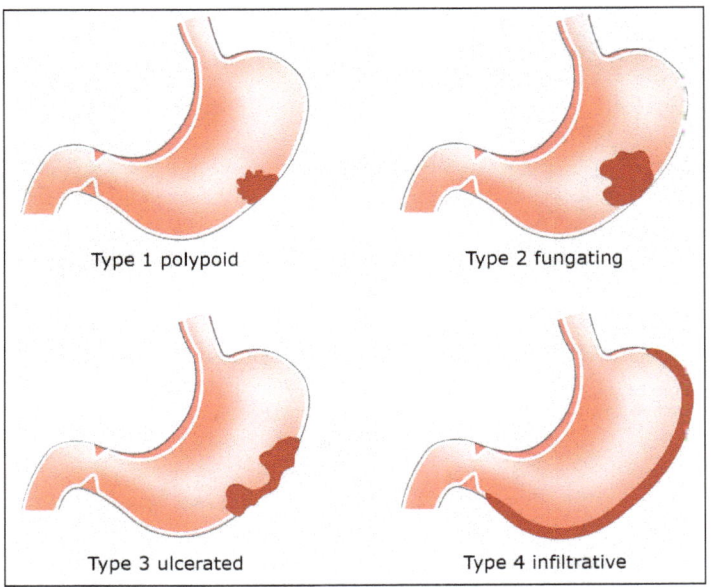

Figure 13.4: Borman Classification.

- Lauren et al described another classification system, dividing gastric cancer into Diffuse type and Intestinal type

Table 13.1: Laurens Classification of Gastric Cancer	
Intestinal Type Adenocarcinoma	Diffuse type Adenocarcinoma
• Enviormental • Affects elderly (M > F) • Associated with H. Pylori Infection, Chronic Atrophic Gastritis, Intestinal Metaplasia & Diet high in Nitrosamines • Arises from Mucosa • Gland forming • Involves Distal Stomach • Hematogenous spread	• Familial • Affects younger population (F > M) • Associated with CDH 1 Gene Mutation • Arises from Lamina Propria • Non Gland forming • Involves Proximal Stomach • Spreads through Sub-Mucosa; Lymphatic metastasis is common; tendency for Transmural spread with Peritoneal metastasis. • Linitus Plastica is a rare form of Diffuse Gastric Cancer

- Japanese classification for gastric cancer: it describes the various lymph node stations in relation to gastric cancer and describes the various surgeries for gastric Ca.

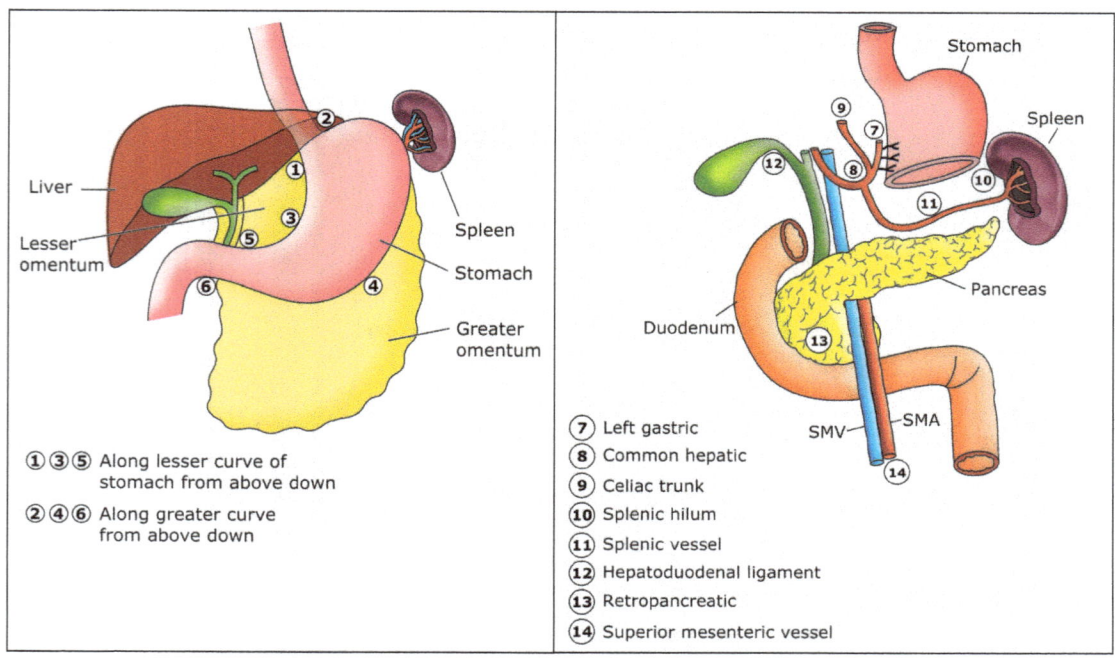

Figure 13.5: Lymph node stations in gastric cancer.

- MSKCC study: it showed the role of staging laparoscopy in gastric Ca post NA therapy.
- Studies comparing D2 vs D1 gastrectomy:
  o Japanese trials have shown advantage of D2 over D1.
  o Dutch trial: it failed to demonstrate advantage of D2 over D1 gastrectomy. Distal pancreatico-splenectomy was routinely performed as a part of D2 gastrectomy which resulted in higher complication rates. However long-term data has shown lower loco-regional recurrence with D2 gastrectomy.
  o British MRC trial: it failed to demonstrate advantage of D2 over D1 gastrectomy. They recommended that distal panceatico-splenectomy should not be routinely performed as a part of D2 gastrectomy.
  o Italian gastric cancer study group trial suggested that D2 gastrectomy may be a better choice in patients with advanced disease and LN metastasis.
  o MA, Cochrane review favor D2 over D1.
  o D2 gastrectomy is now standard of care.
- JCOG 1001 trial: it compared bursectomy vs no bursectomy during D2 gastrectomy for gastric cancer. Bursectomy was not found provide any survival advantage.
- KLASS-01 trial: it showed laparoscopic surgery to be oncologically equivalent to open surgery for early stage 1 gastric Ca.
- REGATTA trial: it compared gastrectomy with CT vs CT alone for advanced gastric Ca. Gastrectomy with CT did not show any survival advantage over CT alone, and hence may not be justified.

COLO-RECTAL CANCERS

- NA therapy in rectal Ca:
    - **German rectal cancer study group trial:** it compared pre-operative vs post-operative CRT in rectal cancers. The regimen consisted of long course 5-FU based CRT. NA-CRT was found to be associated with lower LR. It is a landmark trial which has established the role of long course NA-CRT (NA-LC-CRT) in rectal Ca.
    - **Swedish rectal cancer trial:** it compared pre-operative RT vs surgery alone in rectal cancers. The regimen consisted of short-course 25 Gy RT without CT (NA-SC-RT) in rectal cancer. NA-SC-RT was found to be associated with improved OS and lower LR. It's a landmark trial which has established the role of short-course NA-RT in rectal Ca. Additionally, Swedish rectal cancer trial is the only study to show improved OS (survival advantage) with NA therapy. Rest other trials showed only reduction in LR rates without survival advantage.
    - **Dutch TME trial:** it compared NA-SC-RT followed by TME vs TME alone in rectal cancers. NA-SC-RT was found to be associated with lower LR. It's another landmark trial which has established the role of short-course NA-RT in rectal Ca.
    - **Polish trial and TROG trial:** they compared NA-LC-CRT vs NA-SC-RT in rectal cancer. They found both options to be equivalent.
    - STAR-01 trial, ACCORD trial, AIO-04, FORWAC trial: based on the findings of these trials oxaliplatin is not recommended along with fluoropyrimidine in NA setting. That is capecitabine or 5-FU alone is given along with RT in LC-NA-CRT and not FOLFOX or Cape-OX.
    - Spanish trial, CONTRE trial, EXPERT trial, AVACROSS trial: they studied the role of TNT (total neo-adjuvant therapy) (CT followed by CRT followed by surgery) in rectal cancer. They suggested TNT to be associated with better pCR rates, planned treatment completion rates, with early attack on micrometastasis.
    - PROSPECT trial: the trial studied the role of NA-CT, with only selective use of NA- CRT in rectal Cancer. Pre-operative FOLFOX with selective use of CRT was found to be non-inferior to NA-LC-CRT.
    - RAPIDO trial: Studied the role of SC-RT followed by CT followed by delayed surgery. The authors demonstrated favorable result to suggest this to be considered as a new standard of care in high-risk locally advanced rectal cancer.
    - In general: LC-NA-CRT, SC-NA-RT, and TNT are all validated NA treatment options in rectal cancer. SC-NA-RT is however not advised in T4 tumors.

- MERCURY trial: established role of MRI for local staging of rectal Ca and response assessment post NA therapy.
- Habr-Gama et al described the wait and watch policy following cCR after NA-LC-CRT in rectal cancer. It consists of non-surgical approach in cases which show clinically complete response following NA-CRT.
- Bill Heald et al described the concepts of 'Holy plane (of Heald)' and total mesorectal excision (TME). TME consist of removal of the tumor bearing rectum along with its lymphatic bearing mesorectum by sharp dissection in holy plane of Heald between presacral fascia and mesorectal fascia without breaching the mesorectal fascial envelope. TME has shown to reduce local recurrence rates.

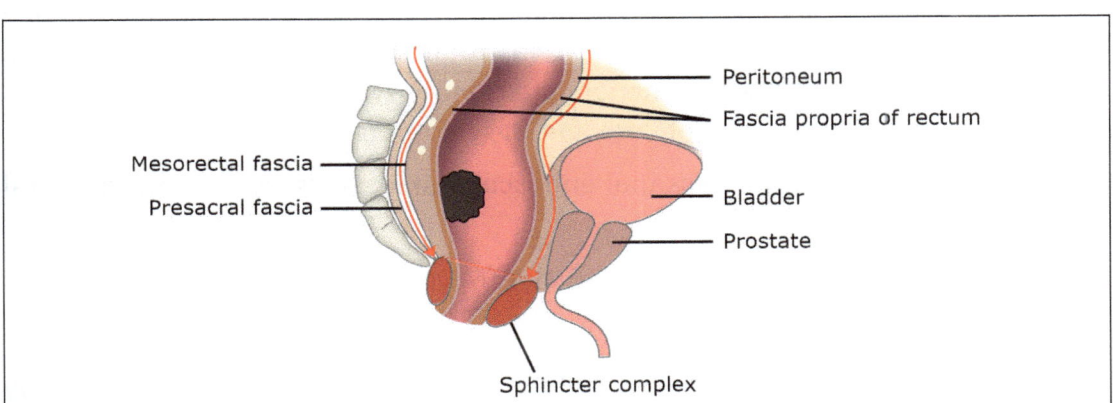

Figure 13.6: Concept of Total Mesorectal excision (TME). The dissection plane posteriorly is in the holy plane of Heald between the Presacral and Mesorectal fascia, Anteriorly once the peritoneal reflection is opened up the dissection is carried between the Fascia Propria of rectum and prostatic capsule through the Denovilliers Fascia.

- Trials which compared laparoscopic surgery vs open surgery for rectal Ca:
    - COLOR-2 trial, CLASSIC trial & COREAN trial: they found laparoscopic surgery to be oncologically equivalent to open surgery with better short-term recovery outcomes (Less blood loss, shorter hospital stay, earlier return of bowel function).
    - ACOSOG trial & ALACART trial: in these trials, criteria of non-inferiority were not met in the laparoscopy group. That is laparoscopic surgery was not found to be equivalent to open surgery, or rather it was found to be inferior to open surgery.
- Trials comparing Robotic surgery vs laparoscopic surgery for rectal cancer:
    - ROLARR trial

        Robotic surgery did not significantly reduce the risk of conversion to open

surgery and it did not confer an advantage in rectal cancer resection.
- COLRAR trial

    In patients with middle or low rectal cancer, robotic-assisted surgery did not significantly improve the TME quality compared with conventional laparoscopic surgery.

- Trials comparing TaTME (trans-anal TME) vs laparoscopic low anterior resection (LAR) for rectal cancer:
  - GRECCAR trial
  - COST 3 trial
- NSABP R-04 trial: it compared abdomino-perineal resection vs sphincter saving surgery (SSS) in rectal cancers. APR was found to be associated with worse body image scores, sexual function and urinary symptoms. Whereas SSS was associated with more weight loss and GI symptoms.
- Trials comparing TEM (transanal endoscopic microsurgery) vs Radical rectal resection:
  - CARTS trial: NA-LC-CRT followed by TEM vs Radical rectal resection
  - TREC trial: NA-SC-RT followed by delayed TEM vs Radical rectal resection
  - STAR-TREC trial: NA-LC-CRT followed by TEM vs NA-SC-RT followed by delayed TEM vs Radical rectal resection
- Adjuvant therapy in rectal Ca:
  - GITSG trial, NSABP trial: based on the findings of these landmark studies adjuvant CRT was being practiced as standard of care in rectal cancers before NA therapy became a norm.
  - EORTC trial, ECOG trial, ADORE trial: these trials are the basis for NCCN's recommendation on administration of adjuvant CT following surgery after NA-LC-CRT therapy in rectal cancers.
- NA therapy in colonic Ca:
  - FOxTROT trial: it studied the role of NA FOLFOX CT in T4b colonic cancer. It was found to result in cancer downstaging with acceptable toxicity.
- COLOR trial, CLASSIC trial & COST trial: they compared laparoscopic surgery vs open surgery for colonic Ca. All three found the oncological outcomes to be equivalent in both groups with patients in the laparoscopic group showing better short-term recovery outcomes (Less blood loss, shorter hospital stay, earlier return of bowel function).

- Turnbull et al described the 'No touch technique' with early ligation of mesenteric vein draining the tumor bearing segment of colon to prevent dissemination of malignant cells. Subsequently JCOG 1006 trail was performed which compared no touch technique vs conventional technique for colonic cancers. It could not prove the superiority of Turnbull technique.

- Hohenberger et al described the concept of complete mesocolic excision with central vascular ligation in surgery for colonic cancer (CME with CVL). The concept is similar to that of TME for rectal cancers and involves sharp dissection in embryonic planes to excise the tumor bearing segment of the colon along with its entire lymphatic drainage. It has been found to result in better LN yield.

- Adjuvant therapy in colonic Ca:
    o NSABP trial established adjuvant 5-FU based CT as standard of care in CRC (regimens used: Mayo clinic regimen, Roswell Park regimen).
    o GERCOR trial: found continuous infusion 5-FU to be equivalent to bolus 5-FU in adjuvant setting in CRC.
    o X-ACT trial: found oral capecitabine to be equivalent to 5-FU in adjuvant setting in CRC.
    o MOSAIC trial: it compared adjuvant 5-FU alone vs 5-FU + oxaliplatin (regimen named as FOLFOX4). Based on the findings of this study FOLFOX was established as the new standard of care.
    o CALGB trial: it studied the effect of addition of irinotecan to 5-FU in the adjuvant setting. It found higher treatment related complications due to irinotecan administration without survival advantage. Hence irinotecan is not recommended in the adjuvant setting.
        ▪ PETACC and French trial also did not find addition of irinotecan to be of any advantage in the adjuvant setting.
    o AVANT trial: it found no advantage of adding bevacizumab in the adjuvant setting. Similarly, cetuximab and panitumumab are also not recommended in the adjuvant setting.
    o IMPACT study and MRC trial, both did not find advantage of administration of adjuvant chemotherapy to stage 2 CRC.
    o ASCO recommendations suggest high risk indications for administration of adjuvant CT in stage 2 CRC.

Table 13.2: Indications for adjuvant chemotherapy in colonic cancer
• T4
• N+
• T3 with high risk features:
– Obstruction or perforation
– LVI: Lymphovascular invasion
– PNI: Perineural invasion
– < 12 lymph nodes sampled
– MSI-high (microsatellite instability); MMR-deficient (mismatch repair gene); MSS (microsatellite stable)

- NIGRO trial: it established the role of CRT in anal Ca (5-FU + mitomycin + RT).

PANCREATIC CANCER

- Criteria for definition of Borderline Resectable Pancreatic Cancer(BRPC):
    - NCCN Criteria:
        - Degree of contact with SMA: </= 180 degree.
        - Degree of contact with SMV-PV: > 180 degree or </= 180 degree with contour irregularity. However, vascular reconstruction is feasible.
    - MD Anderson Criteria:
        - Type A: BRPC as per Anatomical criteria of artery, vein abutment/ encasement
        - Type B: Resectable tumor with questionable extra pancreatic metastatic disease
        - Type C: Resectable tumor with marginal preoperative performance status
- Adjuvant therapy:
    - CRT: GITSG trial studied the role of adjuvant 5-FU based CRT in pancreatic cancer. The study results favored the use of adjuvant CRT. However, the results of the EORTC trial didn't find any advantage.
    - CRT vs CT: ESPAC-1 trial: it is a landmark trial which compared adjuvant 5-FU CT vs 5-FU based CRT in pancreatic cancers. It established adjuvant CT as standard of care.
    - CT: several trials have studied the role of various chemotherapeutic regimens in the adjuvant setting. The important ones are:
        - CONKO-001 trial: it found gemcitabine (Gem) monotherapy to be better than no CT.
        - ESPAC-1 trial: it found 5-FU CT to be better than 5-FU based CRT.
        - ESPAC-3 trial: it found Gem to be equivalent to 5-FU.
        - ESPAC-4 trial: it found Gem-Cap (gemcitabine + Capecitabine) to be better than Gem alone.
        - JASPAC-01 trial: it found S1 to be better than Gem.
        - PRODIGE trial: it found FOLFIRINOX (leucovorine, 5-FU, irinotecan and oxaliplatin) to be better than Gem in good PS patients.
- NA therapy: its role has been established in case of BRPC due to various retrospective studies and RCTs. However, its role in resectable cancers is still being studied.

- ○ Studies evaluating the role of NA therapy in BRPC:
  - ▪ MD Anderson study: it studied regimen consisting of Gem based CRT and found it to be efficacious.
  - ▪ Massachusetts GH experience: they studied regimen consisting of FOLFIRINOX. Although the regimen was found to be relatively toxic, patients were less likely to develop post-operative pancreatic fistula (POPF).
  - ▪ ESPAC-5 trial: it was a four-arm trial which compared NA-Gem-Cap vs NA-FOLFIRINOX vs NA Cap based CRT vs Upfront surgery in patients with BRPC. NA chemotherapy with either Gem-Cap or FOLFIRINOX was found to have the best survival advantage compared to immediate surgery supporting the use of short-course NA-CT in patients with BRPC
  - ▪ PREOPANC trial: it studied the role of Gem based CRT followed by adjuvant Gemcitabine in borderline resectable and resectable pancreatic cancers. NA therapy was found to improve OS.
  - ▪ PREOPANC-2 trial: it is comparing Total NA-FOLFIRINOX vs NA Gem based CRT and adjuvant gemcitabine for resectable and borderline resectable pancreatic cancer.
- ○ Studies evaluating the role of NA therapy in resectable pancreatic cancer.
  - ▪ NEOPAC: NACT: Gem-Ox (gemcitabine + Oxaliplatin) (ongoing).
  - ▪ NEOPA: NACRT: Gem based CRT (ongoing)
  - ▪ NEONAX trial: nab-Paclitaxel plus Gemcitabine (ongoing)
- Palliative CT: several trials have studied the role of various chemotherapeutic regimens in the palliative setting. The important ones are:
  - ○ Landmark study by Burris et al established the role of Gem monotherapy in the palliative setting.
  - ○ MPACT trial: it studied regimen consisting of Gem + albumin bound paclitaxel.
  - ○ Gem-Cap trial: it studied regimen consisting of gemcitabine + Capecitabine.
  - ○ ACCORD-11 trial: it studied regimen consisting of FOLFIRINOX in good PS patient.
  - ○ CONKO-003: it studied regimen consisting of FOLFOX.
- Biliary stenting in distal blocks (Ca HOP, Periampullary Ca): DROP trial found routine biliary drainage to increase the complication rate (especially surgical site infections [SSI]). Various other RCTs, MA and Cochrane review have advised against routine biliary drainage.

○ In general biliary drainage is performed selectively in patients with distal blocks.

Table 13.3: Indication for Pre-operative Biliary stenting in distal blocks
– Cholangitis
– Severe pruritus
– Coagulopathy
– Renal insufficiency
– Poor nutritional status
– Surgery delayed due to any other reason
– When neoadjuvant therapy is being planned in resectable or borderline resectable disease
– When palliation is to be achieved in unresectable disease

- WPD vs PPPD (Whipple's pancreatico-duodenectomy vs Pylorus preserving pancreatico-duodenectomy): RCTs, MA and Cochrane review all have failed to prove one to be better than the other. The final decision on what to perform depends on the surgeon's preference.

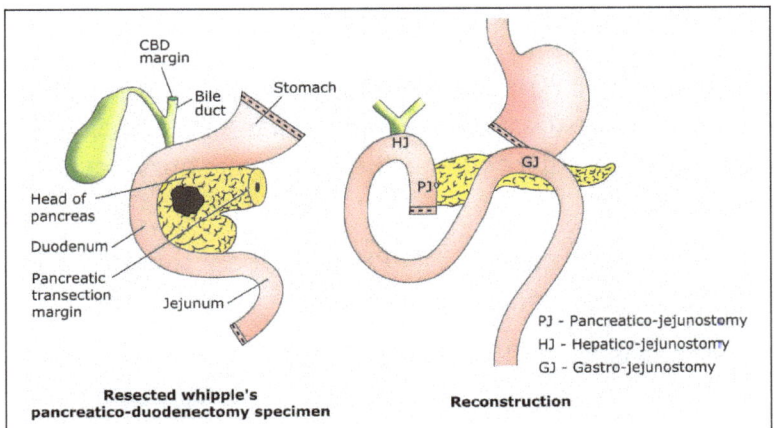

Figure 13.7: Whipple's pancreatico-duodenectomy.

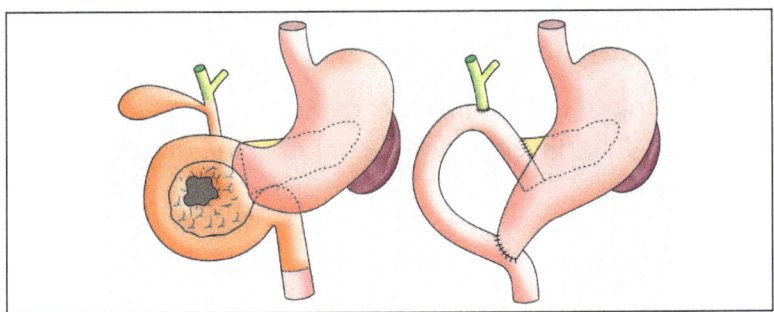

Figure 13.8: Traverso-Longmire pylorus Preserving pancreatico-duodenectomy.

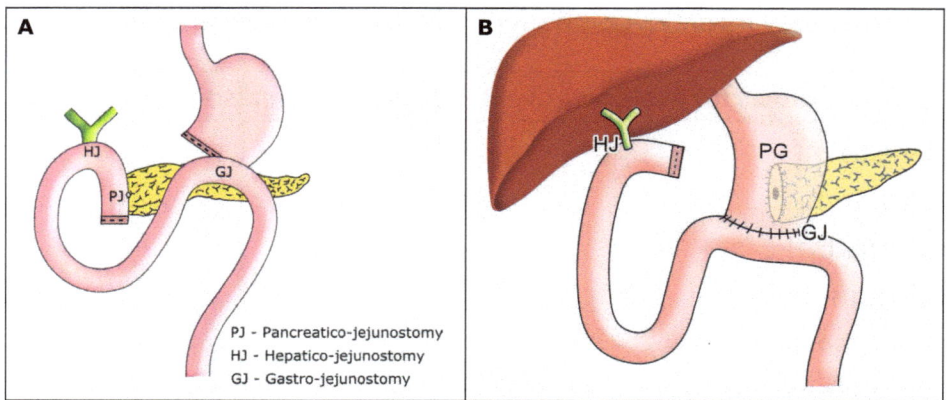

Figure 13.9: (A) Pancreatico-Jejunostomy, (B) Pancreatico-Gastrostomy.

- Pancreatico-jejunostomy vs Pancreatico-gastrostomy:
  - RECOPANC trial: Multicentric RCT which compared PG vs PJ after PD. No significant difference was noted in the rate of grade B/C fistula between the two techniques. PG was found to be associated with increased risk of bleeding events.
  - Similarly, John Hopkins RCT, other RCTs, MA and Cochrane review, all have failed to prove one to be better than the other.
  - Pros of PG: In general PG is considered easier to perform compared to PJ because of the natural approximation of the pancreas and stomach. Additionally, the stomach is well vascularized and the pancreatic enzymes are inactivated by the gastric acid.
  - Cons of PG: higher chance of PPH (post pancreatectomy hemorrhage); pancreatic leak also results in gastric leak.
  - General consensus: Neither technique is better than the other. The final decision lies on the surgeon's preference. Most high-volume centers perform a duct to mucosa PJ.
- Technique of Pancreatico-Enteric anastomosis: Invagination/dunking and their modifications, Duct to mucosa and their modifications:
  - Peng et al described the binding technique of pancreatico- jejunostomy which is a type of dunking/invagination technique. The authors claimed zero POPF in their study.

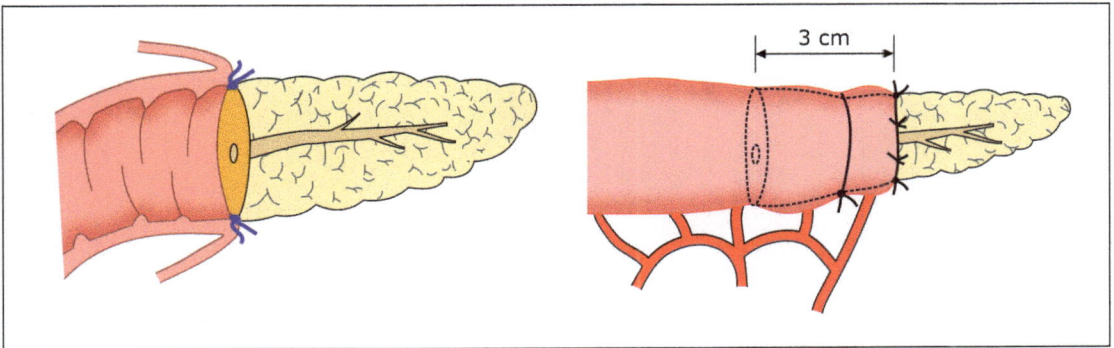

Figure 13.10: Peng's Binding Technique for Pancreatico enteric anastomosis.

- ○ Cattell and Warren described the prototypic Duct-to-mucosa technique of pancreatico-enteric anastomosis.
- ○ Torres et al described the Modified Heidelberg technique which is a modification of the original Duct-to-mucosa technique.

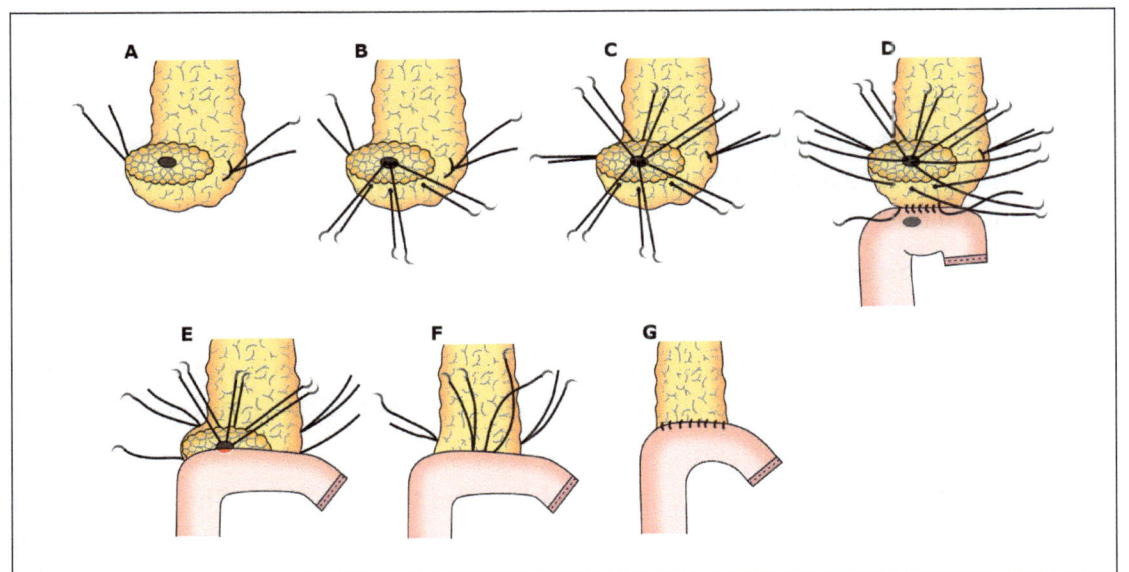

Figure 13.10: Modified Heidelberg technique; in my opinion the difference between Modified Heidelberg technique (MHT) and Cattell-Warren technique (CWT) is that the outer layer of sutures between pancreas and jejunum is Continuous in MHT (as shown in the diagram) and interrupted in CWT.

- ○ Blumgart et al described the Blumgart technique of pancreatico- enteric anastomosis. This technique attempts to achieve both Duct-to-mucosa technique and jejunal overlap of the pancreas.

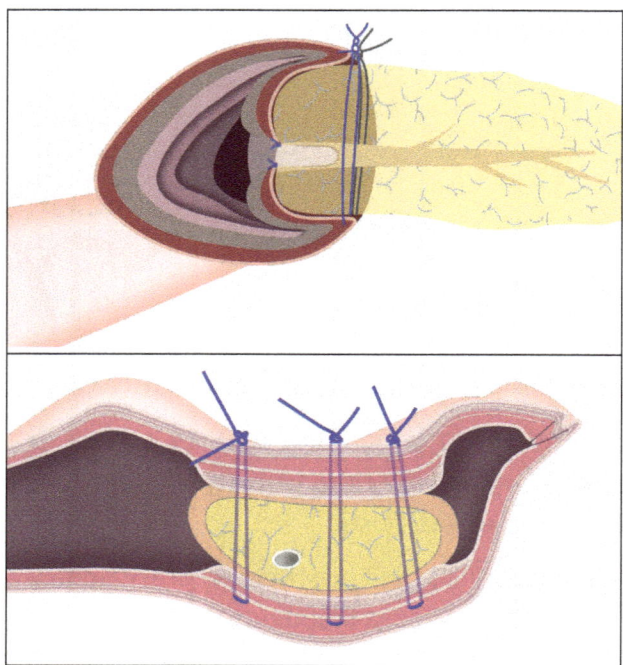

Figure 13.11: Blumgart technique of pancreatico- enteric anastomosis.

- o PANasta trial: This trial compared Cattell Warren technique vs Blumgart technique of pancreatico- jejunostomy. The Blumgart technique did not contribute to a reduction in complication rates compared to the Cattell Warren technique.
- o Dunking technique vs Duct-to-mucosa technique of pancreatico-enteric anastomosis: RCTs, MA and Cochrane review all have showed no difference.
    - In general dunking is preferred when pancreatic duct is not visible due to small size or pancreatic texture is very soft. Many consider Dunking easier to perform.
- o General Consensus: No one technique is better than the other. The final decision lies on the surgeon's preference. Most high-volume centers perform a duct to mucosa PJ.
- Callery et al described the fistula risk score to predict POPF. Factors include: Pathology (periampullary tumor vs Ca HOP), pancreatic duct size, pancreatic texture and blood loss.
- Mungroop et al described the Alternative-fistula risk score to predict POPF. Factors include: pancreatic duct size, pancreatic texture and BMI.
- Extended Lymphadenectomy: no advantage was found by Italian multicenter Lymphadenectomy group study, John Hopkin study, other RCT's and MA.

- LEOPARD 1 trial: it compared minimally invasive distal pancreatectomy (MIDP) vs open distal pancreatectomy (ODP) for carcinoma body of pancreas. MIDP was found to be better than ODP.
- Minimally invasive pancreatico-duodenectomy (MIPD) vs Open pancreatico-duodenectomy (OPD).
  - LEOPARD 2 trial: it compared MIPD vs OPD for carcinoma body of pancreas. The trial had to be prematurely terminated due to higher complication related deaths in the MIPD group.
  - PADULAP trial: Laparoscopic PD was found to be associated with shorter length of hospital stay and favorable postoperative course while being oncologically equivalent.
  - Similarly, GEM RCT by Palanivelu et al found better results with MIPD compared to OPD.
- ISGPS: international study group for pancreatic surgery:
  - It provides guidelines for diagnosis, grading and management of POPF (post-operative pancreatic fistula), PPH (post pancreatectomy hemorrhage) and DGE (delayed gastric emptying).
  - POPF: defined as clinically relevant passage of any measurable volume of drain fluid on or after postoperative day 3 with amylase level > 3 times the upper limit of normal.
    - Biochemical Leak (BL) (previously termed as grade A POPF): it refers to passage of amylase rich drain fluid without any clinical relevance or deviation in the normal postoperative course with no effect on the duration of stay. It is no longer considered as a true pancreatic fistula or post-operative complication.
    - Grade B POPF: it refers to POPF which has resulted in clinically relevant deviation from normal post-operative course.
      - Persistent drainage for > 3 weeks
      - Need for endoscopic, percutaneous or angiographic intervention
      - Presence of signs of infection without organ failure
    - Grade C POPF:
      - Need for re-operation
      - Presence of organ failure
      - Death

- PPH
    - Grade A PPH: early mild bleed (early = bleed within 24 hours of surgery) (mild = small blood loss with Hb drop < 3 gm/dL, without clinical impairment, with need for < 3 units of PRBC).
    - Grade B PPH: early severe bleed or late mild bleed (late = bleed after 24 hours of surgery) (severe = large blood loss with Hb drop > 3 gm/dL, with clinical impairment, with need for > 3 units of PRBC, with need for invasive treatment).
    - Grade C PPH: late severe bleed.

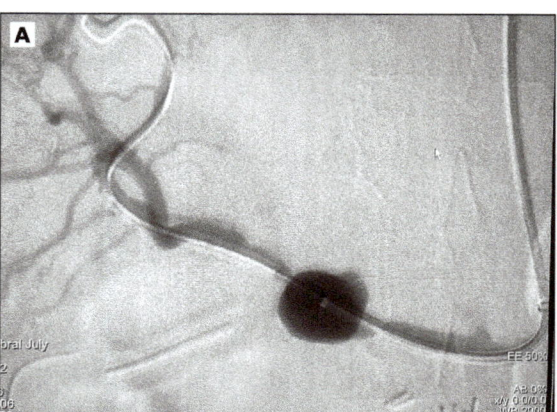 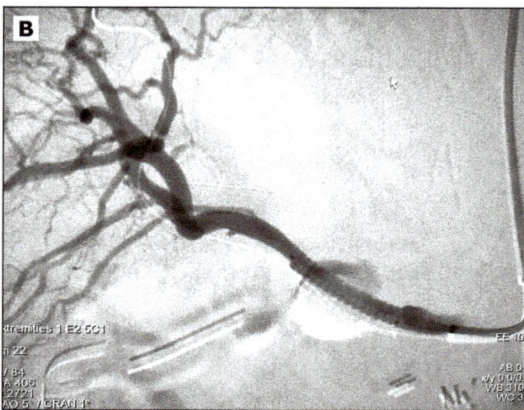

Figure 13.12: Post WPD Pseudoaneurysm arising from Common Hepatic artery; a covered stent was inserted to plug the neck of the pseudoaneurysm. Alternatively, the Interventional Radiologist could use Gel-Foam, Coil or Autologous Cllot.

- DGE: it is defined as need for naso-gastric tube (NG) beyond post-operative day (POD) 3 or inability to tolerate solid diet by POD 7.
    - Grade A: NG needed between POD 4-7 or NG reinserted after POD 3 or inability to tolerate solid diet by POD 7.
    - Grade B: NG needed between POD 8-14 or NG reinserted after POD 7 or inability to tolerate solid diet by POD 14.
    - Grade A: NG need beyond POD 14 or NG reinserted after POD 14 or inability to tolerate solid diet by POD 21.
- Role of Octreotide in preventing POPF: PVS study, MD Anderson, John Hopkin study, all showed no advantage in reducing POPF rates. However, RCT studying the role of Pasireotide in preventing POPF found advantage.
- Strasberg et al described RAMPS (Radical antegrade modular pacreatico-splenectomy) for Ca body of pancreas.

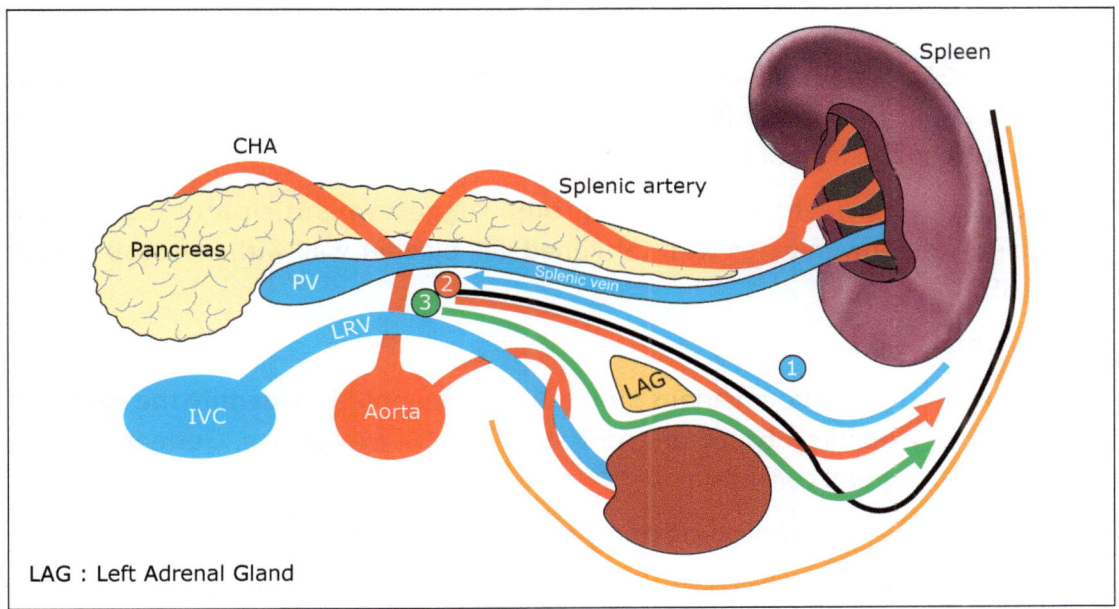

Figure 13.13: Radical Antegrade Modular Pancreatico-Splenectomy (RAMPS): Blue line indicates plane and direction of dissection for conventional Panceriatico-Splenectomy; Red line indicates plane and direction of dissection for Anterior RAMPS; Green line indicates plane and direction of dissection for Posterior RAMPS.

BILIARY CANCER

- The SGPGI group (VK Kapoor et al), GB Pant group (A Aggarwal et al), PGI group (TD Yadav et al), TMH group (Mahesh Goel et al) have contributed immensely to the literature in the field of Ca GB.
- Lucknow approach: the SGPGI group suggested anticipatory extended cholecystectomy in cases with thickened gall bladder wall with low suspicion of Ca GB.
- Incidental Ca GB:
  - Extent of resection: various studies have attempted to identify the extent of surgery required based on the T stage (SGPGI experience, German registry data). General consensus:
    - T1a: simple cholecystectomy suffices
    - T1b: extended cholecystectomy (2 cm hepatic wedge resection)
    - T2: radical cholecystectomy (resection of segment 4b, 5)
  - Port site excision: various studies including that by the MSKCC group suggest that routine port site excision is not mandatory. Whereas others including that by the SGPGI group advocate full thickness skin to peritoneum excision of all four LC port sites. The final decision lies on the surgeon's preference.
- Routine excision of CBD in surgery for Ca GB: not recommended (French multicenter trial).
- Miyazaki et al describe the prototypic method of performing radical cholecystectomy for Ca GB.
- Biliary drainage (BD) in proximal block (hilar cholangiocarcinoma, Ca GB with hilar block).
  - Routine vs Selective BD: studies have not shown routine pre-operative BD (PBD) to be associated with reduction in mortality.
    - Pros of routine PBD: it has been found to be associated with reduction in endotoxinemia, it provides cholangiogram, it improves survival in case of right hepatectomy.
    - Cons: it has been found to be associated with increased risk of septic complications, decreased survival in case of left hepatectomy
    - The Japanese advocate routine PBD and the western groups advocate selective PBD (indications being: sepsis, malnutrition, pruritus, renal failure, prior to PVE, NA therapy).

- In general: PBD is generally indicated when a major hepatectomy is being planned. Surgery is performed once bilirubin is < 3 mg/dl.
  - ERCP with biliary stenting (EBD) vs PTBD vs ENBD:
    - EBD: it is physiological. However there is high risk of cholangitis due to clogging of the stent. Also there is the risk of stent misplacement and migration.
    - PTBD: it is accurate with high success rate. However it is invasive, associated with the risk of vascular and biliary injury. The most important concern is the 5% risk of tumor seeding.
    - ENBD: it is physiological, the risk of cholangitis and cancer dessemination is less. However it is associated with patient discomfort and risk for self removal.
    - General consensus: ENBD > PTBD > EBD
- Makuuchi et al introduced the concept of Portal Vein Eembolization (PVE) as a means for hepatic parenchymal augmentation.
- Nagino et al described the concept of ipsilateral PVE.

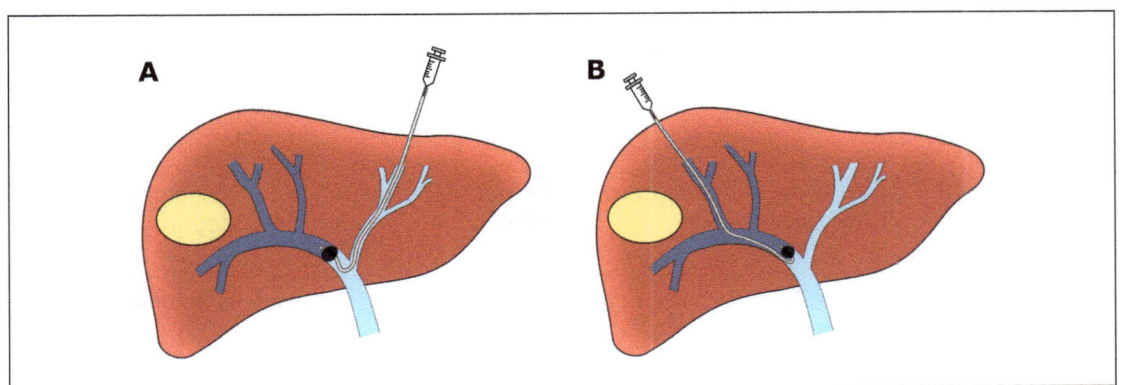

Figure 13.14: Portal Vein Eembolization (PVE); (A) Contralateral PVE, (B) Ipsilateral PVE.

- Extent of resection for hilar cholangioCa: this topic is still controversial. The main reason for this the lack of RCTs.
  - Controversies include:
    - Radical hepatectomy vs parenchyma preserving hepatectomy.
    - Routine caudate lobe resection necessary or not.
    - Extent of hepatic resection for Bismuth Corlette type 1 and 2 tumors.

- The general consensus:
    - Parenchyma preserving hepatectomy is oncologically equivalent to radical right/left hepatectomy/trisectionectomy with less morbidity and mortality. However it is technically challenging, and hence most surgical units prefer performing radical hepatectomy.
    - The main aim of surgery is to achieve R0 resection.
  - Routine caudate lobe resection is recommended.
- Japanese groups (Makucchi et al, Nagino et al, Miyazaki et al, Kawarada et al) have immensely contributed to the literature in the field.
- Karwarada et al described the 'Taj mahal resection.
- Schnitzbauer et al described the concept of Associating Liver Partition and Portal vein Ligation for Staged Hepatectomy (ALPPS).

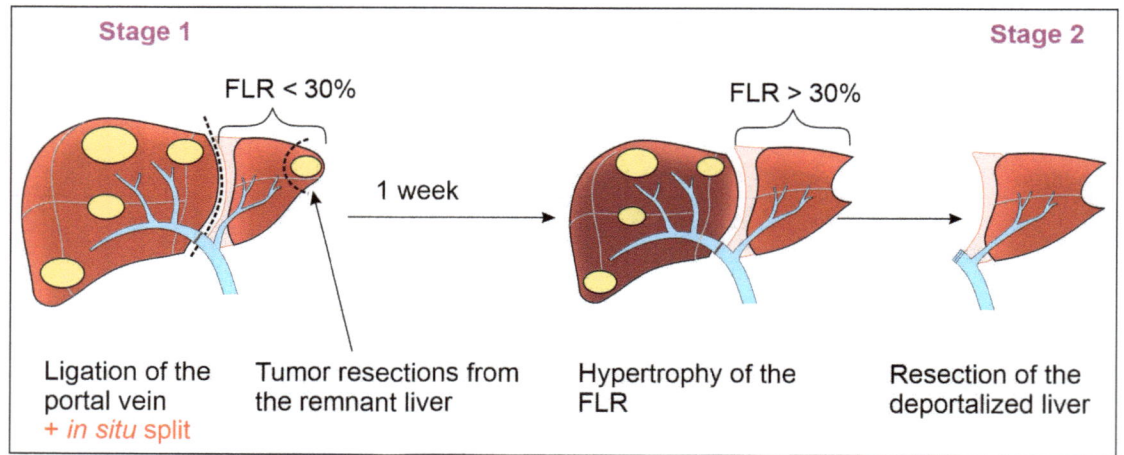

Figure 13.15: Associating Liver Partition and Portal vein Ligation for Staged Hepatectomy (ALPPS).

- Adjuvant therapy: several studies have shown advantage and established the role of adjuvant therapy in biliary cancers. The notable ones are:
    - BILCAP trial: studied the role of adjuvant capecitabine in biliary cancers (cholangioCa, Ca GB).
    - SWOG 0809 trial: studied the role of adjuvant Gem-Cap followed by capecitabinne based CRT in biliary cancers.
    - SGPGI study: studied the role of adjuvant CRT in Ca GB.
- Neo-adjuvant therapy:
    - TMH (Tata Memorial Hospital) study: studied the role of NA gemcitabine

+ oxaliplatin (Gem-Ox) in locally advanced Ca GB. The study results were promising. The authors suggested the **TMH criteria** for NA CT in Ca GB.

Table 13.4: TMH criteria for NA-CT in Locally advanced/Borderline Resectable Ca GB

- Tumor
  - Contiguous liver involvement > 2 cm
  - Involvement of bile duct causing obstructive jaundice (Type I/II block on MRCP/ERCP/PTBD)
  - Radiological/Endoscopic involvement of antropyloric region of stomach, duodenum, hepatic flexure of colon or small intestine
  - i.e. T3–T4 tumors
- Node: Radiological suspicion of lymph node involvement
  - Hepatic artery (Station 8),
  - Hepatoduodenal ligament (Station 12),
  - Retro pancreatic/retroduodenal (Station 13)
  - Size > 1 cm in short axis, round in shape, and heterogenous enhancement on CT/PET scan.
  - i.e. +/> N1
- Vascular involvement: Impingement/involvement (< 180-degree angle) of one or more of the following blood vessels:
  - Common Hepatic Artery and Right & Left Hepatic artery
  - Main Portal vein and Right & Left Portal vein
  - i.e. T4 tumor
- For incidental GBC
  - Residual/Recurrent mass in GB fossa/liver bed
  - N1 nodes as per nodal criteria.
  - Involvement of bile duct causing OJ (Type I/II Block)

- Systemic therapy:
  - ABC-02 trail: studied the role of gemcitabine + oxaliplatin in advanced biliary cancer.
- Mayo clinic described protocol for Liver Transplant in locally advanced Hilar Cholangiocarcinoma.

HEPATO-CELLULAR CANCER & LIVER RESECTION

Hepato-Cellular Cancer

- LI-RADS: Liver Imaging Reporting and Data System is a set of standardized terminology and a classification system for imaging findings in liver lesions. The LI-RADS score for a liver lesion is an indication of its relative risk for HCC.
- RFA vs Surgical resection for HCC:
  - SURF trial: it compared RFA vs surgical resection in early HCC. Both were found to be equivalent.
  - There are several other RCTs and MA which have compared RFA vs surgical resection in early HCC. Most of them have found similar results.
  - However, in general recurrence is more common and treatment related complications is less common with RFA.
- Criteria for liver transplant in HCC:
  - These criteria have been set so as to select patients with CLD and HCC who would achieve favorable long term prognosis with a liver transplant
  - Milan criteria:
    - Single tumor less than or equal to 5 cm in diameter or 1-3 tumor, each less than or equal to 3 cm.
  - Expanded criteria include:
    - UCSF criteria: Single tumor less than or equal to 6.5 cm in diameter or 1-3 tumor, with the largest lesion being less than or equal to 4.5 cm and total diameter of all lesions combined being less than 8.
    - Up-to -7 criteria: sum of total number of tumor and size of the largest tumor in cm being less than 7.
    - Tokyo criteria: 5-5 rule: less than 5 tumors with none individually being more than 5 cm in size.
- Classification system for staging and treatment planning (discussed in detail in chapter 12):
  - BCLC: for HCV related cancers
  - HKLC: for HBV related cancers

Table 13.5: BCLC staging system

o Very early stage (0): single tumor < 2 cm, CTP A, performance status (PS) 0
o Early stage (A): 1-3 nodule each less than 3 cm, CTP A/B, PS 0
o Intermediate stage (B): multinodular, unresectable, CTP A/B, PS 0
o Advanced stage (C): portal vein invasion, extrahepatic spread (nodal and/or distant), CTP A/B, PS 1-2
o Terminal stage (D): CTP C, PS 3-4

- Important guidelines for management of HCC:
    - AASLD: American association for study of liver diseases
    - EASL: European association for study of liver
- SHARP trial: established role of Sorafenib in advanced/metastatic HCC
- Check Mate 040 trial: Nivolumab (anti-PD1 antibody) was found to be effective in advanced HCC progressing on sorafenib.
- KEYNOTE 224 trial: Pembrolizumab was found to be effective in advanced HCC progressing on sorafenib.
- TACTICS trial: it found TACE + Sorafenib to be better than TACE alone for HCC.

Liver Resection

- Belghiti et al: described the Hanging manoever for liver resection.
- Belghiti et al: described the 50-50 criteria for Post Hepatectomy Liver Failure (PHLF): defined as PT < 50% (INR > 1.7) and serum bilirubin > 50 mmol/L (> 2.9 mg/dL) on or after POD 5.
- ISGLS guidelines (international study group for liver surgery): It provides guidelines for diagnosis, grading and management of PHLF (post hepatectomy liver failure), Bile leak.
    - PHLF: defined as a post-operatively acquired deterioration in the ability of liver to maintain its synthetic, excretory and detoxifying functions, which is characterized by raised INR and concomitant hyperbilirubinemia on or after POD five.
        - Grade A PHLF: PHLF resulting in abnormal laboratory parameters without change in the clinical management.
        - Grade B PHLF: PHLF resulting in deviation from the regular clinical course, manageable without invasive treatment.

- Grade C PHLF: PHLF resulting in deviation from the regular clinical course requiring invasive treatment.
  - Bile leak: it is defined as passage of drain fluid with an elevated bilirubin level =/> three times the serum bilirubin level on or after POD 3 or need for radiological or surgical intervention to deal with biliary collection or biliary peritonitis respectively.
    - Grade A Bile leak: Bile leakage requiring no change in the clinical management.
    - Grade B Bile leak: Bile leakage requiring change in the clinical management but not re-laparotomy.
    - Grade C Bile leak: Bile leakage requiring re-laparotomy.

CORROSIVE INJURY

- The Indian contribution in the subject is immense:
  - JIPMER experience (N Ananthkrishnan, V Kate et al)
  - PGI experience (Zargar et al)
  - GB pant experience (A Aggarwal et al)
- Zargar et al described classification system to grade caustic esophageal injury
- Timing of endoscopy: within 24 hours vs between 48-72 hours
  - Early endoscopy allows early grading of injury and appropriate triaging; however, it may underestimate the extent of injury.
  - JIPMER group advocate endoscopy between 48-72 hours. It should not be performed beyond 96 hours due to heightened risk of perforation.
  - Complete examination of the esophagus and stomach by an expert using a flexible endoscopy with minimal insufflation is what is recommended.
- Corticosteroids to prevent stricture: studies and MA have advised against use of steroids as it has not shown to prevent stricture formation. On the contrary it may lead to severe adverse events.
- Role of NG tube: some authors advocate routine placement of NG tube to facilitate enteral nutrition and subsequent dilatation therapy. Others have found it to induce stricture formation. Hence decision regarding need for NG tube should be taken on a case to case basis.
- Esophageal stent insertion: few authors have advocated early stent insertion to prevent stricture formation. However other studies have described drawbacks like stent migration and hyperplastic response. Some studies have found biodegradable stents to be feasible. In general, it is not recommended.
- Early dilatation therapy after injury: not recommended due to risk of perforation.
- Role of Mitomycin C, 5-FU in preventing stricture formation: still experimental with no proven benefit.
- Esophageal resection followed by bypass vs bypass alone at time of Esophago-Coloplasty:
  - Some groups suggest routine resection of the scarred esophagus due concerns of malignancy, mucocele and abscess formation.
  - Opponents of resection suggest that the risk of malignancy is negligible especially in Indian patients where acid injury is more common. Also,

esophageal resection is unnecessarily hazardous.
- Choice of conduit.
    - Right colon vs left colon:
        - Right colon:
            - Advantages: ileo-cecal valve prevents reflux, better size match between ileum and esophagus, cecum may provide reservoir function, option of using left colon is there in case right colon necrosis occurs.
            - Dis-advantage: vascular anatomy of right colon is variable, bulky cecum may become an interference.
        - Left colon:
            - Advantages: vascular anatomy is reliable.
            - Dis-advantage: left colon may be affected by diverticulosis, IMA may be atherosclerotic.
    - JIPMER group suggested the mid-colon esophago-coloplasty. Proposed advantages are no shortage of conduit length and non-reliability on vascular anatomy
- Side to side vs end to end esophago-colic anastomosis: studies suggest side to side esophago-colic anastomosis to be better. Advantages include avoidance of mucocele or abscess formation in the residual esophagus, conduit tip which may be ischemic is not utilized in the anastomosis.
- Route: novel substernal vs native posterior mediastinal: novel substernal route preferred as dangerous dissection in the scarred posterior mediastinum is avoided.
- JIPMER group have described the classification system of pharyngeal strictures and described their management.

NON CIRRHOTIC PORTAL HYPERTENSION

- APASL (Asia Pacific association of study of liver) standardized the definition of EHPVO and NCPF:
    - EHPVO: vascular disease of liver with obstruction of extra hepatic PV with or without involvement of intrahepatic PV or SV or SMV.
        - Additionally portal cavernoma on doppler was a requisite for diagnosis as per Sarin et al.
    - NCPF: disorder of unknown etiology with features of portal HTN, moderate to massive splenomegaly, with or without hypersplenism with preserved LFT and patent PV and HV.
- INASL (Indian national association for study of liver) standardized the definition of portal cavernoma cholangiopathy (previously called as portal biliopathy): abnormality in extra hepatic biliary system with or without abnormality in intrahepatic biliary system in patient with portal cavernoma.
- Sarin et al described the Unifying theory for etiology of NCPH:
    - NCPF: mild recurring thrombotic events involving peripheral portal vein branches in childhood or adolescence.
    - EHPVO: severe, progressive thrombotic event involving main PV in neonatal or early childhood
- The Indian contribution to the field of NCPH is immense:
    - AIIMS experience (S Nandy, P Sahni et al)
    - ILBS experience (SK Sarin et al)
    - SGPGI experience (V K Kapoor et al)
    - GB pant experience (A Aggarwal et al)
    - PGI experience (Mitra et al)
- AIIMS experience: showed the advantage of PSRS in EHPVO and NCPF
- Important guidelines for management of Cirrhotic portal hypertension:
    - AASLD: American association for study of liver diseases
    - EASL: European association for study of liver
    - Baveno consensus

BILE DUCT INJURY

- Timing of cholecystectomy and BDI:
    - There are several studies which have compared early vs late cholecystectomy in acute cholecystitis. The main problem is that the timing (early vs late) has been heterogeneously defined in these studies.
    - Main concern with early surgery is the increased complexity of surgery resulting in higher risk of BDI.
    - ACDC trial: Early surgery (within 24 hours) was found to be superior.
    - Similarly, many other studies, MA and Cochrane review have shown early surgery to be safe, with similar risk of conversion, BDI with shorter length of hospital stay and deceased costs.
    - In clinical practice, LC is done up to 7 days from onset of symptoms or after 6 weeks. LC is preferably avoided in the interval period.
- Safe Cholecystectomy
    - Strasberg et al described the concept of 'critical view of safety (CVS)'. Achieving CVS at time of LC has shown to reduce the risk of BDI.

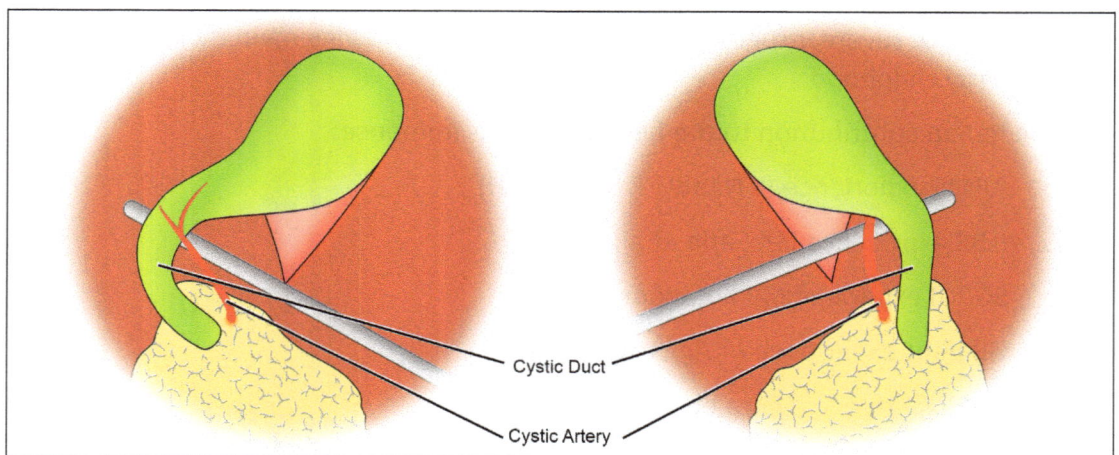

Figure 13.16: Critical View of Safety (CVS), The CVS is confirmed using the Doublet view.

Table 13.6: Criteria required to achieve CVS

- The hepatocystic triangle is cleared of fat and fibrous tissue.
- The lower one third of the gallbladder is separated from the liver to expose the cystic plate.
- Two and only two structures should be seen entering the gallbladder.

- o Similarly, studies have shown that identification of Rouviere's sulcus and limiting the dissection superior to it has also resulted in safer cholecystectomy.
- o V Gupta et al described the concept of R4U line i.e the line joining the Rouviere's sulcus to the umbilical fissure along the base of segment 4 of the liver. Limiting the dissection above this is considered safe.
- o Intra-operative cholangiogram (IOC): routine IOC has not been shown to prevent BDI, it may however help in early identification of BDI. Most surgical units prefer to perform IOC selectively. Studies have shown fluorescence (ICG) cholangiography to be feasible.
- o SAGES described six steps to safe LC:
  - Achieve CVS
  - Understand the potential for aberrant anatomy
  - Use IOC liberally
  - Take time-out prior to clipping or cutting any structure
  - Recognize when the dissection is approaching zone of significant risk and halt before entering the zone
  - Call for help
- The SGPGI group (VK Kapoor et al) has immensely contributed to the literature in the field of BDI
- Classification systems used for BDI:
  - o Bismuth classification of biliary strictures
  - o Strasberg-Bismuth classification of Bile duct injury
  - o Hanover classification
  - o Stewert- Way classification

Table 13.7: Bismuth- Strasberg Classification

- o Type A: Cystic duct stump leak
- o Type B: Ligation of Right posterior sectoral duct
- o Type: C: Bile leak from a divided right posterior sectoral duct
- o Type D: lateral bile duct injury
- o Type E: bile duct strictures resulting from bile duct transection (as classified by Bismuth)

(Continued...)

- E1: stricture in CHD > 2 cm away from hilum
- E2: stricture within 2 cm from the hilum
- E3: Stricture at the hilum; however communication between right and left duct is maintained
- E4: Stricture at the hilum with separation of right and left ducts; i.e. communication between right and left duct is not maintained
- E5: combined stricture of main bile duct and right sectoral duct

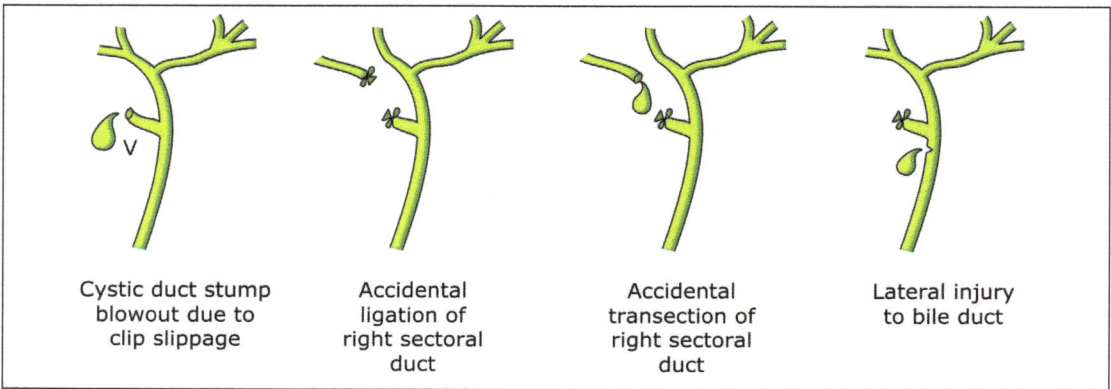

Figure 13.17: Bismuth strasberg classification of bile duct injury.

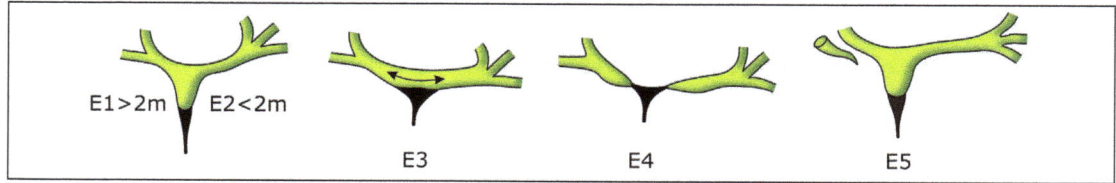

Figure 13.18: Bismuth-Strasberg classification of biliary stricture.

- Davidoff et al: first attempt at repair should be the best attempt as it affects long term outcomes.
- Stewert-Way et al, SGPGI group: described the factors that contribute to the success and failure of biliary reconstruction.
  - Complete pre-operative cholangiogram available or not
  - Intra-abdominal infection controlled or not
  - Level of stricture
  - Number of previous attempts at repair

- Age, Bilirubin and Albumin levels
- Presence of CLD/portal hypertension
- Surgeon experience
- Surgical technique
- Timing of reparative surgery:
    - Immediate (within 72 hours) vs Early (between 4 days and 6 weeks) vs Late repair (after 6 weeks). Remember this classification is arbitrary and there is no standard definition.
    - There is no RCT to compare the various approaches. Additionally, the terminology is not standardized adding to the troubles.
    - Many studies have found early repair to be hazardous, handful have found timing to have no effect on the outcomes and a few have found promising results with early repair.
    - Stewert-Way et al found timing of surgery to be unimportant.
    - Edinburg group reported good results with early repair in selected patients. Mayo-clinic group and John Hopkin group also reported similar results.
    - Danish multicenter study: found early repair to be associated with higher re-stricture rates. French study found similar results.
    - SGPGI group: in general, they advocate delayed repair. However, in an article they suggested that early repair may be considered in patient with ligated/clipped duct after LC when there is no bile leak, no cholangitis with good proximal biliary dilatation.
    - General consensus:
        - Immediate repair at time of primary surgery or at time of referral to tertiary center (within 72 hours) may be considered in select cases where the anatomy is defined and an HPB surgeon with expertise is available.
        - Early repair: although some studies have shown promising results in select cases where there is no intra-abdominal sepsis, it is **generally not preferred.**
        - Delayed repair after 6 weeks is considered the standard of care. It allows for the infection to resolve, inflammation to settle, scar to mature so that the proximal limit becomes well defined.

PANCREATITIS

- Acute Pancreatitis:
  - **Revised Atlanta classification for Acute pancreatitis** (AP)
    - Mild AP: no organ failure, no local/systemic complication
    - Moderate AP: Transient organ failure and/or local/systemic complication
    - Severe AP: persistent organ failure
  - **Determinant based classification for AP**
    - Mild AP: No pancreatic necrosis and no organ failure
    - Moderate AP: sterile pancreatic necrosis and/or transient organ failure
    - Severe AP: infected pancreatic necrosis or persistent organ failure
    - Critical AP: infected pancreatic necrosis and persistent organ failure
  - **PANTER trial:** it compared open necrosectomy vs step-up approach for infected pancreatic necrosis. Minimally invasive step-up approach was found to be better than upfront open surgery. Minimally invasive step-up approach is now considered the standard of care.
  - PYTHON trial: it compared early naso-enteric tube feeding (< 24 hours) vs delayed on demand oral SOS naso-enteric tube feeding (> 72 hours) in acute pancreatitis. Early naso-enteric tube feeding was not found to be superior to delayed on demand oral SOS naso-enteric tube feeding.
  - PROPATRIA trial: Probiotic prophylaxis was not found to reduce the risk of infectious complications in AP. It was associated with an increased risk of mortality.
  - GEPARD study: it established the safety and efficacy of transluminal endoscopic necrosectomy in necrotizing pancreatitis.
  - PENGUIN trial: it compared endoscopic transgastric necrosectomy vs surgical necrosectomy in infected pancreatic necrosis. endoscopic transgastric necrosectomy was found to result in less proinflammatory response.
  - TENSION trial: it compared endoscopic necrosectomy vs surgical step up approach in infected pancreatic necrosis. Both were found to be equivalent.
  - PONCHO trial: it aimed to identify the optimal timing of cholecystectomy in biliary pancreatitis (same admission cholecystectomy vs delayed cholecystectomy). Same admission cholecystectomy was found to be associated with reduced complication rates compared to delayed cholecystectomy.

- Chronic Pancreatitis:
  - Cambridge criteria: for diagnosis and grading of chronic pancreatitis (CP) using ERCP
  - Rosemont criteria: for diagnosis and grading of CP using EUS
  - TIGAR-O classification system for CP:
    - Toxic-metabolic, Idiopathic (tropical CP), Genetic, Auto-immune, Recurrent acute pancreatitis, Obstructive
  - M-ANNHEIM classification system for CP:
    - Multiple risk factors- Alcohol, Nicotine, Nutritional factors, Hereditary factors, Efferent duct obstruction, Immunologic factors, Miscellaneous
  - H Ramesh et al (Cochin) described the ABC classification system for CP
  - Whitcomb et al described the concept of SAPE (sentinel acute pancreatitis event), regarding etiology of CP
  - Indian Pancreatitis Study group studied the epidemiology and symptomatology of chronic pancreatitis in India
  - Mayo Clinic described the HISORT criteria for Auto-immune pancreatitis
  - Zurich series suggested the concept of burn-out in CP
  - ESCAPE trial: it compared the effect of early surgery vs endoscopy first approach on pain in CP. Early surgery was found to result in less pain.
  - Early vs delayed surgery in CP: Various studies have attempted to compare early vs delayed surgery in CP. Early surgery has found to be associated with better pain relief and better preservation of pancreatic function.
  - Trials comparing Pancreatico-duodenectomy vs Begers procedure: both were found to be equivalent with regards to pain relief. Begers procedure was superior with respect to pancreatic exocrine function and quality of life. Also, Begers was associated with lesser morbidity.
  - Trials comparing Begers procedure and Freys procedure: both were found to be comparable in all aspects.

INFLAMMATORY BOWEL DISEASE

- ACT 1 trial: found infliximab to be effective as induction therapy in ulcerative colitis.
- ACT 2 trial: found infliximab to be effective as maintenance therapy in ulcerative colitis.
- ULTRA 1, 2 and 3 trials: found Adalimumab to be effective in moderate to severe ulcerative colitis.
- CYSIF trial: it compared cyclosporine vs infliximab in steroid refractory severe acute ulcerative colitis. Cyclosporine was not found to be superior to infliximab.
- ACCENT 1 trial: found infliximab to be effective as maintenance therapy in Crohn's disease.
- ACCENT 2 trial: found infliximab to be effective as maintenance therapy in fistulizing Crohn's disease.
- GEMINI trial: found Vedolizumab to be effective in Crohn's disease.
- Guidelines for management of IBD:
    - ECCO: European Crohn's colitis organization
    - CCF: Crohn's colitis foundation
- Oxford criteria is used in management of acute severe colitis.
- Jalan's criteria is used for toxic megacolon.
- 2 stage vs 3 stage surgery: there is no RCT to compare them. Generally 2 stage surgery is performed in the elective setting and 3 stage surgery in emergency setting.
- Mucosectomy and hand-sewn IPAA vs stapled IPAA: studies have found neither to be better than the other:
    - Mucosectomy and hand-sewn IPAA:
        - Pro: it removes all diseased mucosa
        - Con: increased chance of incontinence, leak, pelvic sepsis, it is time consuming, there is chance of leaving some diseased mucosa behind
    - Stapled IPAA:
        - Pros: better continence due to preservation of anal transition zone (ATZ), better quality of life
        - Con: risk of cuffitis, dysplasia
    - Generally Stapled IPAA is performed
- J pouch vs S vs W pouch: generally, J pouch is preferred. S pouch may be considered when extra length is required.

OTHERS

- Guidelines for IPMN:
  - Sendai guidelines (2006)
  - Fukuoka guidelines (2012)
  - Revised Fukuoka guidelines (2017)

Table 13.8: Revised Fukuoka guidelines

High-risk stigmata
- Enhancing solid component > 5 mm (strongest association with malignant IPMN)
- Main pancreatic duct ≥ 10 mm
- Obstructive jaundice

Worrisome features
- Cyst ≥ 3 cm
- Thickened and enhancing cyst wall
- Enhancing mural nodule < 5 mm
- Main pancreatic duct 5–9 mm
- Lymphadenopathy
- Abrupt change in caliber of the pancreatic duct with distal pancreatic atrophy
- Cyst growth rate ≥ 5 mm in two years
- Elevated CA 19–9

Treatment
- Resection
  - All main duct IPMNs
  - All other IPMNs with high-risk stigmata
  - All mucinous cystic neoplasms
- Endoscopic ultrasound
  - Cysts with worrisome features
  - All cysts ≥ 3 cm without worrisome features
  - If inconclusive, then close surveillance with alternating MRI and EUS every 3–6 months
  - Strongly consider surgery in young patients

- Neuro-endocrine tumors:
  - PROMID trial: found LAR octreotide to be effective in metastatic NET
  - CLARINET trial: found lanreotide to be effective in metastatic NET
  - NETTER trial: found PRRT (peptide receptor radionuclide therapy) to be effective in advanced NET
- Gastro-intestinal stromal tumors:
  - ACOSOG trial, EORTC trial: established role of adjuvant imatinib in GIST.
  - Scandinavian sarcoma group trial: it compared adjuvant imatinib for 1 year vs 3 year and found advantage with prolonged administration.
  - RTOG 0132 trial: studied the role of NA imatinib in locally advanced GIST and found it to be feasible.
- RECIST: Response Evaluation Criteria In Solid Tumors
  - Complete Response (CR): Disappearance of all target lesions.
  - Partial Response (PR): At least a 30% decrease in the sum of diameters of target lesions, taking as reference the baseline sum of diameters.
  - Progressive Disease (PD): At least a 20% increase in the sum of diameters of target lesions, taking as reference the baseline sum of diameters.
  - Stable Disease (SD): Neither PR nor PD.
- mRECIST: Modified Response Evaluation Criteria In Solid Tumors: used for HCC
  - CR: Disappearance of all arterially enhancing target lesions.
  - PR: At least a 30% decrease in the sum of diameters of arterially enhancing target lesions.
  - PD: At least a 20% increase in the sum of diameters of arterially enhancing target lesions.
  - SD: Neither PR nor PD
- Choi Criteria for GIST to assess response after Imatinib therapy
  - CR: Disappearance of all target lesions.
  - PR: At least a 10% decrease in size of target lesions or 15% decrease in tumor density (in HU).
  - PD: At least a 10% increase in size of target lesions and not meeting criteria of
  - PR with regards to tumor density.
  - SD: Neither PR nor PD

- Morphological Response Criteria by Shindoh et al to assess response of biological therapy on CRCLM.
  - Based on
    - Tumor attenuation
    - Tumor liver interphase
    - Peripheral rim enhancement
  - Optimal response: Tumor becomes homogenous with sharp margins and lacks enhancement.
- Achalasia cardia:
  - Chicago classification used to classify motility disorders
  - Pasricha et al first described POEM for achalasia cardia
  - European Achalasia trial: it compared laparoscopic Hellers myotomy vs pneumatic dilatation in achalasia cardia. It found both treatment modality to be equivalent, however, patients in the PD group required more treatment sessions.
  - RCT comparing laparoscopic Hellers myotomy vs POEM: POEM is not inferior to surgery. However, GERD is more common in POEM group.

Refer to 'CONCISE BIOSTATISTICS MANUAL' written by the author for literature on medical biostatistics. A copy of this book may be requested from the author.

14 Tips for Exam Going Candidates

BEFORE THE EXAMINATION

- Start your preparation well in advance.
- Unlike theory exams where you need to be theoretically strong, practical examination is totally a different ball game where knowledge, vocabulary, confidence and luck, each play an important role. Along with clinical based books also revise standard textbooks.
- Practice by regularly presenting cases to your teachers, senior colleagues and most importantly to your peers. The significance of group discussions cannot be underestimated. Group discussions are possible even if candidates are in different states via use of apps like Skype, Whatsapp and Zoom.
- Make it your daily aim to present at least one case to a teacher and discuss one case with your friends. This will help you improve your fluency, vocabulary and spontaneity.
- Make of list of all probable exam cases and try to present each case atleast twice.
- It is better to make mistakes and realize your weak points before the exams rather than later.
- Practice to make yourself fluent. Make your own format for presenting history and examination, summary and diagnosis without missing any major pertinent points

ONCE EXAM DATES ARE DECLARED

- Book a hotel near the practical exam center and go 2 days before the examination date. Visit the exam center before the day of the exam to confirm the venue so that you don't get a surprise on the day of the exam.
- Do not try to find out the cases kept for exam or the examiner beforehand because it tends to make you biased.
- Keep things that you must carry during practical exam ready:
  - Admit card
  - Identity proof
  - Thesis copy
  - Log Book
  - Instruments – including stethoscope, measuring tape, torch light, rolled X-ray plate for trans-illumination test, Reflex hammer, Gloves
- Sleep well, Pray well

ON DAY OF THE EXAMINATION

- Dress well, dress smartly. Men should preferably wear a light colored shirt, black pant and a clean white well pressed apron along with nicely polished formal black or brown shoes. Please don a well-groomed clean shaven look. A stubble or beard looks good on a magazine cover but not in the examination hall. Ladies may wear a salwar-kameez with dupatta with well groomed hair (avoid keeping your hair open). Both sexes should avoid appearing for the examinations in a jeans, T-shirt, sports shoes with a crumpled apron and untidy hair.
- Attach a badge to your apron clearly mentioning your roll number. Do not mention your name/hospital name.
- Reach the exam center 2 hours prior to the scheduled time.
- Remain calm and pray well.
- Again, my sincere advice to you is to not find out the diagnoses of the exam cases before hand as it may cause you to be biased. A seasoned examiner can easily catch you if you know the diagnosis.
- Once you are allotted your case:
  o Remember be very respectful to the patient and use words like 'aap' rather than 'tu'. You don't want to make the patient angry as an unco-operative patient may be lethal.
  o Do not forget to ask for a female attendant while examining a female patient
  o Ask for a translator, if required.
  o Introduce yourself and get his/her acquaintance.
  o My suggestion would be to ask the patient or his/her relative at the outset 'what do you know about your disease?'. Majority of the times the patient or the relative will have an idea about his/her diagnosis. This will help you ask for pertinent history and look for specific examination findings apart from general points
  o Take history and perform examination in a systematic manner
  o Measure pulse, BP, RR, height, weight, BMI. Do not fake it
  o Do not forget to examine oral cavity, neck nodes, skin, genitals, back and chest
- Once you are done with history and examination of your allotted cases. Write it down on the examination paper. Draw diagrams where necessary (e.g: lump in abdomen)
- Memorize your cases especially the summary and diagnosis/differential diagnosis. At times you may be told to only present your case summary and diagnosis.
- Remember, 'the examiner is always right'

- Greet the examiners with utmost humility and respect. Do not sit until told to. Do not start your presentation unless asked to. Present your case confidently and fluently in a loud and clear voice. But one must not appear over confident or rude. Do not breath heavily or utter incomprehensible words. Many of us have the habit of saying 'Ahh' at the end of each sentence. Practice to stop this habit as it may irritate the examiners.

- Use words like lady and gentleman rather than female and male. Never mention short forms/abbreviations.

- Present your patient's history and examination findings like an essay without mentioning headings like 'chief complaints', 'history of present illness' etc.

- While mentioning diagnosis use words like 'the most probable diagnosis in my case is ….'. Alternatively in cases where you cannot reach a single diagnosis, you may provide a list of differential diagnoses, in which case you can say 'I would like to provide a differential diagnoses for my case, the possibilities are 1, 2, 3 and 4'.

- Once you are done presenting your history, examination, summary and diagnosis, the question that the examiner would tend to ask is 'how would you like to proceed?'. In such an instance, don't jump on to say CT/PET-CT or surgery. A safer answer would be: 'I would first like to review all the available medical records including investigations and treatment given till now. I will then ask for all routine blood investigation and X-ray chest'. Following this you may then proceed with other specific investigation and treatment. Do not forget to mention tumor markers where indicated.

- Stick to your basics. Do not unnecessarily venture to unknown terrains (advanced literature) without having a thorough knowledge of it. It may be counter productive

- Be ready to justify anything that you say.

- When asked a question, answer it straight to the point. Don't hover around it. Do not mention unrelated points just to showcase your knowledge. It irritates the examiner.

- When a question has two or more answers/options, it will be safe to mention all the options, pros and cons of each and what would you do based on your unit protocol. Don't make any controversial statement during exam or be adamant on your point. If you say ABC is the answer to a question but the examiner feels the answer is XYZ, then consider it, it could be a hint. Apologize, alter your answer if required but don't ever argue with an examiner. The examiner is always right.

- If you don't know the answer for any specific question, don't bluff, say 'sorry, I am not able to recollect the answer'. This will help prevent wastage of time

- Remember a specific amount of time is allotted for each candidate. The candidate is the one who should be talking more in this time not the examiner. Answer as many questions as possible. Hence as previously mentioned if you don't know answer to a question, say sorry and proceed to the next.

- Be flexible with your answers.
- No examiner comes with the intention to fail.
- They basically are checking if you are a safe surgeon or not. Hence don't give radical answers. Don't give answers which won't be feasible in normal circumstances. Don't mention surgical options which you won't be able to perform.
- During ward rounds you will generally have post-operative cases and will be asked about what will you do, if a certain complication occurs.
    o For example in a post-operative case of Whipples pancreatico-duodenectomy for carcinoma head of pancreas, you may be asked what will you do if you find blood in drain on post-operative day 7:
    o Your answer should not be 'I will proceed with angioembolization'.
    o A better answer would be: I will clinically evaluate the patient. Inquire for any symptoms and assess mentation. Check airway and breathing and secure them, if necessary. Check pulse, BP, RR, CVP. Look for pallor, auscultate chest and palpate the abdomen and check the drain effluent. Check intake-output chart to see for input, urine and drain output. I would send blood for CBC, cross matching and other tests as deemed necessary. Start resuscitation. Transfuse blood and blood products as required. I shall then counsel/brief the relatives and proceed with a CT angiography to identify the cause of bleeding. If a pseudoaneurysm is identified I would ask for an Interventional Radiology consultation and plan for an angioembolization.
- Long cases and ward rounds will usually decide your fate so perform these well.
- Similarly continue your best performance in the remaining table vivas.
- In the end remember that no piece of paper can decide your future. One day you shall clear all obstacles and pass.

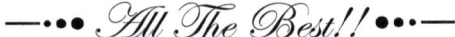

Complication of Important Tables

Table 2.1: Definition of significant weight loss

- Loss of > 10% body weight in 6 months
- Loss of > 7.5% body weight in 3 months
- Loss of > 5% body weight in 1 month
- Loss of > 2% body weight in 1 week

Table 2.2: ECOG/WHO performance scale

0: Fully active; no performance restrictions.

1: Fully ambulatory and able to carry out light work. Strenuous physical activity restricted

2: Capable of all self-care but unable to carry out any other work activities. Up and about > 50% of waking hours.

3: Capable of only limited self-care; confined to bed or chair > 50% of waking hours.

4: Completely disabled; cannot carry out any self-care; totally confined to bed or chair.

Table 2.3: Clinical features suggesting poor nourishment

- Temporal wasting
- Sunken eyes
- Flattened cheeks, Buccal hollow
- Supraclavicular hollow
- Squaring of shoulders
- Prominent scapula
- Prominent intercostal spaces
- Scaphoid abdomen
- Prominent hip bones
- Prominent knee and elbows
- Pedal edema
- Decreased mid arm circumference
- Decreased skin fold thickness

Table 2.4: Stigmata of chronic liver disease (top to bottom)

- Icterus
- Malar erythema
- Fetor hepaticus
- Parotid swelling
- Spider nevi/spider angiomata
- Gynecomastia
- Reduced chest hair
- Reduced axillary hair
- Dupuytren contracture
- Palmar erythema
- Leukonychia
- Flapping tremors/Asterexis
- Abdominal distension
- Caput medusae
- Reduced pubic hair
- Testicular atrophy
- Pedal edema

Table 3.1: Grades of dysphagia (as described by Suguhara et al)

- 1: Able to swallow solid meals with some difficulty
- 2: Able to swallow solid meals but requires liquids along with it
- 3: Able to swallow only semisolid meals
- 4: Able to swallow only liquids
- 5: Able to swallow only saliva
- 6: Unable to swallow anything including saliva

4.1: Zargar Classification

- Grade 1: Only erythema and edema
- Grade 2a: Superficial erosions
- Grade 2b: Deep and/or circumferential ulcers
- Grade 3a: Scattered areas of necrosis
- Grade 3b: Extensive necrosis
- Grade 4: Perforation

Table 4.2: Phases of Caustic Injury

- Acute Necrotic Phase: < 72 Hours
- Ulcerative Granular Phase: 3 days to three weeks
  - Esophagus is the weakest in this phase, hence any intervention is to be avoided during this period
- Cicatrization & Stricturing Phase: 3 weeks to 3 months
  - Its in this phase that the patient starts developing stricture resulting in dysphagia

Table 4.4: Indication for surgery in Corrosive Esophageal Stricture

- Refractory stricture: unable to achieve a luminal diameter of 14 mm over 5 session
- Recurrent stricture: unable to maintain a luminal diameter of 14 mm over 4 weeks or recurrence of dysphagia within 4 weeks of achieving diameter of 14 mm
- Long stricture (> 10 cm), multiple strictures (> 3)
- Failure to pass guidewire across stricture
- Stricture with pseudodiverticulae
- Dilatation related complication

Table 5.1: Laurens Classification of Gastric Cancer

Intestinal Type Adenocarcinoma	Diffuse type Adenocarcinoma
• Enviormental	• Familial
• Affects elderly (M > F)	• Affects younger population (F > M)
• Associated with H. Pylori Infection, Chronic Atrophic Gastritis, Intestinal Metaplasia & Diet high in Nitrosamines	• Associated with CDH 1 Gene Mutation
• Arises from Mucosa	• Arises from Lamina Propria
• Gland forming	• Non Gland forming
• Involves Distal Stomach	• Involves Proximal Stomach
• Hematogenous spread	• Spreads through Sub-Mucosa; Lymphatic metastasis is common; tendency for Transmural spread with Peritoneal metastasis.
	• Linitus Plastica is a rare form of Diffuse Gastric Cancer

Table 5.3: Joensuu Criteria for Gastric GIST

Risk	Size	Mitotic index
Very low	< 2 cm	< 6/50 High power field (HPF)
Low	2.1–5 cm	< 6/50 HPF
Intermediate	2.1–5 cm	> 5/50 HPF
	5.1–10 cm	< 6/50 HPF
High	> 5 cm	AND > 5/50 HPF
	Tumor rupture in itself is a high-risk factor	

Table 5.4: Joensuu Criteria for Non-gastric GIST

Risk	Size	Mitotic index
Very low	< 2 cm	< 6/50 High power field (HPF)
Low	2.1–5 cm	< 6/50 HPF
High	> 5 cm	OR > 5/50 HPF
	Tumor rupture in itself is a high-risk factor	

Table 5.5: WHO Classification of NHL

- Diffuse Large B cell Lymphoma (DLBC): Most common
- Extra nodal marginal Lymphoma (MALToma): 2nd most common
- Follicular cell Lymphoma
- Mantle cell Lymphoma
- Burkitt's Lymphoma

Table 5.6: Lugano classification for staging

Stage	Sub-stage	Description
Stage I		Confined to GI tract
	Stage I1	Confined to mucosa
	Stage I2	Infiltration of sub-mucosa and deeper layers
Stage II		Spread to abdominal lymph nodes (LN)
	Stage II1	Involvement of regional LN
	Stage II2	Involvement of distant abdominal LN
	Stage II E	Infiltration of adjacent organs
Stage IV		Spread to extra-abdominal LN

Table 6.5: WHO Grading system for Neuro Endocrine Tumor

Grade	Mitotic index	Ki-67 index	Differentiation
G1 NET	< 2/10 high power field	< 3%	Well
G2 NET	2–20/10 HPF	3–20%	Well
G3 NET	> 20/10 HPF	> 20%	Well
G3 NEC (NE carcinoma)	> 20/10 HPF	> 20%	Poor

Table 6.6: Todani modification of Alonso Lej classification and its Management

Type	Subtype	Description	Treatment
Type 1		Solitary extrahepatic cyst	Excision with roux-en-y Hepatico-jejunostomy Or Excision and Hepatico-duodenostomy
	A	Cystic	
	B	Saccular	
	C	Fusiform	
	D	Cystic duct dilatation along with CBD dilatation	
Type 2		Extrahepatic supraduodenal diverticula	Excision
Type 3		Choledochocele: intraduodenal diverticula	Endoscopic sphincterotomy Or Surgical transduodenal excision Or Surgical transduodenal sphincteroplasty
Type 4		Multiple extrahepatic cysts with or without intrahepatic cyst	For extrahepatic component: Excision with roux-en-y Hepatico-jejunostomy Or Excision and Hepatico-duodenostomy For intrahepatic component: Hepatic resection
	A	Multiple extrahepatic and intrahepatic cysts	
	B	Multiple extrahepatic cysts	
Type 5		Caroli disease: Multiple intrahepatic cysts	Hepatic resection Liver transplant
Type 6		Isolated dilatation of cystic duct	Excision

Table 7.1: HISORT criteria is used to diagnose Autoimmune pancreatitis

- H: Histology (lympho-plasmacytic sclerosing pancreatitis)
- I: Imaging (sausage shaped pancreas with rim enhancement and narrow duct on CT)
- S: Serology (raised IgG4 levels)
- O: Other organ involvement (OOI). OOI includes Sjogrens syndrome manifesting as dry mouth and eyes.
- RT: Response to steroid therapy

Table 8.1: Child Turcot Pugh score

- Parameters:
  - Bilirubin:
    - 1 point: < 2 mg/dl
    - 2 point: 2–3 mg/dl
    - 3 point: > 3 mg/dl
  - Albumin:
    - 1 point: > 3.5 g/dl
    - 2 point: 2.8–3.5 g/dl
    - 3 point: < 2.8 g/dl
  - INR:
    - 1 point: < 1.7
    - 2 point: 1.7–2.3
    - 3 point: > 2.3
  - Ascites:
    - 1 point: absent
    - 2 point: controlled with medication
    - 3 point: refractory
  - Hepatic encephalopathy:
    - 1 point: none
    - 2 point: grade 1–2
    - 3 point: grade 3–4
- CTP A: score 5–6
- CTP B: score 7–9
- CTP C: score 10–15

Table 8.2: Indication for surgery in NCPH

- Refractory variceal bleed
- Secondary prophylaxis in NCPH
- Symptomatic slpenomegaly, hypersplenism
- Ectopic varices
- Portal biliopathy
- Growth retardation
- Patients from rural areas who lack basic medical facility
- Rare blood group type

Table 9.1: Bismuth- Strasberg Classification

- Type A: Cystic duct stump leak
- Type B: Ligation of Right posterior sectoral duct
- Type: C: Bile leak from a divided right posterior sectoral duct
- Type D: lateral bile duct injury
- Type E: bile duct strictures resulting from bile duct transection (as classified by Bismuth)
    - E1: stricture in CHD > 2 cm away from hilum
    - E2: stricture within 2 cm from the hilum
    - E3: Stricture at the hilum; however communication between right and left duct is maintained
    - E4: Stricture at the hilum with separation of right and left ducts; i.e. communication between right and left duct is not maintained
    - E5: combined stricture of main bile duct and right sectoral duct.

Table 10.1: True-Love and Witts criteria

- Frequency of bloody stools:
  - Mild: upto 4 stools/day with or without blood
  - Moderate: 4–6 stools/day
  - Severe: > 6 bloody stools/day
- Fever:
  - Mild: < 37.5°C
  - Moderate: 37.5–37.8°C
  - Severe: > 37.8°C
- Pulse:
  - Mild: < 90 bpm
  - Moderate: </= 90 bpm
  - Severe: > 90 bpm
- Hemoglobin:
  - Mild: > 11.5 g/dl
  - Moderate: 10.5–11.5 g/dl
  - Severe: < 10.5 g/dl
- ESR:
  - Mild: < 20 mm/h
  - Moderate: 20–30 mm/h
  - Severe: > 30 mm/h
- CRP:
  - Mild: normal
  - Moderate: </= 30 mg/L
  - Severe: > 30 mg/L

Table 10.2: Montreal classification for Crohn's disease

- Age of onset:
  - A1: < 17 years
  - A2: 17–40 years
  - A3: > 40 years
- Location:
  - L1: Terminal ileum with or without cecum
  - L2: Colon
  - L3: Ileum plus colon
  - L4: Proximal small bowel
- Pattern:
  - B1: Non structuring non penetrating
  - B2: Stricturing
  - B3: Penetrating

Table 10.3: Mayo Endoscopic Score

Score	Disease activity	Endoscopic features
0	Normal	None
1	Mild	Erythema, Decreased vascular pattern, Mild friability
2	Moderate	Marked Erythema, Absent vascular pattern, Friability, Erosions
3	Severe	Spontaneous bleeding, Ulceration

Table 10.4: Montreal classification for Ulcerative colitis

- Extent of colitis:
  - E1: ulcerative proctitis: limited to rectum; proximal extent being recto-sigmoid junction
  - E2: left sided colitis: disease limited to the left colon: proximal extent being splenic flexure.
  - E3: extensive colitis: disease extends proximal to the splenic flexure. It includes pancolitis and backwash ileitis.
- Severity of disease:
  - S0: Clinical remission
  - S1: Mild disease as per True Love and Witts criteria (discussed previously)
  - S2: moderate disease as per True Love and Witts criteria
  - S3: severe disease as per True Love and Witts criteria

Table 11.2: Indications for adjuvant chemotherapy in colonic cancer

- T4
- N+
- T3 with high risk features:
  - Obstruction or perforation
  - LVI: Lymphovascular invasion
  - PNI: Perineural invasion
  - < 12 lymph nodes sampled
  - MSI-high (microsatellite instability); MMR-deficient (mismatch repair gene); MSS (microsatellite stable)

Table 13.3: Indication for Pre-operative Biliary stenting in distal blocks

- Cholangitis
- Severe pruritus
- Coagulopathy
- Renal insufficiency
- Poor nutritional status
- Surgery delayed due to any other reason
- When neoadjuvant therapy is being planned in resectable or borderline resectable disease
- When palliation is to be achieved in unresectable disease

Table 13.4: TMH criteria for NA-CT in Locally advanced/Borderline Resectable Ca GB

o Tumor
  o Contiguous liver involvement > 2 cm
  o Involvement of bile duct causing obstructive jaundice (Type I/II block on MRCP/ERCP/PTBD)
  o Radiological/Endoscopic involvement of antropyloric region of stomach, duodenum, hepatic flexure of colon or small intestine
  o i.e. T3–T4 tumors
o Node: Radiological suspicion of lymph node involvement
  o Hepatic artery (Station 8),
  o Hepatoduodenal ligament (Station 12),
  o Retro pancreatic/retroduodenal (Station 13)
  o Size > 1 cm in short axis, round in shape, and heterogenous enhancement on CT/PET scan.
  o i.e. +/> N1
o Vascular involvement: Impingement/involvement (< 180 degree angle) of one or more of the following blood vessels:
  o Common Hepatic Artery and Right & Left Hepatic artery
  o Main Portal vein and Right & Left Portal vein
  o i.e. T4 tumor
o For incidental GBC
  o Residual/Recurrent mass in GB fossa/liver bed
  o N1 nodes as per nodal criteria.
  o Involvement of bile duct causing OJ (Type I/II Block)

Table 13.6: Criteria required to achieve CVS

o The hepatocystic triangle is cleared of fat and fibrous tissue.

o The lower one third of the gallbladder is separated from the liver to expose the cystic plate.

o Two and only two structures should be seen entering the gallbladder.

Table 13.8: Revised Fukuoka guidelines

High-risk stigmata

o Enhancing solid component > 5 mm (strongest association with malignant IPMN)
o Main pancreatic duct ≥ 10 mm
o Obstructive jaundice

Worrisome features

o Cyst ≥3 cm
o Thickened and enhancing cyst wall
o Enhancing mural nodule < 5 mm
o Main pancreatic duct 5–9 mm
o Lymphadenopathy
o Abrupt change in caliber of the pancreatic duct with distal pancreatic atrophy
o Cyst growth rate ≥ 5 mm in two years
o Elevated CA 19–9

Treatment

o Resection
  - All main duct IPMNs
  - All other IPMNs with high-risk stigmata
  - All mucinous cystic neoplasms
o Endoscopic ultrasound
  - Cysts with worrisome features
  - All cysts ≥ 3 cm without worrisome features
  - If inconclusive, then close surveillance with alternating MRI and EUS every 3–6 months
  - Strongly consider surgery in young patients

Table 3.4: AJCC-TNM staging system for esophageal carcinoma

- T stage:
  - T1: Tumor invades submucosa
  - T2: Tumor invades muscularis propria
  - T3: Tumor invades adventitia
  - T4: Tumor invades adjacent structures
- N stage:
  - N1: Metastasis to 1-2 lymph nodes (LN)
  - N2: Metastasis to 3-6 LN
  - N3: Metastasis to 7 or more LN
- M stage:
  - M0: No distant metastasis
  - M1: Distant metastasis present

Table 5.1: AJCC-TNM staging system for Gastric carcinoma

- T stage:
  - T1: Tumor invades submucosa
  - T2: Tumor invades muscularis propria
  - T3: Tumor invades subserosal connective tissue without penetrating through serosa or invading adjacent structures
  - T4: Tumor invades serosa or adjacent structures.
- N stage:
  - N1: Metastasis to 1–2 lymph nodes (LN)
  - N2: Metastasis to 3–6 LN
  - N3: Metastasis to 7 or more LN
- M stage:
  - M0: No distant metastasis
  - M1: Distant metastasis present

Table 6.1: AJCC-TNM staging system for Carcinoma Head of Pancreas

- T stage:
  - T1: Tumor size < 2 cm
  - T2: Tumor size between 2–4 cm
  - T3: Tumor size > 4 cm
  - T4: Tumor involves Celiac axis, SMA, CHA regardless of size
- N stage:
  - N1: Metastasis to 1–3 lymph nodes (LN)
  - N2: Metastasis to 4 or more LN
- M stage:
  - M0: No distant metastasis
  - M1: Distant metastasis present
- Staging:
  - Stage I: T1/T2
  - Stage II: T3/N1
  - Stage III: T4/N2
  - Stage IV: M1

Table 6.2: AJCC-TNM staging system for Carcinoma Gall Bladder

- T stage:
  - T1a: Tumor invades lamina propria
  - T1b: Tumor invades muscular layer (there is no sub-mucosa)
  - T2: Tumor invades perimuscular connective tissue without infiltrating serosa or liver
    - T2a: invasion on peritoneal side
    - T2b: invasion on hepatic side
  - T3: Tumor perforates the serosa and/or invades liver and/or one extra hepatic adjacent organ
  - T4: tumor invades main PV or HA or two or more extra hepatic adjacent organ
- N stage:
  - N1: Metastasis to 1–3 lymph nodes (LN)
  - N2: Metastasis to 4 or more LN
- M stage:
  - M0: No distant metastasis
  - M1: Distant metastasis present
- Staging:
  - Stage I: T1
  - Stage II: T2
  - Stage III: T3/N1
  - Stage IV: T4/N2/M1

Table 6.3: AJCC-TNM staging system for Ampullary Carcinoma

- T stage:
  - T1: Tumor limited to sphincter of Oddi or tumor invades duodenal submucosa
  - T2: Tumor invades duodenal muscularis propria
  - T3: Tumor invades pancreas
  - T4: Tumor involves Celiac axis or SMA
- N stage:
  - N1: Metastasis to 1–3 lymph nodes (LN)
  - N2: Metastasis to 4 or more LN
- M stage:
  - M0: No distant metastasis
  - M1: Distant metastasis present

Table 6.4: AJCC-TNM staging system for Hilar Cholangiocarcinoma

- T stage:
  - T1: Tumor confined to the bile duct wall
  - T2a: Tumor invades beyond bile duct wall to surrounding adipose tissue
  - T2b: Tumor invades adjacent hepatic parenchyma
  - T3: Tumor invades unilateral branches of PV or HA
  - T4: tumor invades
    - Main PV or its branches bilaterally
    - Main HA
    - Unilateral second order biliary radical with involvement of contralateral PV or HA
- N stage:
  - N1: Metastasis to 1–3 lymph nodes (LN)
  - N2: Metastasis to 4 or more LN
- M stage:
  - M0: No distant metastasis
  - M1: Distant metastasis present

Table 11.1: Colo-Rectal cancer is staged as per AJCC-TNM staging system

- T stage:
  - T1: Tumor invades submucosa
  - T2: Tumor invades muscularis propria
  - T3: Tumor invades subserosal connective tissue without penetrating through serosa (visceral peritoneum) or invading adjacent structures
  - T4: Tumor penetrating through serosa +/- invading adjacent structures
- N stage:
  - N1: Metastasis to 1–3 lymph nodes (LN)
  - N2: Metastasis to 4 or more LN
- M stage:
  - M0: No distant metastasis
  - M1: Distant metastasis present
- Stage:
  - Stage I: T1, T2
  - Stage II: T3, T4
  - Stage III: N1, N2
  - Stage IV: M1